OUTSIDE THE ASYLUM

LYNNE JONES

OUTSIDE THE ASYLUM

A Memoir of War, Disaster
and Humanitarian Psychiatry

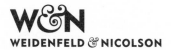
WEIDENFELD & NICOLSON

First published in Great Britain in 2017
by Weidenfeld & Nicolson

10 9 8 7 6 5 4 3 2 1

A CIP catalogue record for this book
is available from the British Library.

HB ISBN   978 1 47460574 8
TPB 978 1 47460575 5

Typeset by Input Data Services Ltd, Somerset

Printed and bound by CPI Group (UK) Ltd, Croydon, CR0 4YY

Weidenfeld & Nicolson

The Orion Publishing Group Ltd
Carmelite House
50 Victoria Embankment
London, EC4Y 0DZ
An Hachette UK Company
www.orionbooks.co.uk

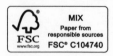

MIX
Paper from
responsible sources
FSC
www.fsc.org   FSC® C104740

For Asmamaw, who shares this story and helps me to see clearly

CONTENTS

CONTENTS

Author's Note

The personal details of all patients discussed in this book have been significantly altered to protect their identity. In many cases stories from more than one person have been composited. Any similarity between any individual patient in this book and any living person is coincidental. On three occasions patients who are already in the public domain have requested that their real names be used: Besnik, Saranda and Fejza. Names of all medical professional colleagues and friends have also been altered, except in five cases where their singular positions do not allow for anonymity (Nkosazana Dlamini, Professor Cerić, Dr Nahim, Baton, Tomaž), and in four cases where the colleagues are deceased (Jill Clark, Dr Hassen, Paul and Kettie). The following friends have consented to their real names being used: Mark, Semir, Narcisa (ch.5), Bini (chs 5 and 6), Peter, Nick, Sabah, Neil and Dina (ch.10), Peter, Larry and MHCE students (ch.12) and Asmamaw (throughout).

To admit any hope of a better world is criminally foolish, as foolish as it is to stop working for it.

Keith Douglas, poet and RAF pilot, 1944

PROLOGUE

Somali border, Ethiopia: September 2007

The *aqal* looks like any other in the refugee camp: bright-blue UNHCR plastic, interwoven with coloured blankets and cloths stretched over a dome constructed of sticks. A thorn fence keeps out wandering livestock, but not the curious onlookers who have crowded into the yard. Dr Asmamaw and I kick off our shoes at the entrance and crawl into the half-darkness, past the used plastic plates, cooking utensils and pots of porridge that fill the patch of earth by the door. The rest of the floor is carpeted with more grubby blankets. Two young men in their early twenties sit upon them. Each is chained by one ankle to the branches that support the dome roof. Their aunt, Amel, crawls in with us.

'I have to chain them,' she explains, 'otherwise Abdullah will get into fights and Usman will get lost.'

I sit beside Usman, take his hand and introduce myself. Aman, my translator, follows precisely.

Usman smiles softly at me and mumbles back a perfect repetition of what I have just said in English: 'Hello I am Lynne, I am Lynne, how are you, are you, are you?'

When I take my hand away, his remains frozen in a half-handshake in mid-air. When I gently put it back on his lap, the hand goes without resistance and stays there. I touch his head and push his chin softly to one side. The chin moves and stops where I stop. I take the other hand, raise it, and then let go. The hand remains in a wave. Usman continues to mutter my name. Abdullah is more responsive, shaking my hand and laughing.

Amel tells me what happened. A year ago the boys were students, living with their parents in Mogadishu. Soldiers from the Union of Islamic Courts came to the house and told the parents the boys had to join their militias. Their parents refused, so the soldiers immediately shot them dead. Abdullah tried to stop the soldiers and they struck him on the head with a gun. He ran bleeding from the house. He told Amel later that he had seen Usman gather his dead mother into his arms. The soldiers ran off. Then the house was shelled and collapsed on Usman, knocking him unconscious. The neighbours dug him out. When he regained consciousness he could no longer speak or take care of himself. He just sat staring and muttering. Sometimes he was completely mute, staying in one position for long periods of time. Abdullah had also changed. He was confused and had constant nightmares.

'Now he reacts to the smallest thing and gets into fights without any reason.' Amel sits beside me in the half-light. Tears run down her face as she talks. 'We all ran away from Mogadishu a few months ago and managed to cross the border and come here. But my husband is in Sweden. He asked me to join him at the beginning of this year, but how can I leave them when they are like this? I have to take care of them.'

'So what happened?'

'He has divorced me. He does not want two crazy people in his family. Now I don't know what to do. The food is not enough. Anyway we are not accustomed to this food. I try and make something. I sell it in the village but they don't pay much, so we are hungry all the time.'

We sit and talk, learning more about the boys and watching Usman. He continues to repeat 'Hello how are you?' and holds his hand in the air. I explain to Amel that I think both boys have mental illnesses caused by a combination of their terrible experiences and the blows to their heads.

'We are going to find a way to help,' I tell her, putting on my sandals.

Asmamaw has already crawled out. I follow, bending low, and am blinded by the bright sunlight as I stand up beside him.

The *aqal* door faces east away from the camp, overlooking scrubby wasteland that stretches towards the border. Plastic bags caught on thorn bushes blow like strange blossoms in the hot wind. Beyond are two low, symmetrical, greyish-brown hills covered in rocks. There is nothing else out there except hyenas, the women in the camp tell me. They can hear them howl at night.

'What do you want to do?' Asmamaw asks.

'What do I want? Hmm . . . skull X-ray, CT scan, some lab work, an immediate end to the conflict in Somalia.'

'I mean right now.' He smiles.

'Get UNHCR to give Amel a larger *aqal* and extra rations. Get them up to the clinic so I can do a full physical examination in daylight. Put both boys on medication that will allow her to unchain them. And let's see if we can sort out a medical evacuation to Addis that would allow investigations.'

'You know that will take weeks. Mental illness is not a priority.'

'I know, but they both had head injuries, let's stress that bit in the referral. I have no idea how much that is contributing to their symptoms.'

We get in the vehicle, and my driver heads up the dirt road between the rows of *aqals*. Every day there are more. The Ethiopian government opened the camp a month ago to cope with a new round of refugees from a new round of fighting in an old and forgotten war.

The old war began in Somalia in 1991 when the government collapsed and plunged the country into years of factional conflict between clan-based warlords. In December 2006 the Ethiopian government joined in, sending their troops to Mogadishu to support a weak transitional government with the immediate effect of galvanising all parties into a new bouts of fighting and atrocities. The violence has been unremitting since, and almost half a million have fled their homes in the last six months. Some of them trekked north through Somaliland and somehow crossed the border to end up here. The camp was built to house five thousand and there are already seven thousand.

We drop Aman off at his family *aqal* and drive to the small corrugated-iron hut that constitutes the medical clinic for the camp. Asmamaw unpadlocks the door and we go into the partitioned space that is his office. It is late and the staff have already gone back to the compound in the village. I still have an hour's drive to Jijiga, where I sleep in the agency house.

I write my notes and file them. Asmamaw goes through to the small ward, basically a dirt-floored room with the same tin walls and five beds. There is one mother with a very tiny new baby. Both are doing fine.

'Why are you working here in a tin hut instead of in some nice private clinic in Addis Ababa?' I ask Asmamaw.

'Where else should a doctor be but with people who need him? I like refugees. I could ask you the same question. These are not your people. Why are you here?'

1: INSIDE THE ASYLUM

I failed in my first attempt to become a psychiatrist. I sat in the boardroom of the Allinton Psychiatric Hospital under the portraits of its nineteenth-century founders. Outside, early summer bluebells bloomed under a copper beech. When the Allinton Lunatic Asylum opened in 1826 'for the accommodation of lunatics selected from the higher classes of society', gardens were considered essential for the 'moral treatment' of patients. Fortunately, they were still there. The gardens were one of the reasons I wanted the job. Fifteen consultants sat around a polished mahogany table looking at me; fourteen of them were men. I knew I was not doing well. No one had asked me the predictable questions for which I had prepared, such as 'Why do you want to do psychiatry?' Or 'What experiences in your year of general practice have you found particularly relevant and useful?' Instead they were focused completely on the less orthodox aspects of my curriculum vitae.

'I see you started off in geography, Dr Jones – what took you into medicine?' A balding man with heavy brows made studying geography sound akin to working in a strip club.

I have friends who can make their path to becoming a doctor sound as if they were singled out by the gods. They read A. J. Cronin's *The Citadel*, where an idealistic Welsh doctor challenges the vanity of private practice in London. Or they had watched *Dr Finlay's Casebook* on TV, where a similarly idealistic young GP saves lives in 1920s Scotland. Or they had seminal experiences in early youth such as their sister's recovery from leukaemia. These experiences set them on a life course which they then pursued without hesitation or deviation.

My career trajectory has been more like a series of circuitous paths, combined with trips down blind alleys, chance meetings and random wanderings. As a six-year-old I loved watching *Emergency Ward 10* on television, where ambulances endlessly pulled into the real forecourt of St Thomas's Hospital in London, and fictional lives were saved while fictional doctors and nurses fell in love, but I wanted to be an archaeologist. I dropped this idea on realising it necessitated studying ancient languages. At ten, after my first flight to Paris, being an air hostess appealed. By fifteen, I was immersed in Shakespeare and Sheridan, and determined to go to drama school and be an actress. But my mother insisted I go to university first. 'And don't study English, the world is full of unemployed English graduates,' she warned me.

So I chose geography. Our parents had taught us to love the outdoors: sending us kayaking, skiing, hiking and walking from an early age. My geography teacher, Jane Skinner, taught me to take pleasure in understanding how the landscape, both natural and human, was formed. Tramping the chalk hills and valleys of the South Downs, mapping villages, tracing their development and interviewing residents about their lives provided a blessed escape from the confinement of a private boarding school for girls. With portable transistor radios clamped to our ears, we listened to Neil Armstrong step onto the moon while staring up at it, camped on a beach in Devon. Geography was the perfect subject for those wanting to know something about everything, but with no special talent for learning everything about one thing in particular.

Studying timber exports from Norway in my first year at Oxford was boring, however. I switched to a new interdisciplinary degree called the Human Sciences. I made the surprising discovery that anthropology taught by Professor Evans-Pritchard and Animal Behaviour taught by Professor Niko Tinbergen and a very young Richard Dawkins were much more interesting than sitting in the pub fretting about who would lead in the drama society's next production of

Hedda Gabler. I loved the idea of spending my life travelling the world trying to observe and understand different peoples and cultures.

The problem was, how to be useful? I come from a family that includes schoolteachers (Welsh grandfather); doctors (mother, father and stepmother); ministers of various faiths (three great-uncles and stepfather); and a step-uncle who had built and driven an ambulance to Spain during the Spanish Civil War and helped Vietnamese Boat People in Hong Kong. Somewhere along the way I had absorbed the idea that life was about doing something you enjoyed and were good at, while also being of service to others. Who did anthropology help?

There are moments of clarity. They stand out in your life like those white signposts with black letters and pointing fingers that suddenly appear at a junction on a country lane, just when you realised you were lost. In my last year at Oxford I saw a documentary called *The Tribe that Hides from Man*. It was about the Villas-Bôas brothers, two geographers and anthropologists, who recognised that remote tribes in Brazil needed shielding from the encroachments of Western civilisation and so became advocates and activists to protect them. They also set up clinics to address the ravages of Western illnesses such as measles. I suddenly realised that if I trained in medicine, I could combine it with anthropology and geography. I could explore the world and be useful at the same time.

I could not attempt to explain all this to the balding man with heavy brows at the Allinton Psychiatric Hospital.

'I thought medicine would be useful.'

'I beg your pardon? Useful?'

I was making medicine sound like a shopping bag.

'In which case, Dr Jones, could I ask why you left medicine altogether for three years to ... ummm,' he glanced down at my CV, 'work in the peace movement?'

This was the heart of the problem. Eccentric degree choices and late entry to medicine are one thing; radical pacifism and a prison record, albeit for non-violent civil disobedience, are another. In 1981 I had resigned from my first job in a busy Liverpool Accident and Emergency department after only ten months, to go and camp outside a military base in protest at the proposed deployment of a new generation of nuclear weapons. My boss, a friendly woman consultant who had taught me a lot, warned me that this was likely to be the end of any medical career.

'I did not feel I had a choice. Health care is surely about dealing with any threat to health. The threat of nuclear war to the wellbeing of us all felt so imminent that it had to take priority.'

'And has the threat gone away?'

'Probably not, but I missed clinical medicine, I realised I did not want to waste my training.'

How to explain that after three years of protests and meetings and public speaking, I was tired of working exclusively on the 'bigger picture'? I was still a committed pacifist but I missed the engagement with individual people and their problems. So I did a year of general practice in Cornwall and discovered that ten minutes was never long enough to hear the whole story. I wanted to understand everything about the person sitting opposite. What really held my attention were the problems in their minds rather than their bodies.

'Given your radical views about non-violence, Dr Jones, my question is would you be prepared to give ECT?' A small man with half-moon glasses and a reddish face looked at me somewhat belligerently. The question took me by surprise. Electroconvulsive therapy is a treatment in which electrodes are applied to a patient's head under anaesthetic in order to induce a seizure. Since its introduction in the 1930s, it has been used to treat a variety of mental disorders and is still controversial, although it has proved effective in treating severe depression. Did he see ECT as a form of violence? If not, why had he asked the question? Perhaps he saw me stirring up dissent among the patients and leading a protest.

'I would be here to learn psychiatry from you, so of course I would give the treatments that you thought appropriate.'

He nodded to himself and asked no further questions. A soft-spoken, friendly-looking man with short black hair said I could leave. They did not appoint me.

'You split the board completely,' a colleague told me later. 'Half of them liked you and half of them hated you. One said he would resign if you were appointed.'

Six months later the black-haired doctor rang me. Apparently one of the appointed doctors needed time to complete his PhD thesis on rat brainwaves. Was I interested in the vacancy? Unfortunately, Unfortunately, the man with half-moon glasses, Dr N., still had concerns about my willingness to give ECT, so I would need to be interviewed again.

In 1973, the year I entered medical school, a psychologist in the United States called David Rosenhan dramatically demonstrated that psychiatrists could not distinguish sanity from insanity. He did this by getting eight normal people to present themselves at different psychiatric hospitals with just one symptom: a mild auditory hallucination. Otherwise they behaved normally. Seven out of the eight were diagnosed as schizophrenic and one as having a manic depressive psychosis. They were all admitted to hospital. Once there, they stopped having the hallucination and reverted to completely normal behaviour. They were recognised as sane by some of their fellow patients, but the staff continued to categorise them as insane, and even when discharged, those with 'schizophrenia' retained the diagnosis of 'schizophrenia in remission'. Meanwhile, other people were demonstrating that psychiatrists rarely agreed with each other when making diagnoses of the same patients. There were particularly strong differences between British and American psychiatrists. The latter had a much broader concept of schizophrenia than their British counterparts.

The validity of the entire psychiatric enterprise was in question from a number of directions. We read Foucault and Szasz and Laing and went to see *One Flew Over the Cuckoo's Nest* and Ken Loach's *Family Life*. We argued over whether psychiatry was an exercise in social control, a bourgeois conspiracy to exile difference; or whether madness was a liberating journey challenging the constrictive insanities of so-called normal life. For a medical student who hated the laboratory it was intoxicating. Far from becoming alienated from psychiatry, I saw it as the one discipline where people read non-medical textbooks, discussed ideas, took an interest in politics, human rights and the world around them, and spent time talking to their patients. A good psychiatrist had to be interested in their patients' lives, not just their diseases.

I spent much of my spare time as a medical student hanging around our local asylums. There was Stoke Park, a turreted castle on a hill above the motorway, once considered a pioneering colony for mentally handicapped children. In 1971 inquiries into its 'slum-like' conditions resulted in both the building of new wards and greater pressure for de-institutionalisation. Glenside was another turreted Victorian Gothic asylum, where Dr Donal Early had pioneered 'industrial therapy'. This was the innovative idea that patients could participate in work within the hospital, earn a small income and learn skills that would help in their rehabilitation and make them employable on discharge. They were constantly short-staffed. Perhaps that was why over-stretched administrators allowed a bunch of inexperienced medical students to come and do movement and psychodrama therapy on their wards, and to help start a group home in the community for some of the longer-term patients.

We knew we were right. Independent life in a cramped, box-like semi-detached villa in a narrow street, rented by Social Services, had to be better than living on a sterile ward in a nineteenth-century lunatic asylum. Surely sleeping in tiny single rooms with views of dustbins or the house opposite, and the daily enforced company of six other ex-patients not chosen by oneself, along with daily responsibilities for shopping and cooking, was preferable to sleeping in dormitories in a large run-down building with meals provided, plus beautiful gardens in which you might wander at will, and the chance to engage in growing vegetables or making furniture?

Two of the transferred patients broke down almost

immediately: one woman found the stress of cooking and taking care of herself too great after living in hospital for two years. She asked to go back. Another man, who had been an inpatient for many years, couldn't cope with the loneliness and confined himself to his room. Nothing would tempt him out. Their experiences taught me that asylums could be just that: asylum.

Dr N.'s concern over my possible refusal to give electroconvulsive therapy was curious, given that he had built his own considerable reputation on challenging the custodial approach to psychiatry: unlocking wards, taking the bars off windows, allowing the sexes to mix and encouraging the psychotherapeutic care of those with psychosis.

Woodside was the Allinton's poor relative, founded some twenty years later to provide an asylum for the county's pauper patients who were cluttering up jails and almshouses. By 1900 it had a thousand patients. In the 1960s it was still, for the most part, a locked institution with seven hundred patients. Dr N., influenced by the libertarian currents of the previous two decades, had worked to open it up. By the time I arrived in the mid-eighties, he had created a therapeutic community within the asylum for acutely disturbed patients. The idea was that, while patients would be given the medical treatments they needed, drugs and ECT – compulsorily if necessary – patient autonomy and independence were fostered through participating in group decision-making and a variety of therapeutic groups. Flattened hierarchies were supposed to create democracy: no one wore uniforms; staff were called by their first names. The 'community' would be brought into the hospital. Relatives could come to group meetings and the patients were encouraged to go out: through recreation, work programmes, day-patient units, sheltered halfway houses.

My day on Larch Ward began with the 'large group' meeting which all staff and patients were expected to attend. Anything could be discussed. According to Dr N. it was a chance for patients to sort out conflicts and difficult treatment choices, confront aberrant behaviours and provide support for each other. I watched in my first week as he skilfully used the group to persuade Enid, a depressed middle-aged woman, to continue her electroconvulsive therapy.

It began in the normal way. Maurice, the charge nurse, read brief notes about the previous day and James as usual raised the problems he was having with his ex-girlfriend. Andy walked in and out of the group three times holding a bag of bananas. Neville and Daniel, both schizophrenic and recovering well from psychotic episodes, asked Dr N. to increase their side-effect medication.

'Birds of a feather,' Andy remarked, getting out a banana and eating it.

'Enid is refusing to go to ECT, she wants to discuss it with you first.' Ray, one of the nurses, came in followed by Enid. She was a plump, sad-looking, middle-aged woman with poorly dyed, thinning blonde hair, wearing a neat flowery dress. She had been made redundant from her job behind the counter of a grocer's shop, and since then she had stopped eating and drinking and worried constantly. She stood facing Dr N.

'I don't want to go. There are a number of things I want to sort out first.'

'It did you a lot of good last time,' Dr N. replied.

'I don't want to go.' Enid was close to tears.

'Enid has a problem.' Dr N. turned to the whole group. 'She needs your help.' He leant back in his chair, eyes closed, one leg crossed over the other, as if to say, this is now no longer up to me.

'You should go, Enid,' Neville said. 'It's good for you.'

'Just like brain massage,' added Daniel, 'very gentle.'

'So will you come along now?' Ray asked Enid.

'I think I will wait and see,' Enid replied, sitting tight on the hard upright chair and clutching at her black patent-leather handbag.

'I know you're frightened of forgetting but that's part of the cure and it does come back.' Daniel sounded very knowing.

Enid clutched her handbag tighter and didn't move.

'I could come with you,' Daniel suggested kindly. By now he had moved across the room and was kneeling by Enid's chair.

'You are holding up the meeting Enid,' Dr N. announced through closed eyes, in a bored voice. 'Is that what you want?'

Andy walked over to Enid, clutching the bag of bananas. 'You should go, you know, it will be all right.' Enid, looking cornered, suddenly stood up and bolted out of the door.

Enid later agreed to her electroconvulsive therapy. I took my turn giving it in the twice-weekly sessions, learning to apply the padded electrodes to the patients' temples after the consultant anaesthetist had given a short-acting anaesthetic and muscle relaxant. The electric shock administered through the electrodes induced a convulsion. Having put on a blood pressure cuff to keep one arm free of muscle relaxant, I watched for the convulsive movement in the fingers, then stopped the current, removed the electrodes, woke the patient and wheeled her into the recovery room of the hospital sick unit. For reasons that no one really understood, the treatment did appear to produce an improvement in mood. Enid stopped fretting, and started eating. In her case there was no noticeable memory loss.

Not everyone was so willing. On one occasion an elderly lady punched me in the face twice, first before she went under anaesthetic and then when she recovered. I felt she had some justification as she was having the treatment against her will.

The tensions inherent in trying to create a 'patient democracy' with acutely ill psychotic patients reflected the contradictions in psychiatry themselves in the mid-eighties. Over at the Allinton in the professorial unit, eager young registrars in tweed jackets and corduroy trousers were busy establishing psychiatry as a bona fide medical discipline. Diagnoses would no longer rest on unprovable theories of causation such as 'childhood trauma' or 'frozen mothers'. They would be based strictly on 'phenomenology', that is, the symptoms that could be observed or were reported, and the course the illness had taken over time. Disease definitions would then rest on these described and agreed patterns of symptoms. As science progressed it could then define the brain pathology underlying the clearly defined symptom clusters. Once that pathology was understood, more refined and targeted biological treatments could be developed. These steps had already been taken with a number of diseases, such as general paresis of the insane, the dementia that accompanied tertiary syphilis; and with epilepsy.

What struck me, however, was that whenever the biological underpinnings did get sorted out, the disease itself stopped being the province of psychiatrists. Those spirochaetes that caused syphilis now got treated with penicillin by specialists in infectious diseases, while epilepsy was primarily the province of neurologists. Psychiatrists were then left with the behavioural and emotional disturbances that accompanied these illnesses, or were still unexplained. I and my fellow trainees took a neuroscience course that year. In between delicately slicing up a greyish-white human brain with its wormlike surface, we took lectures in neurophysiology, neuro-endocrinology and neuropharmacology. One of our lecturers informed us that he envisaged two hundred years hence a specialist for each lobe of the brain, just as now there were specialists for different organs of the body: kidneys, liver, stomach and so on. 'But who then will talk to patients?' He asked. 'Will you be technicians, or psychiatrists?'

The patients that filled Larch and most acute wards suffered from what were called 'functional' psychoses. These were types of madness where the underlying pathology was still not understood, but where the psychopharmacological revolution of the fifties had shown that some drugs could reduce or even remove the symptoms. It was these treatments that had made it possible for patients who previously might have been incarcerated in institutions for years, to leave hospital after a short period of treatment.

Trainee psychiatrists are basically apprentices. We had lectures one day a week and were sent on academic training courses, but mainly we learnt by doing – from our patients, from the nurses and from our seniors, who were supposed to supervise and correct us as we went along. Jack, our senior registrar, who at night played guitar in a small rock band, used some of his working hours to drum into our heads the phenomenological distinctions between the two major functional forms of madness which had been in use since the German psychiatrist Emil Kraepelin identified them in the late nineteenth century. We needed to understand how patients with manic depression, or bipolar disorder as it was now called, could fluctuate between episodes of extreme excitability and episodes of profound depression, and yet have periods of full recovery in between. This differed from schizophrenia, a form of madness in which the patient suffered from hallucinations and disordered thoughts and in which the illness appeared to take a deteriorating course. I loved sorting this out.

There was Graham and Margaret, for example. Graham had been compulsorily admitted from a police cell after they had found him in the early hours one morning, threatening to jump off a bridge into the river below. Twenty-seven-year-old Margaret was admitted on the same evening in a red-silk ballgown, having 'gone crazy' during a party to celebrate passing her exams. Both came to morning meeting the next day. Margaret, still wearing her party dress, walked repeatedly around the room, sometimes stopping in front of a patient to stroke their face, sometimes singing, sometimes simply repeating whatever was said and turning it into a small refrain.

After watching Margaret pace for a couple of minutes Graham stood up.

'I want to die,' he said.

'Die die die die die die,' sang Margaret, circulating the room.

'How do people feel about what Graham has just said?' asked Ray. No one responded. Andy and Neville were snoring loudly, lying back in their armchairs.

'I don't see what good it is being in here painting pictures like at school. I'd rather go home,' said Christine. Christine was a mother and housewife with a chronic depressive illness, whom we had been trying to get home for weeks.

'Go home go home alone alone alone,' went Margaret.

And so it had continued, each patient picking up where the other left off like a chime of hand bells, but no one actually responding or listening to anyone else.

It was not possible to interview Margaret on the first day. She came in and out of the small office where we sat with her mother, slamming the door, sitting down, staring at her mother, getting up, leaving, slamming the door again. Her mother described how her daughter, a trainee accountant, had always been well, except for one period of getting depressed and withdrawn in her last year at college. She had stopped eating and the college had treated her with antidepressants and she had recovered. They thought it was overwork. She had thrown herself into the party arrangements and had a new job lined up. But they had noticed in the last few days she had been more and more irritable and tense. Then at the party she had been asked to make a speech and had started shouting rubbish.

'She was making no sense and shouting at everyone. We were so embarrassed. Her boyfriend tried to calm her down. She just fought him off, so we had to call an ambulance.' The mother began to cry and Margaret started banging her fists on the outside of the glass door.

Graham, in contrast, was completely silent. It was impossible to take a history directly from him either. All we knew was that he was a student. Over the following days we pieced together the story of a shy, solitary, bright boy from a close-knit family who liked reading in his room and had no close friends, but had done well at school. At college, though, things had been different. Everyone seemed cleverer than him. He found it hard to make friends; he joined no clubs, but spent more and more time alone. He became convinced people were talking about him. He would see them eye him when he went to meals in the dining room. He could hear them through the walls of his room at night. He turned up with completely incoherent notes for a seminar. He had chosen physics because he was convinced science could make the world a better place, but he was now sure it was making things worse. He had thought of killing himself, and lay in his room terrified and shouting at unseen visitors. When Jack and I went to assess him, he burst into loud sobbing and clutched Jack round his waist as if drowning.

'Almost certainly a first episode of schizophrenia,' Jack explained to his bewildered parents.

'Will he get better?'

'Yes, probably, if he takes the medication we prescribe.'

'Can he go back to college?'

'Probably best not this year.'

'How long will he need to take medication?'

'It's hard to say. We recommend that he stay on it for quite a while. It will be easier to judge when we see how good his response is.'

When the major tranquillisers had come into use in the fifties and sixties, they appeared to be effective in previously untreatable conditions, like schizophrenia. There had been a hope that understanding their mechanisms of action would help to reveal the underlying disease process itself. If, for example, phenothiazines block the dopamine pathways in the brain, at the same time blocking the frightening thoughts and imaginary voices that occur in schizophrenia, does that mean that excess dopamine causes schizophrenia? Almost certainly not. Margaret, who did not have schizophrenia, and Graham, who probably did, were treated with the same major tranquilliser, which in both cases calmed them down and helped them become more rational.

'We have no idea what we are doing in schizophrenia,' our professor of psychopharmacology told us bluntly, confirming my view that in psychiatry we were still at the stage of giving aspirin for varieties of fever. It was an advance on bloodletting and cupping, but nowhere near a cure for an underlying disease. Even lithium, the drug given to Margaret to stabilise her moods, was not a cure for bipolar disorder.

'Psychiatry is not usually about curing people. It's about making the business of being mentally ill more bearable,' said Jack.

Larch Ward was full of people who found their lives

unbearable. Dr N. had succeeded in creating a large, shifting, somewhat dysfunctional community. Contrary to the popular stereotype, the major conflicts that confronted us were not about locking people up against their will but about persuading patients who had become attached to the unit that they were ready to be discharged. When I told Christine that I completely agreed it was time for her to go home, she burst into tears. 'You are so cruel, doctor,' she said and got up and marched off. Later I found 'Lynne is Cruel' written in large letters in red marker on the wall of the day room.

The other conflicts were over drugs. Again, contrary to stereotype, patients were not angry with us for forcing drugs on them. More often it was over our refusal to prescribe. The most commonly used major tranquillisers had a range of side effects: drowsiness, weight gain and photosensitivity, to name a few. They could also give you some symptoms that were akin to Parkinson's disease, a stiffening of the limbs and a tremor. These uncomfortable feelings could be alleviated with another antiparkinsonian drug which was often routinely administered at the same time as the tranquilliser. The problem was that this side-effect drug had a kick of its own, and had a market value because of this. It was well known that some of the patients were hoarding and selling their side-effect medication. So now it was only prescribed on a case-by-case basis after an examination by the doctor.

One afternoon I was sitting outside, trying to catch up on notes, when Neville came out and started crawling on his hands and knees around the cherry tree, moaning and mumbling to himself. This was his usual response when he was refused biperiden (the side-effect drug). It was hard to concentrate on my notes. 'Academy Award performance, Neville,' I commented as he crawled past me. He got up and started walking normally. I felt rather pleased that my sarcasm had had the desired effect. Then he got out a tobacco tin and hurled it at a car parked on the drive. I cursed myself. Crawling had not bothered anyone but me. The charge nurse Maurice came out and we both ran over to Neville.

'Is that the best you can do?' Maurice asked Neville. 'Now I'll have to get the owner and see if she wants to involve the police.'

Neville began crying, picked up my plastic chair and hurled it across the grass, then walked over to one of the cherry trees, grabbed the branches, which bent under his weight, and began to twist and swing on them. The car owner, a pleasant-looking secretary in a cotton dress, came outside. She stared dejectedly at her car, watched Neville bouncing in a shower of cherry blossom, then shook her head and went inside. I followed her, leaving Maurice to try and disentangle Neville from the cherry tree. As soon as I reached the ward my crash bleep went off. It was Maurice and Bill, the senior nurse. I ran outside again and found them both holding hard onto Neville. He had run to the conveniently located railway bridge and threatened to throw himself off.

'That's it,' Bill said, 'he gets the biperiden,' undermining three months of attempted withdrawal.

'You don't learn psychiatry,' a colleague told me. 'You *become* a psychiatrist – it takes over every aspect of your life, colours every relationship, every book you read.' That spring and summer the only books I read were the textbooks of brain anatomy and neuro-endocrinology necessary to get me through my first-part membership exams. The asylum was my home as well. I slept in the doctors' flat across from the main hospital and watched the cherry blossom give way to the deep green of high summer.

I adjusted. I no longer felt nauseated by the glossy, bright-orange paint used in the hospital reception area. I saw the cheeriness it was meant to denote. I no longer wondered about the thin, drunk man with the tired face who sat next to the bronze statue of the first asylum superintendent, day in day out, with beer cans and cigarette butts piled up around him; nor the grey-haired lady in the baggy dress who sat opposite and picked at her feet. I simply greeted them on my way to the ward. I knew some fundamental shift had taken place when one day, in a large group meeting, we heard a terrible, thin, wailing shriek from outside the open window. It went on and on. No one got up to look at who might be the source of the cry or whether anyone was in trouble. Maurice went over to shut out the sound and we continued the meeting. In the afternoon I did go out to explore. There were no signs of violence, just two men sleeping on the cut grass under the blossoming chestnut trees.

Patients did get better. Within weeks, Graham and Margaret were unrecognisable, transformed back into rational and relatively calm individuals. Christine decided to go home. In her last meeting she got up and went systematically round the room, saying she wanted to thank everyone personally for all their help and support. She shook each person's hand. When she got to Andy dozing in his chair, he looked astonished.

'You don't know that you helped but you did.' She patted his hand.

Trainee psychiatrists do not stay in one place, they rotate. Over the three or four years it takes to pass the examinations that will make them members of the Royal College of Psychiatrists they will usually complete eight six-month attachments to different psychiatric subspecialist units within a given area, the idea being to give them as broad a training experience as possible. That August I moved to Beech Ward to work with chronically ill schizophrenic patients, that group for whom medication was not really working. They had a long experience of coping with new junior staff.

In spite of doing regular on-call duties I had never visited Beech Ward before my first day of working there. I walked down a long, entirely blue corridor: blue paint, blue lino and blue curtains, wondering if some earlier hospital designer had thought this would have a calming effect on patients. If so, the value was lost by what followed when you entered the ward. I thought that Larch had inured me to scuffed walls, scrappy lino and broken furniture, but this was on a different scale. It was a large, well-lit room with long windows running the entire length of one wall. The August sun poured in, picking out the faded wallpaper's ugly brown flower print and showing up the filth on the cream gloss paint.

The ward was divided into three, partly by glass partitions. The first area appeared to be for communal living. There was a piano, a record-player and a television. This last was on, although no one was watching. There was a table-tennis table in the middle of a large carpet. A youngish man with short ginger hair, in a donkey jacket that looked hot for the weather, was patting a ball by himself. I stepped onto the carpet and felt my feet sink into some sort of sogginess. Beyond the living area was one for eating. There was a long table that had stackable plastic chairs piled up on one half. No one had unstacked them despite the fact that lunch had been served and placed on the other half of the table. The patients were simply sitting on other chairs they had pulled up. There were two: a middle-aged woman with long grey hair in plaits and a tall, very thin, middle-aged man in a grubby lumberjack shirt and jeans. Both ate without looking at, or speaking to, each other.

The ginger-haired man looked across at me.

'Are you new? I'm Craig. Would you like to play table tennis?'

'All right,' I said.

No one else seemed to be around and I had no idea what else to do. We started to hit the ball back and forth and the tall man got up and wandered over. His flies were undone and his eyes leaked pus. He watched us for a while, pulled out a packet of cigarettes and lit one, then cleared his throat, spitting out a large gob of greyish phlegm onto the stained and filthy carpet. At this point a tall woman with blonde hair in a bun came in. Her general air of cleanliness and efficiency suggested she was a staff member rather than a patient. She strode up to the middle-aged man and put two tissues in his hand. 'Clean up, Oliver, please.'

Part of rehabilitation consists of teaching patients the habits that make it possible to live in the real world. Oliver started to walk away; the blonde nurse pursued him. 'Oliver, you need to clean up.' Oliver turned and kicked out at her, then suddenly lunged, putting his hands round the woman's neck in a throttle grip, grazing her cheek with his lit cigarette. I dropped my bat and ran over but four other nurses, who appeared out of nowhere, were faster and on him in seconds, unprising his hands and sitting him on a sagging sofa, with a nurse on each side holding him firmly under each arm.

'Hello, I'm the new senior house officer, are you OK?' I asked the nurse.

'Quite all right, I'm Anita.' She smiled. 'It's not as bad as it seems.' She could sense both my consternation and my distaste.

'It's a mess. We've been planning to move for months. There's a new purpose-built unit across the road. Trouble is, every month they tell us one month more. We should be there by September. But that's why nothing gets fixed up here any more.' She went into the tiny office, pushed files off two chairs, mopped ineffectively at some spilt tea.

'Oliver is all right really, but he refuses periodically to take his medication, then he gets agitated. Even on medication he never takes any care of himself. Did you see his teeth?'

I had. They were a mouth full of rotting stumps. 'His eyes didn't look good either.'

'That's because he picks spots on his face and then rubs his eyes and he has this horrible habit of spitting. Anyway, now he has actually proved himself a danger to others we can section him, get him back on medication and perhaps we can persuade him to go to a dentist.'

By 'section', Anita meant using the Mental Health Act to compel Oliver to have treatment. The new 1983 Mental Health Act, introduced a few years earlier, had done much to improve patients' freedoms and make it more difficult to lock people up. But if a patient demonstrated that he was a danger to himself or other people he could, under various 'sections' of the Act, be taken to hospital and kept there for assessment for a month, or for treatment for his mental illness for up to six months. This was the section the ward staff wanted used.

In fact, the majority of patients on Beech were voluntary. Degraded and run-down as it was, it provided some kind of sanctuary. Dr R., the consultant, was trying to minimise dependence on medication and use the same psychodynamic, therapeutic community approaches practised on Larch.

'Chronic schizophrenia can make you greedy, selfish, and destructive,' Dr R. told me in our first meeting. I remained silent, somewhat taken aback. But Dr R. saw such frankness as a necessary starting point. 'This is one place they can come and be accepted when everything else gets too much for them.'

Oliver came into the office a few days later to apologise to Anita.

'I don't want to move to the new building.'

'Why, Oliver? It's going to be lovely, it's got a garden, a dining room, a kitchen and a community room, and you'll have a nice bedroom.'

'It's got gas chambers.'

'Nonsense, Oliver! Look, we'll go over this afternoon and I'll show you. There are no gas chambers, I promise.'

We moved into our beautifully painted new unit that September and had a party to celebrate. There was a band and food. Dr R. insisted on fancy dress. The patients didn't bother but the staff complied. He wore a bishop's robe, I wore a St Trinian's school uniform of tunic, tie, boater and lacy black tights, and Jack was in his Blues Brothers suit. We ate snacks and everyone danced. I was dancing with Diana, a nice woman in her forties who was doing really well compared to most of the others. She was about to be discharged. I had turned away from her for a moment and was briefly dancing with Craig. Even Oliver was sort of shaking from side to side. When I looked back at Diana she was stretched out flat on the floor. Everyone else continued to dance around her.

Sometimes patients lay on the floor in the unit when they simply could not be bothered to continue standing up or go anywhere else. So my first thought was: Why are you lying on the floor, Diana? Then immediately another thought followed: Diana never lies on the floor. I knelt down and felt her pulse. It was going far too rapidly to count: Oh shit! She's fibrillating! The music was still playing and no one else seemed bothered.

'Jack!' I yelled as he whirled past. 'Help! Diana's having a heart attack!' I had already thumped her chest hard with the side of my fist in the hope of jump-starting a normal rhythm. This had never worked for me. Jack and two nurses were beside me in a second.

'Better to move her out of here.'

So we picked her up and somehow carried her to the trolley in the clinical room.

'Can someone get the defibrillator?'

'It's miles away, in the sick unit.' The asylum covered approximately four square miles.

'It would be much quicker to call an ambulance.'

'Then please do it!'

By now Diana had stopped breathing and there was no pulse at all. I pushed her chin up to give mouth-to-mouth, putting my own lips against her clammy skin, while Jack applied the short sharp downward pushes on the chest wall that keep blood circulating. Diana's mouth was full of gunge. No air was going in. I tried scooping it away with a finger. No effect.

'Can someone give me a sucker?'

'We don't have one.'

'What about an airway?'

'Nope, it's all in the sick unit.'

The band was still playing. Jack and I took turns doing compressions. Two ambulance men arrived, much faster than I expected, dumping their boxes on the floor.

'Who's a doctor here?' asked one, hesitantly holding up an endotracheal tube and looking in bewilderment at Dr R.'s red robe and my school tunic and lacy tights.

'I'm the fucking doctor! Please give me the tube and the laryngoscope!'

He handed it over, his look suggesting he knew he was in a madhouse. Amazingly, my old emergency-room habits remained: I was able to insert the laryngoscope and get a clear view of the vocal cords and push the tube in. One ambulance man attached the oxygen and started giving air. Another had already attached the leads from the defibrillator to Diana's chest. We shocked her. Nothing happened. We shocked her again. Her chest rose and fell as the ambulance man rhythmically pressed the air bag. Diana's pupils were in the glassy stare of sudden death. We tried again. Nothing happened.

'Lynne,' Jack said firmly, 'you have to stop now.'

He put an arm out and pulled me momentarily against his shoulder. I remember the feel of his jacket on my forehead. I remember not wanting to turn back to the body. I don't remember which of us said time of death. The ambulance men started packing up. Someone pulled a sheet over Diana. Dr R. said he would talk with the community. I don't remember if the party continued or not. I went home to bed.

At the staff policy meeting that week everyone agreed we needed an accessible defibrillator and equipment to establish a clear airway kept on the ward. One reason for our under-equipped state was that no one could agree on whether or not the asylum was a hospital. Sick patients who needed more intensive nursing care were sent to the sick unit within the hospital, but if they were really unwell, in theory they went to the General Hospital. Psychiatric patients get physically ill like anyone else. Those with chronic mental illnesses get sick more often, because many smoke too much and take less care of themselves. But try getting a bed for a chronic schizophrenic patient on a medical ward. I had spent an hour on the phone the previous week trying to get a patient assessed after he had inexplicably fitted for fifteen minutes. It was only the intervention of the consultant that got him in.

We all went to Diana's memorial. In spite of this grim christening, community life improved, demonstrating that, mad or not, we all respond to the environment in which we live. This was the basis of Samuel Tuke's 'moral' treatment, introduced two hundred years earlier. He had made the radical suggestion that even the severely mentally ill would respond to cleanliness, neatness and comfort in a family-type atmosphere. He had not envisioned the growth of asylums on an industrial scale.

Beech Ward was an attempt to return to this moral order. The chain-smoking and coffee-drinking continued, but people actually avoided dropping their butts on the new carpet. Now that both large and small meetings were held behind closed doors, people wanted to attend them. Because it was a stable community, they worked relatively well. Unselfishness often blossomed. Oliver announced one day that his watch had been stolen but he did not want the police informed 'because we're a family'. He followed up this announcement by bringing a tray of tea to the staff.

I had an office of my own, with potted plants and a view of the garden. The strange thing was that in the old ward I had been around all the time because there was no other space to sit, but the patients had scarcely talked to me. Now they sought me out, came in, sat down in the chair opposite me and just started talking. I had learnt from Jack to stop 'interviewing' and start having conversations, to offer friendship as much as care, and to understand the incredible courage it took for most of them just to get through the day. Craig carefully explained that he was living in three worlds.

'There's the world of outer space, then there's the world of Plutons and Klutons who are fighting one another to death, and there's the world of Beech Ward. Honestly, the stress of it is making me crazy.' He put his hand to his ear and shook his head. His blue eyes took on the unfocused look that meant he was listening to the Plutons.

Craig and Oliver continued to live on Beech after I moved to another unit. Craig jumped off the railway bridge a year later, crushing a vertebra. The emergency departments at the General Hospital put him in a plaster cast and sent him back to the sick unit at Woodside. The nurses called the duty doctor one night. He arrived to find Craig already dead, froth in his mouth, cause unknown. I thought of him lying there in the heavy cast, unable to move, frightened and choking. It was unbearable.

'Well, he wanted to die, didn't he?' a colleague said over lunch.

'No, he did not want to die. He wanted the war in his head to stop. He wanted not to be mad, he wanted a place of his own. I really don't think he wanted to die.' But what I thought of the matter was of no importance. I had rotated on.

Somali border, Ethiopia, September 2007

There's a great jostling crowd at the health centre door this morning. Word has got round that there is a doctor at the camp who treats 'crazy' people. As I try to walk through they grab at me, asking if I can look at this, or this, or this. There's an elderly man who has pushed his paralysed wife up in a wheelbarrow. Mothers clutch their children or hold up infants whose contracted limbs and vacant smiling faces hint at developmental difficulties. There are some muttering young men showing the self-neglect that suggests psychosis, a young woman who is obviously blind, and numerous others on crutches or sticks.

'It's not just mental problems,' the health assistant says. 'It is everything that we cannot treat: paralysis, epilepsy, physical handicap – they all think you will help them.'

It is a biblical scene. I feel a distinct lack of miraculous powers. We try to create some order. The assistant hands out numbered chits and I stand on the steps of the hut and make a small speech, explaining that I will see some people today and the rest at weekly mental health clinics that will run from now on. Then I retreat inside and sit down with one of the clinical nurses to start work.

I am not even supposed to be starting a proper clinic yet. I work for a large international non-governmental organisation, an NGO that provides health care in emergencies. My job here in Ethiopia is to train the government health care staff who run the services for Somali refugees in this camp, to recognise, understand and manage mental health problems. If this can be done right here at the clinic, people will not have to stay chained up or make the long journey to a mental hospital in Addis.

Ethiopia has thirty psychiatrists. They are almost all in the capital and overwhelmed by the demands of treating mental illness in a country of eighty million. When I advertised a job working here in the desert fringes of the country, next to war-torn Somalia, I was not surprised that only three people applied. But one of these is Dr Hassen, a gentle, soft-spoken man with silver hair and a youthful face who comes from

Harar, a beautiful ancient city just down the road. In a previous incarnation he was a professor of physiology. He switched to psychiatry a few years ago and is passionately interested in refugees. He will arrive soon to help me with the training programme and the clinic.

Meanwhile, Usman and Abdullah are already slightly better as a result of the antipsychotic Dr Asmamaw prescribed on my recommendation. They have moved to a bigger *aqal*. Usman is more communicative and washes and dresses himself, and Abdullah is calmer. They are both still chained, but Amel promises that if things continue to improve she will try unchaining them. People at home are often horrified when they hear about chained mental patients, and there's no question it is an abuse. But it is also a sign of care in desperate circumstances, done to protect a relative from getting lost, abused or even killed. Families in flight have sometimes tied up their sick relative as the only means of dragging them across frontiers to safety. Otherwise the individual, not understanding the danger, may refuse to leave. The family won't untie them until they are confident he or she is safe. And newly arrived aid workers need to be cautious. Untying someone before fully understanding the reasons for restraint, without having alternatives to offer, is unwise. This is why I am here. Getting just one person out of chains compensates completely for all my feelings of inadequacy towards the halt, the lame and the blind at the door.

Unfortunately I sometimes lose my clarity of purpose when trying to wash and cook in the evenings. I live in Jijiga, the capital of the Somali region, as far east as you can go in Ethiopia without falling off the map. Tin shacks, cloth-covered *aqals* and stone villas lurk behind high walls along numerous dirt roads like my own. There's a university in a tower block on the eastern edge of the town, and the concrete offices housing regional government as well as the hospital in the centre. Around the corner from us is the very new Ethiopia Millennium Hotel. (Ethiopia's calendar runs seven years behind the rest of the world, and sets this year of 2007 at 2000.)

The town has a quickly-put-up feel that makes it look like the backlot for a cheap Western in Somali costume. People ride around in canopied horse-drawn buggies or three-wheeled *tuk tuks*, and men with guns roam the streets. The men with guns are actually in army uniform. Apparently the prime minister is visiting the region so there are checkpoints everywhere and pat-downs by security men outside restaurants. Someone did try to shoot a politician here a few weeks ago. Whether the shooter was from the Ogaden National Liberation Army to the south or from the war in Somalia to the east, no one knew.

The agency house is in a villa, one block off the main road. When I arrived, the local staff were embarrassed and confused. They didn't know I was coming. They thought the building was just going to be offices. There was no bed, no kitchen, no water, rubbish filled the bath and yard. But the logistician ran around and found stuff in the open-air market that fills the central part of town. Much of it is contraband from Somalia. I now have a bed and sheets. The rubbish has gone from yard and bath. The plumbing does not work but water arrives daily in large metal drums mounted between two shafts and pulled by donkeys. So I can stand in the bath and douse myself from a bucket.

A shiny corrugated-iron kitchen shed appeared out the back a few days ago, but there's still nothing in it. So my boss sent me a very old two-ring gas camping stove that I have set up with a large gas canister, at the far end of the office-cum-dining room. I don't have a phoneline so I go round to the little Internet café on the main road to check mail. Inside, it is full of small boys playing violent video games, not a girl or woman in sight, but the owner shoos two children away to give me a computer. The Internet connection is so slow you can have a short nap while waiting for a page to appear and another while waiting for it to Send. I give up at six o'clock. The owner wants to break his fast, it being Ramadan.

I come home and bang on the high metal gates for the guard to let me in. An armed guard is standard for all NGOs in town, but as he is elderly and alone I do wonder what he would actually do if armed men turned up to kidnap me. I'm looking out for a dog that can bark loudly.

The electricity is still off. By now it's completely dark so I light two newly acquired kerosene lamps and put a large saucepan of water on the stove to boil for tea. I go into my bedroom to do fifteen minutes' yoga. When I come out I can see flickering orange light through the glass section at the top of the office door. I open it very cautiously and see that the kitchen area of the office appears to be on fire. The gas pipe, which turned out to be corroded, has fallen off the gas stove and is blazing away like a blowtorch on the floor. Without thinking, I run over and turn off the gas and it stops. Amazingly, the only damage is melted plastic floor-covering and a scorched wall.

I suddenly realise how lucky it is that the flame didn't melt the short length of pipe and blow up the attached gas canister, the office, and possibly me and the guard. Last year in northern Uganda I walked into a newly built shower in our compound, stood on the wet floor, turned on the tap and got a horrendous electric shock. It strikes me that in this job I am much more likely to be killed in a rather ordinary domestic accident from old appliances or poor wiring than I am to be blown up in a restaurant or taken hostage. I won't think about it. Tonight I am back to heating lentils and water on a smelly kerosene stove outside in the yard.

2: WHY ARE YOU HERE?

I could not find my place in psychiatric practice in Britain. I love psychiatry. I was born curious, and I love the fact that sorting out what's wrong with my patients requires listening and observing intently and enquiring into every aspect of their lives: how they grew up, where they come from, their family background, what happened at school and work, how they get on with others, what happened to upset them. I am never bored with the conversations or stories, however mundane. I also enjoy the arcane game of psychiatric diagnosis, even if I sometimes feel we are debating the number of angels dancing on a pin.

During my training, a patient often seemed to be given one diagnosis on one admission and another on the following, partly depending on the whim of the admitting physician. Graham, for example, came back in as an emergency when I was working on Jameson Ward at the Allinton Hospital during the second year of my rotation. He was living in a bedsit in a shared student house and had found a girlfriend. Things seemed to be going well. But then she dumped him and he stopped studying, eating or going out. His housemates grew concerned at his obvious neglect and at the muttering and cursing that came from his room at night. So they called his GP, who found him weeping and shaking in the corner of his room with a towel around his head to try and keep out the voices. She sent him in as an emergency. The weary house officer on call saw 'previous history of schizophrenia' in the GP letter, but felt that on this occasion he was severely depressed. So he hedged his bets and wrote 'schizo-affective disorder': a composite diagnosis that covered all bases. Graham stayed another month and appeared to make a good recovery. He was sent home to his parents, still taking his medication, and planned to restart college. But then without any warning he went into the garden one day and hanged himself from a tree.

What was clear to me was that psychosis, in all its varied manifestations, was absolutely terrifying for those experiencing it. A patient once explained to me that it was like losing a filtering mechanism in your head. You saw and heard every single thing. Everything was too loud, too bright and it all mattered and felt significant. Perhaps for Graham, once he had recovered full insight and understood his possible prognosis, the prospect of living with severe long-term mental illness seemed unbearable. His death, like Craig's and Diana's before, filled me with anger; but I could not clearly define what my own role should be in response.

There appeared to be two choices. I could join the young men in tweed jackets in the research laboratory, searching for the Holy Grail of the biochemical underpinnings of schizophrenia or the genetics of bipolar disorder, while hustling for research grants and lectureships. Alternatively, I could embrace one of the psychotherapeutic trainings: psychoanalysis or the new, increasingly fashionable, cognitive therapy. But I did not want to choose. Too often I saw colleagues becoming ideologues more interested in fitting a patient to a school of thought than thinking through what the patient needed.

I always felt wrong-footed. I argued with my biologically minded colleagues about the social construction of illness, and the patients' need for care and attention to address their social ills, whatever the science revealed about causation. But when I did a six-month attachment to an outpatient group-therapy unit, I worried that one of the group members who spent each session mumbling, talking and laughing to herself was actively psychotic, and perhaps needed medication. My consultant reprimanded me for my 'activist' attitude, told me that *he* made the diagnoses, and my job was to help run the groups. It was only when I learnt to present any such concerns about the patients as 'my anxieties' that I was allowed to address them.

I also hated what Mrs Thatcher was doing to the National Health Service. Her push to create an internal market was supposed to create a more effective and competitive service. The trouble is that mental patients are rather uncompetitive 'products'. No one really wants them, they are poor advocates for their own needs, so they are very easy to abandon. One summer in the late eighties I worked at a small acute-admission unit attached to the district General Hospital of a busy market town. It was a happy and pleasant place to work. A combination of skilled and friendly nursing staff, good relationships with local GPs, a good social worker and psychologist and hard-working consultants meant that the stigma so often associated with admission to a mental hospital scarcely existed. Because the unit was based in the community it served, large numbers of patients could be managed as outpatients and we could intervene quickly if things broke down. Except that Mrs Thatcher's reforms had frozen the nursing budget, so half our beds were closed, which meant that we spent our review meetings deciding 'who does not need admission'.

How to choose? Alan was an elderly man who got severe recurrent depressions that resolved of their own accord without medication as long as he could be admitted for two or three days. If not, he went downhill quickly and could end up being sectioned because he refused to eat, drink or care for himself. Eleanor was a young mother of twenty-eight who had been depressed for three months. Now she was completely preoccupied with ideas of killing both herself and her children. One of our current inpatients had taken an overdose the previous week when she heard that we planned to transfer her to the Allinton, thirty miles away.

I was learning that good community services are not cheap alternatives to institutional care. They actually require more staff and the back-up of small admission units like ours. This could sometimes be life-saving in the fullest sense of the word.

A community-based unit could provide the intensive support, understanding and involvement needed in a crisis and continue it after discharge, extending it to friends and family. But I did not want to spend my life fighting over beds and resources. It seemed to me the answer was political. I wrote an article about my experiences for a national newspaper. I suggested that spending vast amounts of money on murderous weapons of mass destruction was indicative of a national paranoid psychosis – and that it might be better spent on keeping people alive and well now, rather than killing them later. Apparently it was not so simple. I was told to stick to my patients.

That was the other problem. I had been quite unable to give up politics, although I no longer camped outside a nuclear base. In 1987 the United States and the then USSR signed a treaty to get rid of Intermediate-Range Nuclear Forces: Cruise and Pershing missiles in the UK and Western Europe, and their Soviet cousins the SS-20s. It was the first time the Superpowers had agreed to eliminate a category of weapons and reduce their nuclear arsenals. It felt like a vindication of our campaign.

But that first disarmament treaty shone a bright light on the underlying fracture of Europe. The Marxist historian E. P. Thompson, whose polemics against Cruise missiles had inspired me to join the peace movement in the first place, argued that getting rid of one weapon system was not enough; we had to address the underlying exterminating logic of the Cold War. I agreed. The continuing repression of human rights activists in Eastern Europe justified continuing to maintain nuclear arsenals to defend 'freedom' in the West. These arsenals justified the continuing repression in the Soviet bloc. And these conflicts were also played out in very real hot wars in places like Central America and East Africa.

I spent my holidays in the late eighties travelling to Poland, supporting young people who refused to serve in a Soviet-sponsored army that had imposed martial law on its own people, and to Hungary where students in a democratic movement called Fidesz were challenging the authoritarianism of the state. In my spare time at home I wrote articles about human rights activists in Guatemala who used non-violence to oppose a genocidal US-backed war against the indigenous population; or I helped circulate petitions about a little-known Czech theatre director imprisoned in Prague. By early 1989 I was going out with a Slovene philosopher and writer whom I had met in a cold church in Warsaw, at a seminar hosted by my Polish friends to discuss 'Détente from Below'. Tomaž had been thrown out of the Yugoslav Communist Party for writing a critical book about Stalin. He was now organising demonstrations on behalf of miners on a hunger strike, in a place called Kosovo.

My psychiatric colleagues looked on at all these activities with bemusement. But in my own life medicine and politics had always mixed. My doctor parents had never sat me down and said: Think this or that. Rather, there were givens in our family which were part of the established order of things: the National Health Service, established as my parents qualified, was good, so they were happy to work for it. Apartheid was wrong so we didn't drink South African wine. The Bomb was bad – so we were taken on CND marches in our pushchairs. They belonged to the Howard League, and one of my earliest memories is their excitement when capital punishment was abolished. But it was studying medicine that radicalised me. Simply going onto the wards as a first-year clinical student brought home the inescapable fact that, while everyone is vulnerable to serious disease, you are much more likely to get sick and stay sick if you are poor. On my bookshelf Gandhi, Emma Goldman, Bakunin and Proudhon jostled for space.

This radicalisation was intensified by living with a young black student who had just escaped from South Africa. Nkosazana Dlamini had been the vice-president of the South African Students' Organisation. When its president Steve Biko was killed, she had managed to escape by walking across the border. Bristol Medical School gave her a scholarship and a mutual friend asked if I could give her our spare room. Living with her brought home in an intensely personal way what it meant to live in an unjust and impoverished society. When her brother died suddenly in Soweto and she could not go home, I learnt for the first time what it meant to be a refugee. Influenced by her experience, I joined Anti-Apartheid and helped to get the university to disinvest in its South African shares. That was my first political campaign.

In 1989, after three years at the Allinton and Woodside, I turned off onto another of those meandering side roads that have drawn me all my life. After taking the second part of the exams that would qualify me as a psychiatrist, I got permission to take time off to do doctoral research. I obtained a grant from a large foundation to study the psychological motivations of those non-violent political activists with whom I had worked for the previous decade in Britain, Poland and Guatemala. Asking these activists why they gave up home, work and family to act as they did was a way for me to pull together the diverse threads of my life. For my colleagues at the Allinton, it was yet one more indication of how unsuited I was to the psychiatric profession in Britain. 'I very much doubt you'll return,' said the postgraduate dean gloomily, while granting me leave from the rotational training, 'and if you do, all these periods outside psychiatry will look very bad on your CV.'

But sometimes you arrive at a place where you know you are meant to be. In the highlands of Guatemala I met Maria. She was a courageous indigenous Maya woman who risked her life daily by teaching human rights to her community. In her area, local villagers were refusing to join the government-sponsored 'civilian patrols' that were a method of both militarising and controlling the countryside. She was happy to be interviewed and even happier when she discovered that I was a psychiatrist. Would I please come home with her to see her brother who had been mentally ill for some years?

We took the battered minibus further up into the Quiché highlands, switchbacking over steep-sided pine-covered ridges, then walking the last two miles to the cluster of cane and adobe houses that made up Maria's hamlet. It did not take long to establish that her brother had a severe psychotic depression. He had once taken the two-day bus journey to the mental hospital in Guatemala City but had long ago run out of the medication they gave him. She had not taken him back because they had no money. But now he was obviously severely depressed again, refusing food, and scarcely speaking or moving. This had gone on for months. All I could do was advise that he really did need to return to the hospital and be reassessed. He would benefit from both medication and cognitive therapy, although the latter was unlikely to be available. I listed the possible drugs that I hoped might work, explained their side effects and the nature of the illness, and the things they could do as a family to help him recover and stay well, then gave her money to take him to the city and pay for the drugs.

We walked down the path between small patches of corn, vegetables and fruit trees into the village square. The landscape fell away from the *plaza* and the houses, in fold after fold of blue-grey mountains. Coming towards us was a young woman in a torn *huipil*, stage-lit against this astonishing backdrop by the horizontal afternoon sun. The dirty embroidered blouse had fallen off her shoulder, exposing half her breast. Her skirt too was ragged. Unusually for a Guatemalan woman, her hair was uncombed and unplaited, hanging in dirty threads around her face, which was cut and bleeding. She was crying and shouting. I instinctively went towards her, thinking something terrible had happened. Maria pulled me back, shaking her head and making the familiar gesture of a finger pointed at the head. This was the local 'mad' woman. And then I noticed the small children running after her, laughing and pointing and gathering up small pebbles to hurl at her.

'She is crazy,' Maria said, 'there is nothing you can do.'

'What about her family?'

Maria shrugged.

'She has none.'

I felt a familiar surge of rage, the 'I cannot bear it – this is impossible – we must do something' feeling which is what usually

pushes me into action. I would at least talk to the children. I
stomped over to them as they stood giggling, fascinated by an
irate white woman who obviously could not speak Quiché. I
asked Maria to translate my basic Spanish:

'This lady is sick, you should not hurt her. That will make
her worse. You have to be kind.'

'She shouts at us and she says crazy things. She is a witch!'

'So just leave her alone, then she won't bother you.'

The children giggled some more. It seemed unlikely that
my two-minute homily on being nice to crazy people would
change anything.

The medical anthropology lectures in my psychiatric training had focused on the exotic: the 'culture-bound diseases' such
as 'semen loss syndrome'. Our professors had taught us that
traditional societies coped much better than our own with the
severely ill, and that rates of mental disorder were much lower
there. Yet here in one tiny hamlet in the highlands of rural
Guatemala were two people who had been ill for years and
who were untreated because of poverty or stoned and taunted
because people were afraid or thought they were evil or bewitched. The asylum in Guatemala City was fourteen hours
away by bus. How could it possibly help, and who would want
to be left there, miles from friends or family? It was another of
those finger-pointing signposts in the road. I suddenly understood what I could do: work in remote places like this where
there were no psychiatrists, and try to help. I had no idea how
to do such a thing but I was determined to try and find out.
Then the war began.

My war started while I was cooking dinner on Wednesday, 25
July 1991. Tomaž and I had married in 1990, after my return
from Guatemala. We were now living in Florence while he
studied at the European University Institute and I typed up
interviews for my doctoral thesis. Friends were visiting from
Australia. One of them was reading aloud from the novel he
was writing, while his wife sewed. Outside you could hear the
usual mix of church bells and pigeons cooing. Tomaž was on

the phone to his brother. Then he came into the kitchen and sat quietly, waiting for the conversation to ebb.

'How is everyone in Ljubljana?' I asked.

'It is war,' he said simply. It was the nearest to tears I had ever seen him. There was a shocked, awkward silence, the kind that comes when you realise that while you've been laughing and drinking in the pub, someone outside has just been fatally injured in a car crash. Then we recovered ourselves and begged him to tell us more.

'Stupid,' he said. 'The defence minister announced it on television at seven and then spent two hours in the TV studio, while there are tanks in the street and barricades up, and fighting in the countryside.'

Milošević's ten-day military expedition to Slovenia turned out to be nothing compared to what followed. I think Tomaž's sadness had as much to do with prescience for the future as distress over his family sitting in cellars, wondering if they might be shelled. But I was astonished at the impact the news had on me. For the previous decade I had immersed myself in war, studied it, and lectured on the effects of nuclear weapons and the non-violent alternatives to conflict. I had campaigned against it and lived with the dirtier variety in Guatemala. But this felt personal. It felt like *my* war, particularly as most of my British friends still had difficulty finding Slovenia on a map.

The Balkan wars split the peace movement. Surprising numbers took views such as: 'The death of Tito has unleashed tribal hatreds from the ice chest of Communism', 'The Bosnian war is a civil war between primitive peoples who have been at war for centuries', 'There is nothing to be done but let them fight it out.' Such comments seemed odd, coming from Europeans whose hundreds of years of tribal conflict had stopped only forty years earlier.

Another interpretation was that a hardline Serbian Communist elite had realised they could no longer dominate a democratising Yugoslavia and decided to carve a Greater Serbia from its remnants. Given the ethnically mixed nature of the population across the country, this had to mean displacement and war. When Milošević imposed martial law in Kosovo in the summer of 1990, Tomaž argued that this was a Munich moment and he had to be stopped. But Kosovo was a faraway country about which most people knew nothing.

We went back home to Ljubljana in the summer of 1991, shortly after Milošević had withdrawn the Yugoslav Army from a now independent Slovenia, to concentrate on ethnic cleansing in Croatia. We picked raspberries in the woods and swam in rivers of glass-clear water. Families raked hay in their meadows outside wooden-shuttered, painted stone houses. Churches perched on hilltops. I could imagine the Prince of Ruritania emerging at any moment from a geranium-bedecked inn. It was impossible to believe that real tanks were shelling real people in Osijek, a few hundred kilometres away in Croatia. But journalist friends would call in on their way to and from various front lines, reporting the growing brutality. 'War is good business, we will all be famous now,' said our friend Ervin.

The Bosnian war began in spring 1992. Bosnians voted for independence from the remaining rump of Yugoslavia. The European Union and the United States recognised the new country. Bosnian Serbs declared their own mini-state and began killing and expelling non-Serbs from the areas they controlled. The rest of the world watched. Every day there were more reports of killing. The library in Sarajevo was shelled; there was a massacre of people queuing for bread.

Fragments of war continued to wash up on the margins of our lives in Ljubljana that summer. A journalist friend was killed in Sarajevo, one of eight journalists killed in the country that year. I began to work as a volunteer in the new refugee camps in Ljubljana. They were full of escapees from the north Bosnian town of Prijedor and its surrounding villages. They had tried non-violence. When the Serbian and Yugoslav Federal Army took over the town, the Muslims and Croats complied with requests to hand in all their weapons including hunting rifles, and to mark their houses with white flags. Mass dismissals from jobs followed, along with campaigns of vilification.

Next came arbitrary arrests, rapes, the expulsion of women and children, and the imprisonment, torture and massacre of men.

The anarchist and pacifist beliefs that had framed my life for the previous two decades no longer made any sense. I had always believed the writer Kingsley Martin's point that to defeat Fascism by military means we must become Fascist ourselves. But I could not think of any non-violent strategies that could stop genocide – for this is what the horrors had become. The Serbs had inherited the troops and weaponry of the fourth-strongest army in Europe, the Yugoslav Federal Army. So the arms embargo, imposed on all sides, had simply set this advantage in stone, giving them the muscle and the ability to cleanse non-Serbs with impunity from the regions they claimed. However, the Bosnian Army around Sarajevo was fighting back and that city, with its mixed population of Serbs, Croats and Muslims, had still not fallen. For the first time in my life I understood that there are situations where the only way to stop violence is by using violence, and that what the Bosnians needed was military assistance. I signed a public declaration calling for the lifting of the arms embargo, so that the Bosnians could arm and defend themselves.

When we returned to Britain that autumn, I spent eight weeks writing an essay trying to explain why military support for the Bosnians was needed. I sat in our tiny cottage in Cambridge tearing up draft after draft. The activity required such a rethinking of every speech I had ever given that I became physically ill with the effort: sore throat, headache, stomach ache, my whole body rebelled. The fundamental principle at stake was my pacifist belief that all human lives are of equal value and that therefore one life could not be taken to save another. This meant one was pushed into developing active non-violent means to protect life and human dignity when they were threatened.

The problem is that active non-violent resistance works best when there is something that can be withheld from those who have violence at their disposal. It may be the withdrawal of labour, as had occurred with Solidarity in Poland. It may be consent to govern, as had brought down the totalitarian East European regimes. It could be refusal to join a government militia, like Maria and her friends in Guatemala. In these situations the population under attack has value, which acts as some restraint on the use of violence by the attackers. But if a people have no value and the aggressor's sole objective is their removal by expulsion or death, there are no limits on the use of violence, especially when the victims have been demonised and presented as a threat to that aggressor's wellbeing. The only hope is an observing moral world: other peoples and states who are moved to care about what is happening, who see themselves as somehow responsible and implicated – and so act to restrain the aggression.

No one acted when the Nazis liquidated the Warsaw Ghetto. No one was acting to restrain the Serbs in Bosnia. Indeed, it had been clear since the London International Conference on the Former Yugoslavia in the summer of 1992 that my government hoped for a quick victory for the Serbs and the division of Bosnia between Croatia and Serbia, so that the inconvenient moral problem of a beleaguered Muslim population would simply disappear.

'I am against war,' I wrote. 'That is why I wish to stop it. The fact is that even limited actions – such as effective sanctions, a genuine air-exclusion zone, secure corridors for the delivery of humanitarian relief, or the arrest and trial of war criminals – are impossible without at least the threat of force.' The article was published in a peace movement journal and I lost half my friends overnight.

The drip, drip, drip of devastation from Bosnia continued. Tomaž and I became socially dangerous. Dinner parties in Cambridge with people uninvolved in the Balkans were awkward affairs. People would fret over whether they should bring up the war or not: to do so risked everyone getting upset. After all, it was scarcely a subject for wit or banter. How do you mix concentration camps and starvation in Sarajevo with comments on the nice white wine from Sainsbury's? Yet not to do so would seem callous.

I felt both envious and resentful of those who neither knew nor cared. I stopped writing to friends because all my letters sounded so didactic or despairing – either a lecture or a rant – that I couldn't bear to think of others reading them. I had nothing personal, amusing or intimate to say about the war, or anything else. Tomaž also grew angrier and gloomier by the day, furious at what he saw as the willed ignorance of both the British media and the government. Sometimes I felt he saw me, his British wife, as part of the problem. Not surprisingly, the war was not good for our marriage. Although we agreed on the politics, we argued over what to do. Tomaž hated listening to the news. One morning he hurled his small radio across the room, incensed at the stupidity of a particular interviewer giving the Bosnian Serb leader, psychiatrist Dr Radovan Karadžić, yet more airtime. I preferred the pseudo-knowledge that came with the bulletins, even though listening made me angry and depressed.

I grieved for that optimistic self of the previous decade. I had been naive and arrogant but I had felt a hopefulness that, with enough of us engaged, we could shift something. Words like 'empowerment' rolled off the tongue so easily. Now, when a shift was really needed, I no longer had that sense of possibility. The basic optimism that had coloured most of my life seemed to be seeping away. I wanted to do something. But that was another point of disagreement between us.

If I see a problem I am someone who needs to be up against it. If it's nuclear weapons I want to be camping outside the base; if it's psychosis I want to be there with my patient; if it's human rights abuses in Guatemala I want to be interviewing and writing about those being abused. Tomaž felt that action was too often a substitute for thought. 'What are you going for?' he asked me, when I had suggested I might join a planned peace camp on the border of Kuwait, during the first Gulf War. 'It is foolishness and vanity. You are going so you can act, so that people can see you acting, so that you don't have to think.

You will be too busy to contemplate the real value of what you are doing. This is the easiest thing. This way you don't have to stay here and think about what really can be done. These peace camps cannot possibly stop the war. It is here that things must change. And doesn't it matter that I need you?' I had seen the logic of his argument. I also felt touched at being wanted. But now, having argued for military intervention, I felt I had a responsibility to work in Bosnia and share the consequences. This time Tomaž did not see it as foolish but said simply: 'You are my wife. I wish you would not go.'

So we compromised. In 1993 I put aside my thesis for a few weeks and went back to Ljubljana to the refugee camps where I had volunteered the previous summer. According to the Slovene friends, Bosnian teenage boys had since developed a sort of criminal culture in the camp. There they were, stuck out beyond the motorway on a half-built industrial estate in a wasteland of wintry fields. Families shared huts that had previously been the homes of Bosnian summer workers. There was no school, and the boys refused to participate in the offer of sports or clubs.

'They just sit around watching TV or make occasional forays to steal things like food supplies from the canteen,' a local doctor told me. 'All they want is cigarettes, money and girls.' Goga, my boss, thought it would be useful if I tried to start some groups. Perhaps the boys would be able to discuss their feelings.

My psychiatric training had included a fair amount of group work. There was six months of out-patient group therapy; and every unit in which I had worked ran 'small' and 'large' groups for patients, and support groups for staff. So I felt I could manage something. Except that the boys had no interest in any kind of group discussion about their problems. They agreed to come only when I asked for help with mine. I said I needed a crash course on Bosnian history and culture and asked if they could provide it. They agreed, and to my astonishment twenty turned up for the first meeting. We sat, tightly squashed together, in a hut that served as a club room and smelt of sweaty feet.

'Before you begin I want to ask you a question,' a tall boy said aggressively. 'You're English. I want to know what you think of your Foreign Secretary, Douglas Hurd?'

Trainee psychiatrists attend 'T groups'. The idea of these training groups is that they can both learn about psychodynamic group processes and discuss feelings arising from work-related issues. Ours had not worked very well. The excellent consultant psychotherapist in charge could not get past our reluctance to share any significant feelings in this strained and artificial atmosphere. This was partly because, however sensitive he may have been, he belonged to the supervising group whose evaluations would determine our future careers.

I never brought up Diana's death; a friend of mine never mentioned the anxieties and miseries that were making them contemplate resignation from the training rotation. As the training years progressed we got into the habit of all going for lunch at the pub beforehand, where we would laugh, gossip and moan about work, giving ourselves all the support and ventilation space we needed. Then we would reluctantly drag ourselves back to the 'group' to go through the motions of meaningful interpersonal discussion. We were reminded that this was not the place to discuss politics or even ward events – instead we should focus on our 'feelings' about them. Our supervisor remained opaque, never sharing a word about himself. Confronted with the Bosnian teenager's question, he would have immediately replied: 'Why is it important to you to know?'

'I don't know him personally,' I said to the Bosnian boy, 'but if you are referring to his policy towards Bosnia, I disagree with it. Indeed, I am deeply ashamed of it. That is one of the reasons I am here with you.' The boys nodded and the group was allowed to continue.

The next time I walked down the muddy track to the camp I found a non-violent protest going on. A bunch of boys had locked themselves into the club room and put all the furniture in the yard outside. They were staging an occupation, shouting to all passers-by about their treatment in the camp.

'Once I get the key back they'll be forbidden from using the club again! Ever! They are nothing but trouble!' the camp administrator shouted at me. I went in search of some other boys to see what we could negotiate. A large group was having coffee in a family room and begged me to come in. I sat down and they poured out all their grievances in a torrent.

'Srebrenica is about to fall, what are you in the West going to do about that?'

'Let it happen, as always!' one of them answered.

'We should be there, not here – we should be fighting.'

'No one wants us, the camp administrator never stops hassling us about noise.'

'We don't have a town anymore.'

'We don't have a country. We don't belong any where.'

'We don't even have a room.'

It went on like this for about half an hour.

'I have a suggestion,' I ventured, in a brief pause.

There was silence.

'I can't do anything about Srebrenica or the West's stupidity, you know that, and you know how I feel. But perhaps I can help you to negotiate with the camp administrator to agree to any of your needs that are reasonable.'

So that was what we did. Lisa, who ran the group with me, and I and a group of ten boys moved to a nearby café to discuss non-violent negotiating strategies. Getting the boys briefly outside the camp made all the difference. They came up with a list of their needs, of things they wanted to do in the room, arrangements for the key and rules for the club. They weren't evicted.

The children taught me to be completely flexible. I abandoned many of the formal rules I had been taught at home about leaving the external world outside the room, about fixed boundaries, regular attendance and precise times. With no school and nothing to do, these teenagers rarely knew what day of the week it was or what time. So Lisa and I would run around alerting them on group days and they would drift in.

No subject was off-limits, and if they asked me my own views, I answered honestly. They taught me a great deal about Bosnia and in doing so discussed their feelings for their country, their home towns and their dead or missing relatives, and got into intense arguments about politics and the war. The girls had their own group in which we had equally intense discussions about what it meant to be a Muslim girl, and relationships with boys. It didn't seem to matter that we did not always agree – they rarely did with each other – and my openness gave them more confidence. I didn't see it as a therapy group. They were grieving, angry and frustrated at camp life but their experiences did not appear to have made them sick. My work was as much about restoring respect for their views, their autonomy and their normal life as about dealing with any intrapsychic angst.

When I came home after two months, Tomaž told me he had met someone else and wanted to separate. So I was free to work in Bosnia after all. After some months of weeping, I pulled myself together and got a job with an aid agency in Sarajevo.

Somali border, Ethiopia, October 2007

Aman, my translator, wants me to see a woman whom he sometimes hears shouting at night. He has found out where she lives
and takes me there. When we arrive I find a heartbreaking scene:
a little girl of seven sits bolt upright against one side of the shelter
nervously watching an emaciated woman stretched out on a thin
cotton mattress on the other side. The woman wears only a torn
cotton shift. She has a great tangled mass of uncovered hair that
sways around her narrow face. Somali women always cover their
hair with a small scarf even in the privacy of their own homes. It's
the first time I've seen a woman with uncovered hair in the camp.
She cannot keep still: she sits up, she lies down, she buries her face
in her hands, runs her hands through her hair, shakes her head. All
the while she mutters, sings, moans and shouts to herself.

Aman tries to translate exactly, speaking in the first person,
as I have taught him:

'Oh God what will happen? Why have you done this to
me? What will happen? Why have you done this? My father,
my husband . . .' Aman breaks off. 'Sometimes it makes sense,
sometimes I just don't understand it – it is just a rush of words,
it is too fast, I cannot translate.'

A small two-year-old boy sits close to his mother, watching her.
He is dressed in a grey woollen sweatshirt pulled over torn red
trousers. His face is dirty and tear-stained, his eyes large, bewildered and frightened. He places one tiny hand on his mother's
leg as if to calm her, until she brushes it away in irritation. A
middle-aged man comes in and sits next to us. He introduces
himself as Saidu, and the disturbed woman as Amina, his sister.
'She's been like this for two years. She hardly sleeps. She won't eat
much. We don't need to chain her, she is too frightened to go out.'

The problem first began three years ago. Amina was always
a volatile, moody person: sometimes up and excitable, sometimes very down and miserable. But she brought up her first
daughter without difficulty. Then in one round of the fighting
in Mogadishu, her husband and her father were both killed in
front of her. She was knocked unconscious.

When she woke up in hospital she was violent, incoherent and screaming at people. She was pregnant at the time. Her brother took her home, untreated. They somehow managed to look after her and the symptoms subsided. But eight months later, immediately after the birth of her son, she became sick again in a similar way: singing, shouting, and irritable. It has been unremitting until now. Like many others, Amina's brother decided to flee Mogadishu when one of the factions in the conflict, the Islamic Courts Union, began forcibly recruiting in his part of town. They reached this camp a few months ago. All his time is taken up with her care and protection.

Amina lies down for a moment. The boy again tries to snuggle up close, tucking himself under one flaccid arm, but Amina pushes him away. Saidu scoops the boy into his arms. At least the children have one loving relative, but mother is mother even when she is so sick. I move across to see if I can make contact. Amina has her back to me.

'Amina, can I help you?' I ask. Aman translates and she turns a face of such misery and pain towards me, wet with tears, that I could weep with her myself, but she stares past me and turns away, the brief moment of connection gone. I sit watching and listening some more.

'I think she has something we call bipolar disorder, and we can treat it.' I then explain in detail to Saidu how the illness fits with how she appears now, and her ups and downs before she was sick; how stressful events such as witnessing deaths, and the hormonal changes of childbirth, can trigger episodes. 'We will start her on medication; we have to get her daughter into school. It's not good for the children to be with her every moment when she's so sick.'

Saidu comes back with me to the clinic to pick up some medicine. I explain about possible side effects and promise I will call again the next day to see how Amina is. In the last few days the news from Somalia has been really bad. It is hard to see what can bring this to an end, but it gets little coverage in the Western media. Asmamaw asks me why the world cares so little about some wars and so much about others. I cannot give an answer. I have the same question about some diseases.

3: ON A FRONT LINE

Sarajevo, 1994

When a well-known news reporter climbed the steep hill above the Kosevo Hospital in the centre of Sarajevo to find out what was happening in the kindergarten at the top, she did not stay long. I know this because I followed in her footsteps a few months later and Dr M. told me what happened.

'She asked if there were any children. I told her, "No, not any more." Then she asked if we had any raped women? I said, "No." "Well, traumatised soldiers perhaps?" I explained that this was now the home of seventy patients with chronic schizophrenia, of all nationalities, we are a multi-ethnic community. She went off without filming anything or talking to any of us.'

I followed Dr M. into the two downstairs classrooms where the mental patients of no interest to the journalist lay and dozed on cots, or stared at the ceiling. They had an extraordinary story. When the Bosnian war began in April 1992, Dr M. had helped look after 350 patients at a big psychiatric institution outside the city. Bosnian Serb forces had occupied that area and all non-Serb doctors like herself had been forced to leave that May. The patients were evicted the following month. Seventy of them had somehow found their own way across front lines and into the besieged city, where they had been housed in this kindergarten. Dr M. knew all of them by name. For the first two winters of war they had not had heating or beds and slept on the floor. There was no bomb shelter either, but often the patients ignored the shelling and went outside.

She was amazed none had been killed. She was sorry they

had to be in hospital. They did have psychotropic drugs and none were acutely ill, but their families were either a long way away or could not cope. The biggest problems were lice, gastro-enteritis and a lack of anything to do. She had no materials or staff for rehabilitation. 'We have just one group discussion a day and television in the evening, so they are all becoming institutionalised.'

'What do you need?'

'Underwear, socks, shoes, bedlinen, fruit and vegetables.'

We wandered back to the front door and looked down over the shattered but still beautiful city. We could see the parliament and the minaret of the sixteenth-century mosque next door. We could make out the line of elegant nineteenth-century mansions below the Kosevo Hospital. There was a park opposite that had been turned into allotments for vegetables. Most of the trees had been cut down for fuel, but the remaining ones blazed red and yellow in the afternoon sunlight.

Dr M. pointed out her home, which was visible in the Serb-occupied territory across the river. She had lost it at the beginning of the war and worked without pay for almost three years. Now, like her patients, she depended on humanitarian aid and the meals provided by the hospital for those on duty. I thought about my patients Oliver and Craig back on Beech Ward in Woodside, and wondered if they would have found their way across two front lines in a war. I found it very moving that one of the last remnants of this multi-ethnic country was a community of evacuated asylum patients living in a kindergarten.

Taking care of hospitalised mental patients was not really part of my job at that moment. It was my first position with an international NGO and they had not given me a job description. Patrick, the friendly director of their Bosnian programme, had told me in a brief telephone interview that I was to give some lectures on mental health and run some training groups for social workers. Otherwise, I should make myself useful to any other agency wanting mental health support. This vagueness was a good thing, as I had no training whatsoever in front-line psychiatry. I was making it up as I went along.

A bomb exploded in the open-air market in the centre of
Sarajevo in February 1994. It instantly killed sixty-nine and
wounded two hundred. This outraged the Western powers
enough for them to threaten airstrikes on the Bosnian Serbs.
Realising that for once the West was serious, the Serbs placed
their heavy weapons under UN control and agreed to open
certain 'humanitarian' corridors for supplies to the besieged
cities of Sarajevo, Goražde, Žepa and Srebrenica. These were
now declared to be 'safe havens'. NATO started to patrol the
airspace and threatened to bomb 'either warring party' for any
transgression.

This meant that in the autumn I could fly into Sarajevo from
the Croatian capital Zagreb on a Russian Yak 4C. I was given
a 'blue card', a little piece of plastic from the United Nations
High Commission for Refugees (UNHCR), stating that I was
'operational assessment staff, consultant to an international
NGO'. The card was the magic talisman. Courteous, mono-
syllabic Scandinavians in blue helmets allowed me through
the gate of the UN compound into a strange world of army
barracks, large satellite dishes and white containers pretending to be offices. A Swedish medical officer gave me a severe
telling-off when I went for a shot. Did I not know there was
hepatitis A in Sarajevo at present? Why had I not got a yellow
card stating what previous shots I had been given? I felt inadequate. I hadn't expected things to be so organised: staff cars
to drive me around, free health care, shopping at the PX shops
for whisky and tobacco. I was suddenly part of an occupying
elite. I could see how this might become addictive.

Flying into the city took slightly longer than planned. There
was fog. The Bosnian Serbs could not make up their minds
whether to sell Sarajevo airport to the UN or shoot at incoming planes, and they were, as usual, bargaining and shooting at
the same time. Once flights were available, aid workers were
third in the queue after troops and diplomats, but ahead of
journalists. So I sat in a cold tent chewing my fingernails. I

was weighed down with food and the reading materials requested by my employers, and suffocating in my flak jacket. If anyone had pushed me over I would have had to lie prostrate on the ground like a medieval knight in armour until someone picked me up again. Once on the flight, I took 10 milligrams of temazepam, and fell asleep with my head on the shoulder of a young Swedish diplomat. I awoke to bright sunlight, beautiful mountains and small villages in wooded valleys below. Two journalists were telling 'how I survived the war' stories.

The plane started its descent and some of us, including me, put on our helmets. 'Why lose your head if you don't have to?' said one of the journalists. 'Sit on your flak jacket,' another advised me. 'They're shooting from the ground.' Then we were on the ground and there was Patrick, standing in the autumn sun in a sweatshirt and baseball cap, hand outstretched to greet me. I felt overdressed and rather foolish.

The agency housed me on the third floor of a beautiful turn-of-the-century mansion in Hapsburg Empire style, with porticoes and curlicues. Inside was a well-provided apartment with two reception rooms, high ceilings, heavy drapes, plush furniture, a freezer, three televisions and two cookers, one electric and one gas. But I had the strange sensation of living *on* this apartment rather than in it. Water did not come out of the taps. It came from the bottles and pans and assorted containers that filled the kitchen and bathroom. Electricity was intermittent. After spending my first three nights blundering about, searching for candles and matches, I learnt to place them just inside the front door. I kept food cold on the balcony, cooked on the small kerosene camping heater provided by the agency, and huddled in the corners of rooms under blankets to keep warm. It was a bit like the peace camp at Greenham.

In some strange way I felt that all my life had been a preparation for living in this besieged late-twentieth-century European city. Standing to strip-wash in the freezing bathroom, I had a vivid memory of myself at nine with six other shivering girls in an equally icy communal bathroom at school. Matron was teaching us the correct technique: remove pyjama top, take flannel, do face, ears, neck, chest, underarms; take flannel in one hand, flick to back, catch corner with other hand, pull diagonally in both directions to wash back. Dry top half, replace pyjama top, remove bottoms, take a second flannel to wash lower half. Bath: Tuesdays, Thursdays and Saturdays or Mondays, Wednesdays and Fridays, no baths on Sundays.

No baths here in Sarajevo at all, unless I chose to plunge into my carefully hoarded cold bathwater and use it all at once.

Then Aleks would arrive to pick me up in the minibus, doing a rapid circuit of the city to gather up other staff. The foggy early mornings made it safer; even so, he accelerated over the streets exposed to sniper view. I liked Aleks, a Serb from a Bosnian government anti-terrorist unit before he joined the agency. He made me feel secure.

The office itself was in one of the shattered glass tower blocks next to the Holiday Inn. After climbing eleven floors I had an excellent view of what everyone called 'Sniper Alley'. This was the main road running along this side of the river. It lay in direct view of the front line that followed the hills on the other side, and then snaked down through the Jewish cemetery. Sometimes there was a burst of gunfire from the hills. On my first day I watched as down in the street below everyone suddenly stopped moving: a freeze-frame in a motion picture as they paused at the edge of the road. The UN anti-sniping unit, one of their tanks placed across every major junction on this side of town, remained motionless and silent. Then one girl made a run for it, reaching the other side of the road without difficulty. The firing stopped. People carried on as if nothing had happened. Kenan, one of our drivers, wandered in clutching hot coffee.

'You do know just opening the blinds makes you an easy target for snipers.' After this I kept them shut.

My immediate boss was Narcisa. Slim and chic, formerly a dermatologist, she ran the psychosocial project with her partner, Semir. He had trained as an oncologist before serving two years on the front line. His best friend had died in his arms and he had lost many others. His commander gave him six months off.

Narcisa and Semir looked rather like brother and sister. Both had short dark hair, large eyes and delicate pale faces. But while Semir wore jeans and an old padded jacket, Narcisa was dressed elegantly in a pre-war suit and nylons. My other colleagues were Yelena, the social worker, and Zara, my translator. Everyone had the gaunt and shadowed look that I associated with most of the long-term residents of the city. Plump faces and new clothes were a good way of picking out newcomers. All three women began the day by carefully applying eye makeup at their desks. I learnt to do likewise. Wearing this much makeup was an entirely new experience for me, but I now felt naked without it.

The topics 'Making up at work' along with 'Making coffee before starting work' occupied an entire staff meeting during my first week. Patrick felt that as a professional organisation, 'war or no war,' people should be at their desks by 8.30 sharp, not mixing up Nescafé and sugar in the kitchen.

'If you want coffee first you should get here at 8.15 before work, or wait for coffee-break at ten.'

'The drivers cannot start earlier,' Aleks said. 'It is not safe, for one thing.'

'All Bosnians start the day with coffee and conversation.'

'That may be, but this is an international organisation. I have already relaxed a number of rules. I have not, for example, complained about any of the women washing their hair in the kitchen in their lunch break.' The office had lights and hot water from a generator, which no one had at home. 'I draw the line at makeup, though. Please do not make up at your desk. You should do it at home before work.'

'It's impossible. The light is much better here than in our flats.'

It was not resolved. Everyone continued to make coffee in the kitchen before we scuttled off to our desks, where we continued to hastily apply makeup before settling down to work.

Learning how to live in a besieged city required new skills. Learning how to be a useful mental health practitioner meant continuing the flexibility I had begun to acquire in Slovenia. When I presented myself to Professor Cerić, the head of social psychiatry at the Kosevo Hospital, he immediately asked me to set up a support group for the twenty-two remaining psychiatrists working there. I asked if that was appropriate, pointing out that I was rather junior compared to him and his colleagues, and had had none of their experiences.

'Exactly why you will be perfect! We need an outsider, someone untouched by the war, like yourself. We do not take time for ourselves.'

I remembered meeting with a Bosnian refugee psychiatrist in Croatia the previous year. She told me that the British Institute of Group Analysis had run a training group in Sarajevo. She had been in the group with Radovan Karadžić and his wife until a month before the war. 'Karadžić was such a nothing I didn't notice him.' No one discussed politics in that group and apparently no one had any idea of what Karadžić had in mind for his colleagues. I told Professor Cerić I had only limited experience and had no formal training in group analysis myself. I could not run a group of this kind.

'We are not looking for group analysis,' Cerić said quite sharply.

I wondered if he shared my thoughts that a therapeutic training process which failed to notice that a group member had plans for the elimination of his Muslim co-workers and the rest of the Muslim population in the country, possibly lacked something essential. I felt too shy to ask. The professor sat under a wall full of framed certificates. There was also a small cartoon in which an angry woman accosted her psychiatrist: 'My problem, doctor, is neither psychosis nor neurosis, it is just that I exist day after day in grim reality!'

'We simply want a place where we can talk about what is happening day to day and offer more support to one another,' Professor Cerić added. 'I think we need this. You will facilitate.'

My favourite group was a self-help group for young women.

Another international agency asked me to run this at one of their drop-in 'counselling centres' in town. The young women, mostly in their late teens and twenties, came up with a list of topics they wanted to discuss during our weeks together:

1. Women/job/baby.
2. Talking with men about sex, or not?
3. Marriage, or not?
4. Do we need to be married to have a baby?
5. Is closeness to parents good, or not?
6. Can women be happy in marriage?
7. Homosexuality.
8. Husband as 'boss', or not?
9. Love.
10. He loves her but she is just a friend, and vice versa.
11. He loves her but he is afraid.
12. Is it good to stay with someone who does not love you any more?
13. What makes a good marriage?
14. What happens after divorce?

But often we ended up with something quite different, depending on what was bothering them at the time. The war had created a completely new situation for these young women and they were feeling their way through it. One difficult question was 'Sex with boys, or not?'

'I want to experience everything and everything is going faster than usual. Girls are freer, open, we are running for our lives and sometimes it is too fast and you fall,' said nineteen-year-old Belma.

'Yes, and girls do things they would never normally do, because there may be no tomorrow,' twenty-year-old Amra added.

'They go and catch an UNPROFOR soldier for ten Deutschmarks. I wouldn't, but I have heard of it.'

'I don't believe it,' said one of the younger girls.

'It's true. It's wrong, it's a shame!' Belma came in.

'I had a boyfriend, a regular relationship. We went out, but we did not sleep together. Then I broke it off because I did not like him very much. I didn't give it much thought, but he was quite upset because he cared more for me than I for him. Then I heard that he died at the front, and I feel really bad. Not so much because I want to be with him again, but that I stopped it. I feel I caused him suffering and that was unpatriotic – no, I don't mean that – just not fair on him, he was about to die and I hurt him.'

'Look at us,' said Amra. 'We think more about the boys' thoughts and feelings, but you cannot stay with someone just because you pity them. You must be honest.'

'Boyfriends don't respect us enough any more. I went out with a boy. I liked him but on our first date he asked if I would sleep with him. I was shocked. He said, "Well, I don't know if I will be alive or dead tomorrow, so why not now?" I told him first of all there are plenty of sexually transmitted diseases in Sarajevo; secondly, it's just not right on a first meeting. Then he said, "I cannot imagine how you can refuse, there are plenty of prettier girls in Sarajevo." After that he would not even say hello to me in the street. I feel completely miserable. He really thought I was that kind of girl.' The speaker looked fifteen and was on the edge of tears. The girl next to her put an arm round her.

'Believe me, there are plenty of men like him in the city. They only think about themselves. War is a great excuse for them,' said Belma.

'I don't know who is guiltier, war or men. Plenty of girls do say yes, so men are losing respect for girls in general.'

'But before the war lots of girls slept with men after parties,' another girl chipped in. 'You cannot say it is bad. I and my boyfriend just try to make one another happy, because who knows if we will be alive tomorrow? We just want to avoid conflict.'

'I hope,' I said mildly, as we wound up, 'that if you're deciding to sleep with someone new, or even someone you know, that you are all using a condom.' I knew they had already had lectures on the topic from other staff but thought it was an opportune moment to reinforce the message.

'Do you know how disgusting a Bosnian condom is?' Amra laughed. 'And there is no lubricant in the city. Anywhere!'

I think these groups worked well because the Bosnians asked for them and decided on the topics they wanted. But not everyone wanted the psychosocial support we offered. My predecessor at my agency had decided that Bosnian social workers needed 'group support'. Twice a week I went out to the social welfare office, in a small wooden hut set between the grim Tito-era apartment blocks of Novi Grad. Before the war it had been cheap accommodation for workers. Now it was a desolate front line. In the wasteland outside there was a sort of market run entirely by elderly women in too-thin coats and with too much makeup barely hiding haggard faces. Each one had in front of her a small tea towel on top of which she had arranged bits of her life for sale: small pieces of valuable jewellery, a pair of good shoes, a kitchen appliance, a plastic doll, a few tomatoes, some books, some linen; nothing anyone actually needed. No one was buying anything.

'Don't photograph me,' one woman said.

'I am so sorry, I want to show people at home what is happening here.'

'Go to the Residence and photograph the President. He is dining well and getting fat!'

The social workers were distinctly ambivalent about our programme. When I had first arrived we went around asking them what topics they would like to discuss in these groups. A few of them wanted more discussion on the psychological topics that I addressed in the formal lectures, such as grief and stress, but others were more concerned about obtaining cleaning materials and dealing with headlice.

'How can you expect any psychological problems to be solved when there is no food? When I spend all day with people who want food and I have none to give. Do you understand who gets food in this city? The army, the government, and Bosnians with NGO jobs.' Elena, the head social worker, glared directly at Semir, Zara and me. 'And those with friends in the West,' she went on. 'The other ninety per cent are struggling, especially since they closed the Red Cross kitchens. Oh yes, they say there is food in the shops, but who can buy it? Who has marks any more?'

Me, I thought. The attack felt warranted. The rationing system in the city was a constant source of complaint: fat café owners and black-marketeers got the same rations as frail, impoverished old ladies and nursing mothers. With our blue cards, we international humanitarian workers and Bosnian NGO staff were protected. We mostly ate at the UN canteen, using coupons to buy cooked lunches and otherwise unattainable luxuries like yoghurt and bananas flown in on UN planes. I got through my lunch coupons fast as Semir and Narcisa were broke and were paid only at the end of each month. The only way I could handle the discrepancy between my own and their salaries was to share everything I had. I mostly avoided thinking about the discrepancy between myself and 90 per cent of the population. Not today.

Elena was too thin and yet rather glamorous, with poorly dyed red hair, stretch pants and a floaty black and gold top. She did not want the support group.

'Outsiders contribute nothing because they do not understand the situation. We support each other and we know all we need to know!' She and her colleagues looked at me with tired, tired faces and I felt an overwhelming sense of uselessness.

I was intensely aware that I was with people whose lived experience of the mental health effects of war outweighed anything the textbooks had taught me, and often contradicted it. For example I had been taught that women were more vulnerable to depression, stress disorders and attempted suicide. Professor Cerić and his colleagues were seeing a hundred and fifty outpatients a day.

'Where are the women?' I asked.

'They have no time to get sick,' Cerić said. 'Too busy taking care of the children and trying to find food and water.'

It was young men who lay listlessly on the iron bedsteads in the intensive care unit, staring at the ceiling.

'Attempted suicides,' said Cerić.

This unit made the old Beech Ward, where I had begun almost a decade previously, seem like a luxury hotel. There was dirty, torn lino on the floor, dirty undecorated walls, and dirty broken windows. Empty plastic bottles were lined up in rows against the walls. Water was spilt on the floor. No nurses were present.

Apparently everyone, staff included, had done better psychologically in the first two years of the war. When the shelling was intense the suicide rate had fallen. But now that things were slightly easier, the suicide rate had increased again, along with depression and other stress effects like post-traumatic stress disorder and reactive psychoses. They used drug treatments, Cerić explained. 'We have all become very biological.' No one wanted to take the risk of attending regularly for psychotherapy. Fourteen high-explosive shells had fallen on the psychiatric unit alone. It was better to stay safe indoors and take drugs.

These did not always work. Another part of my job was meeting with social workers assisting in the collective centres for displaced people, so that they could discuss cases that particularly worried them. For instance, there was a man who had developed an obsessional routine with prayers and beads that had to be done six or seven times a day in different spots in the centre before he felt all right. It upset everyone else. Two visits to the psychiatric clinic plus medication had not resolved it, but now that he had a new girlfriend he felt better – what did I think? I thought it was a nice example of how successful relationships can often be more helpful than drugs.

However, another case of an old man who woke early every morning and wept, but would not eat or speak and now moved only very slowly, did sound as if he needed a proper psychiatric assessment. Any number of diagnoses were possible: depression, hypothyroidism, Parkinson's, dementia. The social worker said she had no time to take the patient to the clinic. She wished the psychiatrist would come to them. It was not a bad idea. Indeed, Professor Cerić had told me that war might finally give him the opportunity to do something he had planned for years: train GPs to do more psychiatry and finally get community mental health services out of the hospital and into the community.

Nor had my training prepared me for dealing with grief and loss on this scale. For the first time in my life I was living in a society where every single person had lost someone or something. The full horror emerged through matter-of-fact, quietly spoken statements such as:

'My mother is dead, a heart attack, because of the war.'

'My father had a stroke.'

'My house is on the other side, I can see it from where we live now, we lost everything. We live with my grandparents.'

'My brother was killed at the front.'

'My boyfriend was in a camp, we have heard nothing.'

'I was wounded twice.'

'The house fell on us.'

'I spent five months in a cellar, not daring to go out.'

'My sister was killed fetching water . . . fetching food . . . taking some air . . . crossing the road . . .'

'My professor lost his leg standing in the street.'

One afternoon, Semir and Narcisa took me to the soldiers' graveyard. It was in the Muslim part of town, in the park where Semir had played as a child. It was one of those smoky, misty November afternoons. We walked up the hill past four soldiers digging a new grave, towards two rows of entirely fresh graves. Chrysanthemums, Michaelmas daisies, late marigolds caught the afternoon light. The park was full of Semir and Narcisa's dead friends. 'He died a month ago . . . he died last year . . .' They never complained.

I was learning that grief does not progress through the seemingly organised stages presented in my textbooks – of denial, anger, sadness, bargaining and so on. On the contrary, it has a thousand faces. One of the most common here was a kind of respectful reticence, a recognition that everyone had similar experiences and that it was best not to burden friends and neighbours with yours, because doing so amplified the grief of both, rather than diminishing it.

And I realised that, just as Professor Cerić had predicted, I did have a role as an outsider. The most important conversations occurred when I was just hanging out, making up at work, standing in the office kitchen, sitting in a café. Because nothing bad had happened to me, people felt it was all right to burden me. I could listen. So I did.

When I wasn't working I wandered the city. Sarajevo was full of 'corners'. You climbed a flight of steps or wound your way down a hill and suddenly you were in another community: old brick and timber houses with steep tiled roofs huddled together along narrow streets. Here was a small mosque with a wooden fence, a minaret, a flower-filled garden. There was a man with two or three goats wandering down the middle of the cobbled road. There were whole streets where cars had collapsed in on themselves from neglect, tyres flat and windows broken.

There was rubbish everywhere, not much paper litter but piles of tin cans, old clothes and rags. There were always stray mongrels and their puppies, and sometimes old people scavenging in the rubbish. It was supposed to be collected by the UN, but it often sat for days until it was burnt in metal containers. Then the air would be filled with acrid smoke, adding to the feeling of decay. Many of the houses' façades were blistered and pockmarked from shrapnel, or had massive shell holes. No one had the money to take care of their upkeep. In the city centre was some of the loveliest Secessionist architecture I had seen, but the plaster wreaths and garlands that fronted the buildings were broken, and the faces and masks stared down with sooty eyes from shattered cornices. The city appeared to be weeping.

But some of the small shops had new shutters and newly tiled roofs, a sign of hopefulness that contrasted with the gutted buildings. And in the early evenings the streets were packed with people. Someone had set up a stall selling Korans and beads. Families bought chips and ice-cream to eat as they strolled and greeted friends. Off-duty soldiers strolled along with their arms slung round their girlfriends' shoulders. I usually sat and wrote letters in the garden of a favourite café. It had a vine-covered terrace looking over what used to be a small outdoor cinema. The rusted remains of metal seating still formed a semicircle in front of a ruined proscenium arch. Sparrows took a dust bath in a newly turned patch of earth where the café owner was growing vegetables. In the late afternoon, the light put a sheen on the domes of the mosque next door and I could hear the bells from the Catholic cathedral along the street. It was quite impossible to believe that there were men with guns in the hills around us, trying to decide whom they might shoot.

The strangest thing was that I didn't feel afraid. By November random shellings were a more or less daily occurrence and I found it hard to make sense of this lack of fear. It was not courage, because it required absolutely no conscious effort on my part. I would hear the sounds: the crackle of sniper fire; the crack and boom of outgoing shells, a longer thud for incoming. It was as if I believed myself to be encased in transparent armour-plating. I could not imagine it touching me, so it would not do so. An irrational sense of personal specialness and immunity.

This magical thinking was helped greatly by the normality of everyone else's behaviour. We might be walking to lunch, or I might be sitting in Professor Cerić's office talking. There would be the thud of a shell landing somewhere, but people would continue walking or talking as if nothing had happened. So I did the same. One evening I was visiting Semir and Narcisa at their apartment. When I came out the thud was close enough to make me contemplate going back inside. But then I thought: If I go in, when do I come out again? So I kept on walking home, distracting myself with the breathtaking beauty of a city lit only by moonlight. The modern flats where Semir and Narcisa lived rose like ziggurats, juxtaposed against the city centre with its clustered roofs, spires and pale minarets, all surrounded by the black silhouettes of hills, entrancing and eerie at the same time, especially as there was no roar of traffic. I reached home safely.

This detachment was very useful. It meant I could walk to work and sit in the social centres and cold welfare offices. I took obvious precautions like avoiding known sniper spots. Eleven were wounded and one killed on the tram running beside the river during my first days in the city. The worrying aspect was a kind of numbing. I could not shake off that feeling of detachment. The intake of breath still came if I heard of someone killed, or saw the pictures on the evening news, but the oddest thing was how the television footage of other people's tragedies was somehow more real and upsetting than my own reality, which felt increasingly like a movie.

As the shelling increased again, denial became more difficult. I knew we had moved into a new phase when Aleks told me not to wear my seatbelt because the danger from being trapped in the car under sniper fire now outweighed the dangers of driving fast. Cars travelling at 60 kilometres an hour were not so vulnerable. The problem was that every time the Bosnian Army had a success in another part of the country, Serb forces punished Sarajevo with more shells and sniping. At work people spent whole staff meetings talking about the increasing dangers. A curious mixture of jubilation and anxiety prevailed. On the one hand everyone was happy with the victories, but the Bosnian men also realised it meant an increased likelihood of being recalled into the army. In the previous week fifteen Bosnian UNHCR staff had made use of their blue cards to leave Sarajevo for good. Semir said he thought about leaving but could not imagine what he would say to his son.

'I couldn't stand being a refugee, treated like a "thing", in some country,' Milica, a psychologist friend, told me. Milica's mother was Serb and her father Bulgarian.

'But it is too much – we're exhausted – abnormal food for three years. Sometimes you just don't care if you stay alive, you see people who don't bother to run for safety when they should. They kill you inside, step by step. You feel nervous, confused, you start to forget things, you become depressed, aggressive. Initially you can fight it. Then the depressions become longer, but this isn't classic depression. Nothing bad has happened. Yet I have no good feelings. I am shaking inside. It's a kind of hopeless, helpless feeling. We all fight this desperation in our own way, allergies, breathing, it has to be expressed in some way.'

Everyone I knew in Sarajevo was tired. What was astonishing was that, in spite of the exhaustion, the quiet non-violent resistance continued. This was the biggest paradox. Having become an advocate of military intervention, I was now a witness to an extraordinary act of mass non-violent defiance. Karadžić's stated aim was to take Sarajevo, to make it the capital of a Serbian Bosnia. This meant terrifying non-Serb Bosnians into leaving the city, as had successfully happened in so many towns in the north. The Sarajevo suburbs of Ilidža and Grbavica had fallen to the Serbs and non-Serbs had been driven out, but the rest of the city remained the mixed community it had been for five hundred years.

Narcisa, Milica and all my friends moaned about the increasing corruption, the black market, the power of the various militias, the growing religiosity of the various ethnic communities, the fact that government elites had sent their own children abroad. Still they put on their makeup and smartest clothes and went to work without fail, every single day. Professor Cerić told me he had taken not a single day off work since April 1992. He felt he couldn't leave, or everyone else would follow. All the hospital doctors had worked without pay for two years. They got breakfast at the clinic, and lunch and dinner if they were on duty. Otherwise, they depended on humanitarian aid or relatives abroad. When Cerić lost his house to the Serbs at the beginning of the war, he moved to his brother's apartment and grew tomatoes on the windowsill.

'But you know what? This teaches you how little you need from modern life. You just need basics. There used to be a lot of cardiovascular problems here and obesity. All that has disappeared. I myself lost thirty-three kilos.' He made the siege of Sarajevo sound like a superior diet club.

Young people promenaded the streets at night, crowded into discos like the Cotton Club below my flat, and insisted on a cultural life. 'It's a kind of defiance,' Semir explained, 'to show them they cannot destroy this city.' One night I sat in at a sandbagged Obala Gallery beside the river attending a film festival organised by the British Ambassador, Robert Barnett. The Bosnians cheered and cheered when Mark Cousins, the visiting director of the Edinburgh Film Festival, said, 'This is the most beautiful cinema I have ever seen.' Far from being annihilated, Bosnian dignity under fire captured global attention and there were increasing calls for 'something to be done'.

The trouble was that the 'something being done' at that moment was the provision of humanitarian assistance. Some of the most powerful armies in the world had become relief workers. There was now an extraordinary and expensive UN air service running flights in and out of the city, bringing in supplies and aid workers like myself, while convoys of aid drove along supposedly protected 'blue routes' to besieged towns and enclaves around Bosnia. So when cries for military intervention grew too loud in Britain, the Foreign Minister Douglas Hurd was able to say that any Western military action taken would harm the aid effort, the aid workers and the peacekeepers protecting them, so nothing more could be done.

This presented me with a dilemma. I had decided that I had a moral responsibility to do relief work in Bosnia because I was ashamed of my government's inaction, and their apparent wish for the Bosnian government's defeat. Prime Minister Major had phoned Bosnian Prime Minister Izetbegović recently to tell him to stop a successful Bosnian offensive around Bihać, a city in the north-west of the country. However, as an aid worker I was part of the humanitarian effort, which my government used as the excuse for avoiding definitive military intervention. Arguably, my presence here, far from assisting all my Bosnian friends, actually prevented them from obtaining the military assistance they needed to have a chance of surviving and winning this war.

I was not the only one debating whether our humanitarian presence in the country might be making things worse. An embattled Bosnian town commander in Goražde asked a visiting journalist in 1992: 'Send a message to your governments, thank them for their food and medicines. Tell them that at least we will die with full stomachs.' It was the aid agencies that were clearest and most outspoken about this 'humanitarianisation' of the conflict. Alain Destexhe, Secretary General of Médecins Sans Frontières, wrote bluntly that same year: 'UN troops and humanitarian organisations are being made the alibi for the lack of political action.' He argued that 'humanitarianism will find itself in the dock with the accused . . . a companion to the territorial conquest and ethnic cleansing, even to a certain extent making them possible'.

Elena, the gaunt and glamorous social worker whom I had come to admire, put it to me succinctly: 'Do you understand how terrible this war is? Do you know who is to blame? The West should be ashamed! You talk about psychological problems. Huh! Eighty per cent of our psychological problems would be solved in one instant if your government would act to lift the siege of this city!'

1995

I resolved my moral dilemma by going home. I decided to combine political advocacy in Britain with short trips back to Bosnia.

The Bosnians launched a full-scale offensive to liberate Sarajevo in June 1995. They were defeated, and the shelling of the city returned to the intensity of 1992. In response to threats of punitive airstrikes, the Serbs took UN peacekeepers hostage and used them as human shields at military targets. In July 1995 Srebrenica fell. Twenty-five thousand Muslim civilians were deported and eight thousand Muslim men and boys were massacred. Žepa was taken and non-Serbs were executed, Goražde and Sarajevo were next in line. While Western politicians agonised over which particular brand of inaction was appropriate at this point, my every spare moment was taken up with meetings and demonstrations calling for military intervention.

My clinical work in Britain formed an odd counterpoint to my political concerns. By now I was the senior registrar at a busy outpatient clinic for children and adolescents in a large county town. I drove back and forth to work through the beauties of an English summer. Plum and apple blossomed; I assessed suicidal teenagers. There seemed to be an epidemic of adolescent overdoses: young girls who played Russian roulette with their lives by reaching for the pill bottle whenever there was a crisis. I talked to anorexic teenagers whose existence centred on every calorie consumed. I treated young psychotics and learnt to identify and help autistic children. I ran groups for children who were sexually abused, and groups for parents who could not manage their children's behaviour. I learnt how to do play therapy, cognitive therapy and systemic family therapy and how to 'intervene' in emergencies.

One day a mother and son came to see me. He was a plump, awkward fourteen-year-old with blond hair and a reddish complexion, who twiddled his thumbs and stared at the floor. His mother wanted me to do something because he was causing trouble at school. As we talked, it emerged that his father had regularly and viciously beaten the boy since he was three. He used a belt, or occasionally a piece from a wooden chair. No, the mother didn't like it, but she had no idea how to stop it. She said she'd thought of reporting it, but was frightened that they would lose their home. Sometimes she wished the father dead. I told her I was now obliged to report it myself, but that the law would protect her and Social Services would help. So I intervened. I called Social Services who, with the police, interviewed the boy and then arrested the father, putting an injunction on him so that he was banned from the home. I felt pleased and uncomfortable at the same time.

Child maltreatment is associated with so many adult

pathologies. Children who are beaten may turn into beaters themselves. After ten years of abuse, the child was now protected. But there was no question that I had helped break up the family.

On 29 August the Serbs bombed the marketplace in Sarajevo again, killing forty-one civilians. I heard the news on the radio as I drove to work. I could not stop crying so had to pull the car over and stare at the fields of ripe wheat beside the road until I had composed myself. On 30 August, after three years of asking, we got what we wished. I caught a newspaper billboard saying 'NATO Bombs Serbs' and a wave of emotions swept over me: instinctual disgust at the word 'bombing', immediately replaced by a mixture of amazement, relief, horror, followed by guilt at my relief. NATO had begun Operation Deliberate Force and was bombing Serb military positions and their supporting infrastructure. Friends who had been in Bosnia with me rang to say they were 'quietly cheering'. I finally got through to Narcisa and Semir, who told me they were 'dancing in the streets'. Within weeks, the siege of Sarajevo was lifted, Croat and Bosnian forces went on the offensive to retake territory, and the Serbs sued for peace.

It was a bad peace. The Dayton Peace Agreement, brokered by Richard Holbrooke, the US Assistant Secretary of State for European Affairs, partitioned the country and rewarded the Bosnian Serbs with Republika Srpska, a large part of the territory that they had ethnically cleansed during the previous three years. It remained completely unclear how and when indicted war criminals like General Mladić and Radovan Karadžić would be arrested; or how non-Serb refugees would ever be allowed to return to homes that Serbs now occupied. 'Humanitarian military intervention' on behalf of 'innocent civilians' had brought an end to the war but failed to challenge the Fascist ideology that had started it.

I went back to Sarajevo for a conference in the spring of 1996. I stayed with Semir and Narcisa, now married and full of plans for the future. Semir was almost unrecognisable in a beautifully cut Italian suit and tie, telling me, 'I always used to dress like this before the war!' He had restarted his training as an oncologist. Narcisa planned to combine motherhood with training as a psychiatrist. We ate in a newly reopened Italian restaurant. They were the only Bosnians in there apart from the staff.

'There are more foreigners here than during the Olympic Games,' Semir remarked.

The international humanitarian community and the new governing civil and military elites had arrived in full force. Traffic jams of white vehicles indicated the new order of things. Now that there was no shelling, life in Sarajevo had become very comfortable for those with Deutschmarks. There were art shows, new bars and discos everywhere. The shops were full of electronic goods, Italian clothes, German food. The rubble and debris were just a blur beyond the shiny reflections from the new plate-glass windows. Yet the reality of most people's lives was grim. There was no industry. There was massive un-employment. Those who had jobs were still scarcely paid.

'A lot of people are dying now,' Semir said. It was as if the peace had allowed some weakening of resistance. A friend of his had suddenly developed a non-Hodgkin's lymphoma at thirty-four. There was an increased rate of suicide among the elderly, depressed because children who had gone abroad had still not returned home.

When I called on Professor Cerić, he looked and sounded exhausted. He had been ill, he felt nobody had absorbed how desperate the situation was. There was a new cartoon on his wall. It showed two almost identical pictures side by side. In both, a middle-aged couple walked down the steps of a public building, weeping and saying, 'Never again.' The only differ-ence was that in one the sign above the building said 'Holocaust Museum', and in the other, 'Bosnian Museum'.

'Will freedom be able to sing in the way that those who fought for freedom did?' Semir asked me at dinner, quoting the poet Branko Miljković: 'Now substitute the word peace,' he said.

Somali border, Ethiopia, November 2007

Jijiga is a town with an edge. We drive up the road past the hospital, cross a small stream, pass a guard post where a soldier, recognising the Toyota, lowers the rope with a wave, and suddenly there is empty space. Rocky pastures roll east towards the border. The vast quietness has the same seductive power as the open sea. It will take at least an hour on the bumpy dirt road to reach the refugee camp. All I can do is stare out of the window.

The emptiness is illusory. Irregular patches of wheat, corn, barley and *khat* break up the terrain. Occasional clusters of cloth-covered *aqals*, identical to the homes in the refugee camp, are enclosed by cactus fences and stone walls. Sometimes there are a few trees. The flocks of delightful black-faced sheep look exactly as if they have pulled black socks over their heads and are about to rob a bank. For no reason that anyone can give me they are called 'one K' sheep and are only found here in eastern Ethiopia. I love this time of day. The white horizontal light of early morning outlines the sheep and their attendant herders, and flattens the hills. A squat, solitary, white-washed mud-brick building casts a deep shadow.

I spent part of my first few weeks talking to Somali mothers about the difficulties they have rearing their babies in the camp. In September this was still a new refugee camp with relatively few international NGO workers, so the white lady in the big car was the major attraction. This made it very difficult to talk to one person at a time. I did try.

Hoden, one of the traditional birth attendants who works at the clinic, let me sit on a mat within a shaded area in her relatively large fenced compound. Within half an hour there were forty to fifty people – men, women and children – all crowding around and joining in the discussion. Some thought I might be 'making a distribution' or 'writing a list' and wanted to be sure they were not left out. If you're a refugee, feelings of powerlessness and exclusion are so great that finding out what any list is for, and whether it's appropriate to your particular needs, is secondary to making sure you are on it. One woman said I should send her to America, half a dozen asked for medicines. Mostly they just wanted to join in the discussion.

So I gave up my idea of individual interviews. 'Look,' I said, 'first of all I know there are so many things you need but I personally don't have those things to give you and that is not why I am here. I am happy for you to tell me about those needs, but all I can do is pass them on to the right people. I am here to learn about how you raise your children, and I would like Somali mothers to teach me. I would like to hear from as many as possible, but I can only manage five at a time. If the rest of you want to sit round the outside and listen, please do, but please don't interrupt the group.'

Hoden identified five women and we made a small circle. The rest pressed close to listen. Sometimes the roar of conversation beyond the group was so great it was hard to think, but my five mothers didn't seem bothered in any way and were happy to talk. We had to break for prayers at noon, but everyone came back to talk more. At the end they asked what would come of my conversations. When I explained that I hoped to start mother and baby groups, they all clapped. This was despite the fact that most still had no bed nets, no soap, and no school for their children.

In those first weeks I understood nothing. I was, as always, completely dependent upon my translator and on this occasion things were not going well. Translation for mental health requires an extraordinary combination of skills. Translators are interlocutors with the community, cultural interpreters, co-therapists. They must have the ability to keep their thoughts to themselves and literally translate the person speaking – not easy where psychosis is concerned. At other times they have to guide me through some cultural maze and stop me from blundering. Mostly I've been lucky and made friends with an extraordinary group of individuals across the world: Zara in Bosnia, Bini in Kosovo, Adam in Chad, Dan in Sierra Leone.

Faraax was different. A local Ethiopian Somali schoolteacher, he found it quite impossible to put his own thoughts and feelings aside. In our first week he started shouting at one middle-aged woman in the group because she didn't answer the question.

'What is she saying, Faraax? I'm interested in everything she says, even if she does not answer my question.'

'She is diverting, always diverting.'

'I am very interested in diversions – please don't shout at her!'

'No, it is too complicated, you won't understand.' He harangued her some more. When talking with me alone he was anxious to show off his English and used long, complicated, mostly incorrect words where short ones would do. I struggled to understand him. Sometimes he was simply wrong and would not be corrected.

'All psychologists are very conservative,' he remarked one day as we drove home. I puzzled over this, not feeling the description fitted me, exactly.

'What do you mean by conservative?'

'They like to find out things, learn new things.'

'Perhaps you mean "curious"?'

'No, absolutely not! I have read books. The word is conservative.'

Faraax had fourteen children, the youngest a few months old. He told me it was the Prophet's instructions, a gift from God and his wife's wish. I wondered mildly what instructions the Prophet might issue at that moment, faced with a population explosion, no water in eastern Ethiopia and starvation all around. I knew such thoughts could not be shared with Faraax. I needed to find another translator.

Aman is completely fluent in English because he used to live in London. He got to London on foot and by boat and bus, travelling up through Sudan and Libya, then entered Europe via Italy. He stayed for almost a year, living with relatives. But he was deported back to Somalia after being picked up without papers. He followed his family to this camp. He is intelligent, funny, empathetic and very glad to have a job. We get on well and all the women like him.

We have developed a routine. People in the camp are now

accustomed to the car and no longer mob me when I arrive, although supplicants still thrust small scraps of paper in my hand saying, 'My son is handicapped, please send him to Europe,' or 'Please contact my family in Kenya.' Mostly women crowd round, saying, 'Leena Leena, we want to teach you too, when will you visit us?' I choose a particular woman and sit in her enclosure on a mat. As soon as we begin talking, other women press into the compound and I invite them to join in, until there's a group of five. After that, I ask newcomers simply to listen. If they feel something significant is missing they can tell me at the end.

All the families I meet in the camp have been under fire in Mogadishu. Most have lost close relatives: killed in shelling, or from being in the wrong place at the wrong time, like Rumiye's grandfather who 'was crossing the road when another group caught him and slaughtered him'. Or families simply separated in the panic. Many have been refugees for fifteen years, fleeing Mogadishu every time there was fighting. One mother told me she had run away from her home twenty-four times, another thirty. In 2006, when Ethiopia invaded and the fighting escalated, all of them were bombed and shelled. Not many have husbands with them. The adult men remained in Mogadishu. 'He has a second wife,' or 'He was killed,' or 'He is lost, or 'We got separated,' they say vaguely. I am left with a mental image of a capital city filled with lost men, clutching Kalashnikovs, wandering among the ruins, looking for their absent families.

The striking thing is that when I ask these women what bothers or upsets them most, it is not their memories or feelings about those terrible events but the stresses of day-to-day living with seven thousand other refugees. They are mostly urban women: market traders, nurses, office workers, who mourn a city which, they insist, was filled with palm trees and ocean breezes, not hot dusty air; where there was pasta, rice and sorghum to eat, not World Food Programme corn and oil; where they had room for their large families, not tiny stuffy *aqals*; where there were no scorpions or hyenas.

'There is no shade.'

'There is not enough water.'

'Three families share a pit latrine.'

'And no one keeps them clean.'

'We are new; we come from different places and don't understand one another.'

'Everyone is isolated in their own home, we cannot help each other.'

'We manage with God's help, and no one else.'

This is a lesson I've had to learn a hundred times. If you do not address the miseries of the present, they will always trump the horrors of the past.

4: TRAUMA TALES

At the beginning of the First World War, my grandfather Gwilym Jones, a twenty-year-old schoolteacher from the valleys of South Wales, volunteered for the Royal Army Medical Corps. For the first two years he was a medical orderly and stretcher-bearer at Ypres, where some of the fiercest fighting took place. I imagine him, knee-deep in the waterlogged trenches, struggling with five others to lift and carry a wounded man back to the regimental aid post; or staggering back through shell holes, trying not to trip on the rotting bodies of the already dead, trying not to think about the next round of shelling or shrapnel. I picture him kneeling down in the mud with his small supply of field dressings, hoping to stem the bleeding in a punctured chest or shattered limb. I think of his exhaustion as this went on day after day, until he too was invalided out and almost died of staphylococcal septicaemia.

I have to imagine this because he never talked about it. The only story he told me was that he and my maternal grandfather – a Viennese Jewish businessman and an officer in the Austro-Hungarian Army – discovered that they had both been on the Italian front at the same time, but on opposite sides. Gwilym had been sent to Italy after recovering from the septicaemia. So it was mere chance that one had not killed the other, and that I was here at all. He told my father the briefest facts and there are no surviving diaries or letters. But those years of immersion in death and dying did not appear to cause lasting mental scars. My father described him as a happy man with a keen intellect and a passion for education and radical politics.

There were no moods or nightmares, no violence or substance abuse. The only time he got drunk was when Labour won the election in 1929.

My father's war was much easier, though not without incident. Just before he went up to Cambridge to read medicine, in the summer of 1942, he went cycling with a friend in the West Country. One day in Cornwall they were buzzed by a German fighter plane. They jumped off their bikes and hid behind a large granite gatepost. When the fighter turned and came back in the other direction, they skipped behind the other side of the post. He remembered the noise and the little puffs in the dust on the road. 'I wasn't frightened, I just could not believe it,' he told me sixty years later.

A second lucky escape occurred in 1944 when he was living with Uncle Idris, a vicar in London. One Sunday morning he was sleeping in the vicarage and woke to find most of the ceiling on his bed. A V2 rocket had come down on the almshouses across the garden, killing forty or fifty people instantly. He remembered the absolute devastation. He tried to help but felt rather useless compared to the professionals. In spite of both these near-misses, he had no memories of being afraid at the time, nor was he troubled by them afterwards. My mother didn't find the Blitz particularly upsetting either. At the height of the raids on London she recorded in her diary, with precise detail, the state of her dog's health and the births of various puppies, but nothing about being regularly bombed or sleeping in an air-raid shelter in the garden.

This was not what was expected. Before the Second World War the government had worried that bombing might cause widespread panic. Experts predicted more than four million mental cases in the first six months. As it turned out, the number of psychiatric casualties was much lower. A 1941 article in the *Journal of Abnormal and Social Psychology* described the 'imperturbability of the majority of the population' and their remarkable 'acclimatization even to heavy raids at night. A considerable proportion manage to sleep through the terrific racket.' There were fewer neurosis cases than expected and a quarter of those with pre-existing neurotic trends had actually improved. 'In general, the psychological disorders attributable to raids seem to be considerably less serious than the social disorganization consequent on the destruction of so many homes and personal belongings, the disruption of communications, and the difficulties of feeding, evacuation, etc.'

This unexpected resilience seems to have been due to a British government policy decision to treat civilian psychiatric cases in a particular way. When they arrived at emergency rooms they were met with sympathy, given hot tea and reassurance. 'They were all told that their reaction was due to fear, that that fear was one they shared with all other patients and the first aid workers, and that it was important that they should return to their normal work and resist the temptation to exaggerate the experiences through which they had passed,' Dr Henry Wilson wrote in the *Lancet* in 1942. He treated 134 patients with reactions ranging from acute emotional disturbance to stupor and hysterical paraplegia. All of them could be discharged within twenty-four hours and only six needed further treatment over the next nine months.

By the time I got to Sarajevo in 1994, caught up in the third European war of the twentieth century, attitudes had changed. The predictions of mass psychological casualties were the same. The difference was the interest and attention given to one particular diagnosis: post-traumatic stress disorder or PTSD, and its potentially dire long-term consequences. Some writers suggested that more than a million Bosnians had post-traumatic stress and that this was going to be the main public health issue for a generation.

Post-traumatic stress disorder did not exist when I was a medical student in the 1970s. In line with the newly published ninth edition of the *International Classification of Diseases* (ICD), we were taught to recognise acute reactions to stress, which were defined as 'very transient disorders of any severity or nature which occur in individuals without any apparent mental disorder in response to exceptional physical or mental stress, such as natural catastrophe or battle, and which subside in a few days'.

They could take the form of strong emotional reactions such as panic, fear or depression, or behaviour disturbance such as agitation, or fugue states in which the person appeared numb, absent or dazed. If the condition persisted and was not associated with a pre-existing disorder, it was called an 'adjustment reaction'. The emphasis was on 'normality' and 'reaction'.

The general view was that prolonged complaints after any accident or disaster often had more to do with the possibly unconscious wish for compensation rather than continuing distress. We were encouraged to read the classic 1961 paper on 'accident neurosis' by the British neurologist Henry Miller. It warned us to watch out for 'the patient slumping forward with head in hands during a consultation, requesting a glass of water'. The attitude might well be one of 'martyred gloom', but also 'very much on the defensive, exuding hostility especially at any suggestion that his condition might be improving'.

I was quite unaware of the lobbying going on across the Atlantic, where doctors treating Vietnam veterans and Holocaust survivors had found common ground with those working with victims of rape and sexual abuse. These advocates argued that many in their client groups had suffered for many years, and that the diagnoses they had been given such as depression, anxiety, substance abuse or personality disorder neither encompassed nor addressed their particular needs. They proposed the inclusion of an entirely new disorder in the soon to be released third edition of the *Diagnostic and Statistical Manual, DSM III*.

Post-traumatic stress disorder was distinctive in this manual because it included a cause in the description of the problem. The diagnosis could be made only if someone had been exposed to a catastrophic event outside the normal range of human experience. The identifying symptoms included some form of re-experiencing of that event in the form of nightmares, intrusive thoughts or actual flashbacks, when the individual might feel as if the whole experience was occurring again. Consequently, they would try to avoid any situations, or persons, or conversations that might remind them of the event and trigger these frightening episodes. Such efforts to avoid thinking about it could lead to a numbing of the emotions. The person might complain that they no longer felt anything. Finally, there was increased alertness and jumpiness.

The first time I heard the term 'PTSD' used was in 1985 when some psychologist colleagues rushed off to provide psychological counselling in Bradford after a fire killed fifty-six and injured more than two hundred. Then suddenly PTSD was everywhere. A flash fire killed thirty-one people at King's Cross Station; a plane fell out of the air onto the small Scottish town of Lockerbie killing all 259 on board and eleven on the ground; police mismanaged the football fans at Hillsborough and ninety-six people were crushed to death. On every occasion the comforting voice of the newscaster assured us that professional counsellors were on hand.

I can recall having traumatic symptoms myself on a couple of occasions. The first time was as a medical student, when the thirteen-year-old girl from whom I was taking an admission history had simply keeled over in front of me and stopped breathing. I immediately started mouth-to-mouth resuscitation. But then she haemorrhaged from her mouth, covering me with blood and making further action impossible until I was swept out of the way by the crash team. The girl died of an incurable haemorrhagic disease. I could not get the physical experience out of my mind for the next two weeks. I replayed it and replayed it in technicolour detail, seeing her pale face and tasting her blood. I tried sharing the experience with a couple of sympathetic friends but that made the memory more intense. So I just kept busy and filled my mind with other things and it eventually faded of its own accord. The same 'intrusive recollections' – as I had now learnt to call them – occurred after Diana's sudden death on the dance floor at Woodside. They too faded after a few days.

The explanation I worked out for myself at the time was that such upsetting and unusual experiences, both of which involved life and death and engaged multiple senses – sight, smell, touch, taste – created a particularly intense and unforgettable memory. It felt as if my mind needed to keep re-examining the disturbing sensations until they made sense, lost their novelty value and could fade away. Was this an illness? I thought not, and was very glad no one had labelled it as such on the two occasions when I experienced it.

But the general public felt otherwise. They had learnt from a media with a growing taste for 'trauma stories' that any potentially life-threatening event required professional assistance. Dire consequences for mental health would follow if this was not provided.

One night during my child psychiatry training, when I was on duty for emergencies, I was asked to come in and see a sixteen-year-old who had been struck by lightning. She and her boyfriend had taken shelter under a large solitary tree in a local park during a thunderstorm. The bolt had gone through the tree, into her boyfriend, stopping his heart and giving her a second-degree burn on her side. A passer-by had done CPR on the boy, who survived and was in intensive care. She was on the paediatric ward.

'It's early days for a psychiatric assessment,' I remonstrated with the admitting physician.

'Her mother is insisting that she is "traumatised" and needs a psychiatrist.'

So I sat beside the bed of a drowsy, tearful teenager who told me she felt guilty because her boyfriend had been trying to teach her not to be afraid of thunder. That was why they had gone out when the storm began. Now she was terrified she had killed him.

'Has no one told you he's fine?'

'Yes, but they won't let me see him.'

'Get in the chair,' I said, pulling up a wheelchair. Off we went to the intensive care unit, where her now conscious boyfriend was equally pleased to see her. Neither showed any residual psychiatric effects in the coming months or had any need to see me again.

I did see children for whom the diagnosis seemed appropriate. In the mid-nineties I interned in a specialised clinic in

London where children who had experienced or witnessed violence, such as the murder of their mothers, came for treatment. In my own clinic I saw sexually abused children whose memories of the abuse, and the chaos of their current lives, drove them to make repeated attempts on their own lives. But I was curious about the growing hold this one diagnosis had on the professional and public imagination. Perhaps it was because PTSD was a diagnosis without stigma.

The rise of biological psychiatry and the attempt to present mental illnesses as brain diseases had still not removed the taint of moral and personal failing associated with the majority of psychiatric disorders. But here was a disorder that came packaged with a clear-cut cause, that was obviously not the patient's fault, and which set them in the sympathetic and dramatic light of victimhood. Here was a diagnosis that could be taken as a badge of suffering. In situations where victimhood was questionable, as for example with Vietnam veterans who had returned from an unpopular war, or with the policemen whose methods of crowd control had contributed to the deaths of the ninety-six at Hillsborough, the diagnosis transformed possible perpetrators into sufferers requiring compassion. Meanwhile, those treating PTSD could be seen as responsive and empathetic to public distress. PTSD gave psychiatrists a glamorous role in the emergency room and on the front line of a disaster that had nothing to do with their usual emergency calls: calming and controlling a 'crazy' person, listening to the miseries of a battered wife, arranging detoxification for someone high on amphetamines, or sorting out yet another teenager overdosing on paracetamol because of a bust-up with her boyfriend.

Researchers invented new instruments to measure the newly described cluster of traumatic symptoms. The predicted rates in different populations and the possible treatments were all debated in new journals and discussed at the international meetings of the new societies set up to explore the new diagnosis.

All this activity was not confined to European and American psychiatric clinics. The rising interest in PTSD coincided with a growing media interest in humanitarian affairs. The Rector of Bergen University told the assembled delegates at the 1993 meeting of the European Society for Traumatic Stress Studies that 'the opening up of Eastern Europe and the Bosnian war provides a wonderful laboratory for our work'. The Bosnian psychologists sitting beside me winced. They had been flown in from the Sarajevo section of that 'laboratory' by UNICEF. In 1994 there were seven humanitarian agencies running counselling centres in Sarajevo. Other agencies, like the one for which I then worked, were engaged in training staff in the recognition and identification of traumatic symptoms and their appropriate treatment in various kinds of individual, family or group therapy. 'We come for the light, the heat and the company, not for the psychological counselling,' my Bosnian women friends told me. 'All Bosnians have a personal psychologist: she is called your best friend.'

What immediately struck all of us living under siege at that time was the irrelevance of calling anything 'post-'. Another problem was judging the significance of particular symptoms. One researcher found that 95 per cent of a sample of 364 displaced Bosnian children living in collective centres met the criteria for PTSD. But he wondered if, in the midst of continuing conflict, some of those symptoms might be adaptive.

The children had been repeatedly shelled during the two-month research period. The hypervigilance that made a child startle at a sudden sound could actually keep them alert enough to take cover. Researchers in other war zones such as northern Sri Lanka found large numbers of those who had experienced aerial bombardment had symptoms of PTSD. But those affected did not regard themselves as psychiatrically unwell. They saw the symptoms as an inevitable consequence of war. In many war zones the population needed 'sensitisation' by Western health experts to realise that they had a mental disorder requiring treatment.

By the late nineties I was caught up in an increasingly vitriolic debate within the mental health profession. One side argued that the 'inventors' of PTSD pathologised normal stress reactions and undermined people's natural coping abilities. The imposition of the diagnosis was another example of cultural imperialism. There was no evidence that any of the various counselling treatments on offer worked.

On the other side, the advocates of the diagnosis insisted that 'trauma denial' was preventing millions of sufferers getting the medical help they needed. 'To make a drama out of trauma is fully justified,' wrote Dr Fokko de Vries in the *Lancet* in 1998, defending a humanitarian counselling programme in Bosnia. 'The absence of proof that counselling helps should not be seen as proof that counselling is useless. Absence of proof does not equal proof of absence. [. . .] Mental health programmes are relatively cheap. The human suffering that can be relieved by them is in my opinion priceless.'

'Dr Vries alludes variably to suffering and to trauma as if they were interchangeable. Surely we must be clear that suffering per se is not pathology,' wrote back Dr Derek Summerfield. This was the heart of the issue. PTSD had become a signifier for all the moral, social and political evils of war. To say that people did not have PTSD appeared, to some, to be saying that they had not suffered. This suddenly became clear to me during a postwar mental health conference in Sarajevo. Dr Summerfield had been invited. He suggested that the long-term rates of PTSD in the city might not be all that high.

'How can you say that?' a local psychiatrist snapped back. 'Have you any idea what we have suffered in this city?'

The trouble is that if you reduce the moral, social, economic and political complexities of a conflict to a disease category that can be universally applied, this appears to suggest that there is a simple medical fix to all the miseries caused. One medical fix that was gaining in popularity at that time was 'critical incident stress debriefing'. This was first developed for use with fire-fighters, paramedics and other front-line workers exposed to extremely stressful events. The idea was that a trained facilitator – possibly a co-worker – could help their peers process the thoughts and feelings associated with the 'critical incident' or 'traumatic event' by going through a series of structured steps.

This would be done in a group or individually. First they were asked to describe what had happened in order to make the incident come alive again. After this they examined their thoughts, what they were thinking at the time of the event, their reactions, particularly the worst part of the event for them personally, and the symptoms they experienced, physical and mental. This was followed by education to explain the normality of these reactions and provide advice on managing stress. At the end of the session the facilitator summarised what had happened and helped the individual or group put the event behind them and come back into the present. It was emphasised that debriefing was not psychotherapy, but a method for reducing normal stress reactions to a terrible event. The suggestion was that not only would this have the immediate effect of reducing acute distress but it could actually prevent the development of later, more severe, traumatic reactions. There was no definitive evidence to prove that this happened. But, as with all new treatments, there were many believers.

I began to understand why 'trauma counselling' was so attractive to the donors who funded humanitarian programmes. It required very little in the way of capital resources, medications or highly specialised staff. Local people could apparently be trained in the recognition of both PTSD and its prevention by appropriate counselling techniques in a matter of days or weeks. Interventions like debriefing could be given to whole populations without bothering to sort out who was sick and who was well. Undertaking such a programme showed that something immediate was being done to address people's misery on a large scale. No need, then, to engage in the more difficult and awkward questions of how to stop the conflict causing the misery and how to get justice or reparations for those affected. At that trauma conference in Bergen, a group of us including the Bosnian psychologists, Dr Summerfield and myself had suggested to the assembled delegates that we adopt a motion stating that 'we recognise that we have an ethical duty to address not just the effects of massive trauma but also its causes and perpetrators'. The motion went on to condemn the actions of a fellow psychiatrist, Dr Radovan Karadžić, the leader of the Bosnian Serbs.

The delegates were opposed. They argued that it was 'too political'. A bland motion condemning all war as bad for one's mental health was adopted instead.

Goražde, 1997

In the winter of 1997 I was still trying to figure out my own position on the diagnosis. By then I was working for another international NGO, in a small town in south-east Bosnia. Goražde had had a terrible war, under siege from Bosnian Serb forces for four years. The population had lived without running water, no power, scarce food, constant sniping and regular periods of bombardment. The town had almost fallen in the spring of 1994. The Bosnian Serbs only withdrew because of the threat of NATO airstrikes. When I arrived in December 1996 it was sunk in fog, gloom and mud. The Dayton Peace Agreement had left Bosnian Muslim Goražde as an isolated urban enclave, still surrounded by the territory of the other entity, Republika Srpska. The story of the war could be seen in the shattered roofs, some with tarpaulin still stretched over shell holes; in the homemade waterwheels floating on the River Drina that had been used to generate electricity; in the foot-bridge running under the main bridge that had given people cover from snipers.

I lived with two other agency staff in one of the three-storey villas huddled between the north side of the Drina and the wooded hillside. We bathed in chlorinated river water that we heated in pots on the stove. There was electricity, but still no street lights. You took your life in your hands if you walked along the main road at night, hoping you wouldn't break your leg in a pothole, fall in the mud or get run over by one of the Portuguese or French tanks that made up the UN peace-monitoring battalions. There was mass unemployment. Most of the town's population had worked in the armaments factory, now closed, or in the now inaccessible industrial suburbs of Kopači, or Serb Goražde, as it was now called.

The town had had no psychiatrist for four years. A local GP had done what she could. My job was to run a mental health clinic in the small hospital on the south side of the river. The hospital director gave me a room in the freshly whitewashed outpatient clinic. We furnished it with a desk, some chairs and a lockable filing cabinet for notes. After he announced on local radio that I would run clinics on Tuesdays and Thursdays there was a queue of patients waiting outside the clinic door each morning. They were aged from six to seventy and had problems ranging from sleeplessness to schizophrenia, severe bipolar disorder and Huntington's chorea. Very few would have been helped by a diagnosis of PTSD. Some had had their problems for years. Some were the previously sick and vulnerable, tipped back into illness by the war.

Elderly Mrs Babić was not at all interested in giving me a history. She sat solidly in her headscarf and cardigan, waving her arm at me in the peculiar gesture older women had in this area, a cross between beckoning someone to come close and throwing a lasso. 'I can't sleep, I can't sleep, please give me some medicine!' she said repeatedly. I told her that in England patients complained that doctors were too brief and did not listen. It was a first for me to be told that I was taking too long. This produced a small half-smile. Her niece persuaded her to be patient and answer my questions. Between them they explained that she had suffered a bout of agitated and depressed behaviour a few years previously and had recovered after a spell in hospital. But the kidnapping of her son in the middle of the war had made her very disturbed again. She was sent to Sarajevo and put on antipsychotic medicine. She had been quite calm for the last year. But recently, with the war over but her son still not returned, she had stopped doing the housework or eating, sleeping or enjoying coffee with her friends.

Mrs Babić pulled out a dirty plastic bag that contained a

mass of different drugs. There were the antipsychotics from the hospital in Sarajevo, small glass vials of intramuscular diazepam from the emergency room here, the small blue pills a friend had given her, plus yet more white pills from a local doctor. She took all of these intermittently but none of them helped. I explained that I thought the stress of the war and missing her son had made her depressed again and that the right drugs might help. But it was a good idea to take drugs from just one doctor so as not to get confused, and not to take any given for friends. We made a plan as to how to reduce her antipsychotic drug slowly and switch her over to antidepressants. Mrs Babić reluctantly let me swap these for the unnecessary pills in her bag.

Mrs Babić did not have PTSD, but the ex-soldiers and ex-prisoners who came to see me did. There was Nedjad, who used to live in Foča and was imprisoned at the start of the war along with many of the Muslim men in that town. He had been tortured for a year by Bosnian Serbs he had once regarded as friends and neighbours. Then he was released and had fought on the front line and been wounded in his shoulder. It was still not right. He had nightmares every night. They were always the same: he was back in prison and being abused. He did not want to tell me how, but there was no escape. He managed to do a part-time job as a cleaner in the hospital. He had heard that there was an ex-prisoners' group, but he did not want to go. The idea of listening to the terrible experiences of others and being asked to share his own made him feel worse. He preferred trying to forget the past by listening to music, drinking, and taking diazepam. During the war, on the front line, he had taken 50 milligrams a day, like so many other soldiers. Now he was trying to cut down.

The town was drowning in a sea of tranquillisers. Almost everyone I saw was taking diazepam as a matter of course, obtained from a doctor or a friend. The aid agencies had delivered the drugs in large quantities during the war and many were now dependent, particularly people with PTSD. And if you couldn't find diazepam there was biperiden – the same side-effect drug that was traded at Woodside – that could be dissolved in alcohol to get high.

I also saw some children with clear cases of PTSD. They had all witnessed the death of someone close at hand. Elvira had watched three men blown up at the door of her shelter. One had survived, faceless, and begged for water. He had bled onto her. On another occasion she had been with three friends when they were hit by a grenade. Two had died instantly and a third lost her leg. Elvira had stood helpless in the middle of the street while her friend cried for help. Four years later she continued to have nightmares every night and awoke in tears. In the day she felt strangely detached. She could not control her moods. Sometimes she would be happy, sometimes inexplicably angry.

But most of the problems people brought to the clinic simply did not fit this pattern of symptoms. The war had produced many other kinds of difficulty. Sophia stammered and could not get her sentences out since being evacuated and separated from her parents at the outbreak of the war. Mirsad wet his bed and soiled his clothes at school. His mother beat him because of this, but even so Mirsad could not bear to let his mother out of his sight. They lived with three other families in five rooms and could see their old apartment in Kopači every time they went past it on the bus. It was now occupied by Serbs.

The most common problem among the ex-soldiers was chest pain. Bojan arrived one morning at the clinic short of breath, pale and trembling with anxiety. A short, chubby, middle-aged man, slightly balding with close-cropped blond hair, he sat down and talked without stopping.

The problem had begun during the war. After the funeral of a close friend who had died fighting on the front line, Bojan had collapsed with chest pain. Everyone thought he was having a heart attack. He had been sent to Sarajevo and put in intensive care with chest monitors, and had had blood tests. Then after a few days they had told him it was his 'nerves', and sent him back to his unit in Goražde. Since then he'd had frequent attacks of chest pain and was still terrified of dying of a heart attack as his father had done before him, dropping dead suddenly at sixty. He took diazepam but it didn't stop the pain, and he had heard from others the drug caused problems.

He wanted to stop the diazepam, but when he tried he felt worse. No, he did not have nightmares or any painful memories from the war. He missed his friend and many others who had died. He liked visiting the graves and talking about them. He wished he could talk about them more, but people had put the past behind them and did not want to hear about the war. He ate and slept well, he enjoyed the company of his twelve-year-old son and his wife. He played football. He was a bricklayer and there was plenty of work. But he was angry, angry with the doctors who had implanted the idea of a heart attack, angry with other doctors who had given him drugs that didn't work, and angry with everyone for the way things were.

In the wars of the latter half of the nineteenth century and the early twentieth, cardiac problems with no organic explanation were among the most common causes of invalidity. They were given various names: 'Da Costa's syndrome' after the doctor who first described the condition during the American Civil War, 'soldiers' heart', 'irritable heart' and later 'disordered action of the heart'.

The symptoms were similar to Bojan's and the other ex-soldiers that I saw in the town: the feeling of the heart beating too fast, pain in the heart area and shortness of breath. In the late nineteenth century it was thought that the strapping carrying the soldiers' packs put pressure on the heart and constricted the blood supply. During the First World War special cardiac hospitals were created. When doctors recognised the psychogenic origins of the problem they switched the name again, to 'effort syndrome'. In late-twentieth-century Goražde heart disease was one of the commonest forms of mortality, particularly among middle-aged Bosnian men. Everyone lived on a diet of coffee, high-fat food and tobacco. I didn't find it at all surprising that people's anxieties should focus around their hearts.

Some of my colleagues at home argued that the PTSD construct should be adjusted to include all post-conflict reactions in both adults and children. I saw no value in this approach. Diagnosis is supposed to be a means of labelling a problem clearly, so that you can communicate briefly with others what pattern of symptoms you are seeing and what they might expect. The label given should also allow you to predict the course of the illness, its prognosis and treatment. A patient who has a persistent cough and is diagnosed with pulmonary tuberculosis requires a quite different treatment from a patient with the cough of a chronic smoker.

Using 'post-traumatic stress disorder' to account for all post-conflict psychological problems seemed to me akin to using the term 'cough' for all chest problems. The end result of such an approach was that you gave the psychological equivalent of cough mixture: the ubiquitous undefined 'counselling'.

Mirsad's bed-wetting and soiling responded very well to tried and tested behavioural methods. He kept a 'star chart', pasting little gold stars into his exercise book every time he had a dry night. A certain number of stars earned a small reward. I encouraged his mother not to spank him when he was wet, but to give lots of praise when he was dry. Mirsad became less clingy and his mother less frantic. Sophia's stammer got better with music, singing and play therapy. With Nedjad I had to find meaningful ways to discuss his experiences and help him make sense of them, so that he no longer needed to drown the memories in tranquillisers. The men with chest pain responded well to a simple mixture of education, breathing exercises and relaxation. After a year or more of being told they had 'nerves' or 'The pain is in your imagination', or 'You're crazy, there is nothing wrong with you', hearing a doctor say, 'The pain is real, but it is not dangerous and there are physical things you can do to make it go away' was very appealing. They felt better after doing the relaxation and breathing exercises, so some of them kept coming.

Not all. Some of the soldiers would come once or twice. Then they would disappear for weeks, then turn up again. I would meet them in the small market where I bought beans and sausage, or on the central bridge over the Drina where everyone promenaded as a warm spring turned the river blue. Or they would gather at the Coco or the Pyramid – the two discos in town – and sit on the cheap plastic chairs under ugly fluorescent light, drinking vodka and exchanging prescriptions and rumours. Would Goražde be handed to Republika Srpska in some partition deal? Or would it be the launching point for a new offensive? I had no idea. I had taken to joining them in the disco. I had quite given up trying to preserve the rigid boundaries demanded by psychotherapists back home. In this small isolated community there was no way to shut myself away from my patients without insulting them. I had also learnt that while half of them were reluctant to come and see me in any formal setting, either alone or in a group, they were very happy to all shout at me at once while very loud music was playing.

Some had other solutions. One of my patients with chest pain was a middle-aged man who had lost his twelve-year-old daughter in the last year of the war. She had been playing outside when she was hit by a grenade. He had taken responsibility for cleaning her body and organising the funeral. Since then he had often had a severe stabbing pain around his heart. The cardiologist had examined him and told him to come and see me as they could find 'nothing wrong'. He wondered if it was connected to his daughter's death. He had never cried as he believed it would be wrong to do so.

'The grave will fill with water and the child will drown – it will be a burden for her and she will not be happy in paradise.'

'I think your heart aches with grief,' I said.

This made sense to him, but he still preferred not to talk about it. This was the Islamic way, he explained. I could not see how insisting on the ventilation of feelings and the overt expression of emotion so beloved of Western psychotherapy could help if it went against the grain of what he believed to be right. I told him I did think three years was too long to be in this kind of pain and I wondered what the local religious leader, the *Hodža* advised. He agreed to see him and later sent me a note saying he had quite recovered.

The most difficult problem I faced did not fit into any

diagnostic categories. It was violence. Mothers beat their children in overcrowded collection centres, drunken husbands beat their wives. Families fought over kitchen space. On one occasion I was called to see a young woman displaced from Foča who had jumped into the Drina after her sister-in-law accused her of stealing food. I could reassure her that she was not going mad, and offer to meet with all the family to help mediate the conflict, but I could not offer what she really needed: new accommodation or the possibility of returning home.

The violence was also directed outwards. Nedjad was furious at the local police, who he felt had had a cushy war while he had been in prison and then on the front line. Now they had jobs and swaggered around in their uniforms while he had no work. On one visit Nedjad told me he had thought about killing one of them. I did not know how to assess dangerousness in this context. If I used the criteria I had been taught at home, I had to worry about most of the young men in the town. They were angry, resentful, irritable and on drugs of various kinds. They had access to lethal weapons and had spent the previous four years trying to kill people in order to survive. Luckily they did not all come to see me, but I had to make decisions about the ones that did. I hoped that insisting Nedjad locked up his gun with a friend and allowing him to regularly ventilate his feelings to me would be sufficient, while we tried to address the more difficult symptoms of flashbacks and drug dependence.

What came across from all these young men was a feeling of waste, betrayal and hopelessness. They felt that nothing was finished. This was neither peace nor war, so there was no point in trying to restart their lives, as who knew when the war might start again? Anyway, with 90 per cent unemployment in the town, where would they find work? If they left, where would they go? And what were they fighting for if they then abandoned the town they had saved? It was not just the ex-soldiers who felt like this. The atmosphere of uncertainty infected everyone. Nothing was quite worth it. People found it hard to take the initiative, make up their minds, make a decision. Simple questions such as 'What time can you manage an appointment?' were often met with something I called the 'Goražde sigh': a long exhalation of breath, followed by a silence and a half-smile.

But to call the community 'traumatised' was to do the town a gross disservice. It missed the point. Goražde had not been struck down by some psychopathological post-conflict plague. It was still under social and economic siege. In those first few months of 1997 the Goražde bus to Sarajevo was held up at gunpoint and all the passengers robbed. A man was kidnapped, threatened with execution by having a plastic bag put over his head, then left tied to a tree while his truck was stolen. On another occasion a truck driver was knocked out while driving after being hit on the head with a rock. The Serb police refused to let him be moved to hospital until he had paid a 500-Deutschmark fine for losing control of his vehicle and hitting two cars. Shop owners no longer felt they could bring in goods, children stopped going to sports events, families did not visit their relatives.

The Dayton Peace Agreement supposedly guaranteed freedom of movement and the right to return home. It was clear to me that enforcing these provisions would do more than any single mental health programme to address people's psychological distress. Freedom of movement could jump-start Goražde's economy and break the community's feelings of isolation. If people could return to the homes from which they had been expelled they would no longer quarrel over kitchen space.

There were moments when things worked out. Mrs Babić came in one morning and kissed me on the cheek. Her niece told me she was up and about doing the housework and enjoying family life again. There was Alija, a slight, gentle elderly man who had stayed on his farm in the mountains throughout the war supplying the army with food. When the war ended he had suddenly felt there was no more point to his life. We met regularly to talk. Things improved slowly. I did a home visit one day, driving up above the river valley between small orchards, meadows and vegetable plots. Plum blossomed in every garden. Alija showed me his hives where he kept bees and gave me a large jar of honey. At the next appointment I took him to one of the big development agencies to suggest they use him to train others in beekeeping. They loved the idea and so did he. I had never seen him so cheerful.

I had learnt not to suggest to my patients that they do this or that or go here or there to solve the innumerable problems that beset them. Such ideas would simply elicit the Goražde sigh. Anyway, how to decide which of the plethora of international agencies to approach? The most effective thing was to take the first step together, to introduce people and show that it could be done. The truth is that I really enjoyed this kind of direct action. I felt that things were shifting, just an inch or two.

After my contract with the agency finished, I stayed in Goražde another year doing research on how children made sense of the conflict. They confirmed what my clinical experience had taught me and what Anna Freud discovered in her nursery in London during the Second World War. Children can cope with the fears of bombing and sniping if their parents are present and coping well. Many Bosnian children had vivid, intrusive memories, but very few saw them as a sign of illness. Some even hung on to them 'because we should not forget the past'. I learnt that there were things that were worse than war. One of the sickest children had regarded wartime as one of the happiest periods of her life because her abusive father had been away on the front line. It was his return after the war and his continuing violence towards her and her mother that had led to misery and an overdose. When her mother divorced and found her own place to live, the daughter recovered.

By now I had developed an allergy to the word 'trauma'. The term was on everyone's lips and yet told one nothing. One problem was that the word itself had become meaningless through overuse. So when colleagues or friends at home said 'Poor you, dealing with all that trauma,' I had to stop myself saying bitingly: 'Please define your terms. Are you referring to the events – torture, shelling, kidnapping or whatever, to which people have been exposed? Or are you referring to their reactions to these events? And if the latter, are you talking about their physical or mental reactions? And are you talking about normal or abnormal reactions, because that *one* word is now used for all of the above.'

The problem was not helped by resorting to dictionaries. The *Oxford English Dictionary* enshrined the ambiguity. It acknowledged that the word originates with the Greeks and meant a 'wound, or external bodily injury in general', then explained that today's definition includes both 'physical and mental injury' and the 'states or conditions caused by these'.

The revision of the *DSM* classification in 1994 added to the confusion. The definition of a 'triggering event' was broadened. According to *DSM IV* you no longer had to be directly exposed to an extreme stressor that would cause distress in anyone to qualify for the diagnosis of PTSD. The stressor could be anything that you personally found extremely distressing. Indeed, your exposure might even be second-hand. You might have heard about the event from a friend or witnessed it on television. This meant that the same diagnosis was now being used for a woman traumatised by having hot tea split over her in a smart hotel, for children who had become terrified after watching a ghost story on TV, teachers who faced investigations for incompetence, and soldiers or civilians who had seen their friends blown up or been raped or tortured in prison.

Derek Summerfield filed the newspaper cuttings and kept me posted. My favourite was the 'pet psychiatrist' who diagnosed 'the canine equivalent of PTSD after a car crash'. The dog had stopped winning championships and become a jittery, irritable wreck. He had lost value as a stud. Damages were awarded. It was interesting how many of these cases in Britain and America led to successful compensation claims. I sensed the ghost of Dr Henry Miller laughing at us all. It felt like an insult to Nedjad and Elvira to use the same diagnosis.

But by 1998 my patients, and the town, were recovering. Goražde had brightened and opened up. Houses and apartment blocks were painted in vivid colours, checkpoints had disappeared from the road. A jam factory started up, a sports centre opened, teams came to play, people were travelling again. Nedjad stopped me in the street and told me how well he felt. He now had a girlfriend. They hoped to get married. A warm, loving relationship had proved the most effective therapy. I sat on the balcony of my apartment by the river and watched children with brightly coloured nylon rucksacks run past on their way to school. My landlord was tending his bees. Swallows and martins nested in the burnt and deserted house next door. At night you could hear nightingales. You could almost forget there had been a war. It had moved south, to Kosovo.

In October 1998 I followed it there. A doctor running a small children's charity rang me up and asked if I would go to Kosovo to set up emergency mobile medical clinics. The idea was to give displaced Albanians access to primary health care and mental health at the same time. My lack of this kind of managerial experience mattered less to him than the fact that I had been visiting Kosovo intermittently since my honeymoon there with Tomaž in 1990. I knew my way around, had friends there, and I possessed a visa for the Federal Republic of Yugoslavia.

Jijiga, Ethiopia, December 2007

On Saturday afternoon Asmamaw invites me to his house. I catch a horse buggy to the other side of town. Half a dozen other staff and drivers from the camp are already sitting on thin cotton mattresses on the floor. Asmamaw urges me to sit beside him. A television plays in the corner but no one is watching. They are chewing *khat*, smoking, and drinking sweet sodas. There's a woman making coffee over hot coals in a small metal container. The door of the windowless living room is open, making a bright white rectangle of the sunlit yard outside. Conversation flickers between the Somali of the drivers and the Amharic of the camp staff. Sometimes no one talks at all.

Asmamaw offers me some *khat*, the Somalis nod their enthusiasm. Everyone chews it in this part of Ethiopia in much the same way as we drink coffee. You can buy fresh bunches of the leaves for five birr on every street corner. The waist-high green shrub grows in small plots all along the dirt road between here and the camp. It has displaced the fruit trees that used to grow on the mountainsides around Dire Dawa. The woman who owns the largest garage in Jijiga and the New Millennium Hotel got rich exporting planeloads from this scrubby desert area to the rest of the world.

Melkamu insists I take the freshest and youngest of the bright-green leaves from the end of the twig, these being the most potent. I pick a small cluster, roll them between my fingers and place them as prompted between my cheek and my teeth. I chew gently. It tastes the way you would expect green leaves to taste: green. Someone offers me a swig of 7Up. I sit back and wait. Nothing happens.

'I don't notice anything at all,' I say after about thirty minutes of contemplation. The smell of fresh coffee drifts across as the woman pours and passes the tiny cups.

'It takes time,' Melkamu says. 'You have to chew it regularly for a few weeks at least.' The Somalis smile and nod and offer me more. I shake my head.

'What would your parents say if they knew you were chewing

khat on the Somali border?' Asmamaw asks me.

'My mother has long ago given up worrying. She views me as being on some kind of extended gap year and is still waiting for me to get a proper job. My father is dead.'

'I am sorry.'

'He died two years ago. He was eighty and had had a good life. He said to my stepsister a few days before he died that he was "past his sell-by date"! But I still miss him. What about your parents? Would they approve?'

'My mother does not like it, but she knows it is part of our life, something we do when we are together. My father never chewed *khat*. He is dead, like yours.'

'Now it is my turn to say sorry.'

'Don't worry, it was a long time ago. I was twelve.'

'That's very young to lose a father. How did he die?'

'He was a soldier. He was thirty-six. It was a war. He was killed not so far from here. We don't know the place exactly. The body was never found.' Asmamaw's face is still and impassive, impossible to read. No one else is paying attention.

'This would be under Mengistu, or Emperor Haile Selassie?' I am struggling to marshal the few bits of Ethiopian history that I know. Asmamaw smiles.

'Mengistu Haile Mariam's Derg deposed Haile Selassie in 1974. In 1977 we were at war with Somalia. They came almost all the way to Dire Dawa. If the Soviets had not switched sides, perhaps they would have gone further.'

Over the course of the afternoon Asmamaw tells me about his childhood. He grew up on a military base in a small village near Harar. His father Sisay was a sergeant, the chief mechanic for a small unit of commandos. The unit officers had been trained by the Americans and Israelis, who backed Ethiopia at that time. The father Asmamaw describes is a gentle man who never raised his voice, loved his friends, read and wrote poems and told his son not to be a soldier. They had a one-room house divided by a curtain. Asmamaw and his three sisters shared one bed, his parents the other.

Asmamaw saw it as an easy life. He went to school. There

was clean water from a tap twelve metres from the house. He had clothes and enough to eat. In the same compound there were other families with twelve children who struggled. He saw fathers who drank and beat their wives. This never happened in his home. The hardest thing was that his father was posted on the Somali border and could not return often. Asmamaw remembers always waiting.

The war with Somalia began in 1977 when its president, General Siad Barre, turned his tacit support for a disgruntled Somali liberation movement in eastern Ethiopia into a full-scale invasion, with the aim of creating a Greater Somalia. Jijiga was taken and much of the surrounding area. Somali tanks reached Dire Dawa and Harar. Sisay's unit, trapped behind enemy lines on the border, realised any attempt to return to base would be hopeless. They decided instead to drive into Somalia, trek south for days and then double back to Addis. Once reunited with his own side, Sisay was astounded to be told to hand in his M14 rifle in exchange for a Kalashnikov and to be given an East German IFA vehicle in exchange for his American jeep. The Soviet Union and Cuba had calculated that Mengistu's Derg offered better chances for influence in East Africa than Barre's fractured Somalia. The switch changed the course of the war and cost Sisay his life.

It was a chaotic time. Asmamaw saw planes flying from Dire Dawa every day and heard the boom of heavy weapons. There was a curfew. There was shooting around the town on most days between local troops and the Western Somali Liberation Front. Sisay came home for one night in August. He told Asmamaw, 'I am a soldier. I can die at any time – be a father for your sisters, help your mother, study hard.' He embraced the boy and left around eight in the evening. That was the last time Asmamaw saw him.

Deaths on the base were always announced to the assembled families on Sunday mornings. That Sunday in October they called out 'Sisay Yigeremu' and five others. The previous week some of Asmamaw's friends had lost their fathers, so he thought: Now it's my turn. He cried. 'Ethiopians are silent in love and cry and shout loudly at death,' he explained to me. 'That is our tradition: all day and night you cry.' And following the tradition, they put mattresses on the floor and sat there as relatives, friends and neighbours visited over the following days. Even people who had lost fathers and husbands in previous weeks came. Then, life had to go on.

I ask Asmamaw if this experience of war and losing a loved and admired father 'traumatised' him, but he could not understand the term. He never experienced traumatic symptoms but he thought of his father all the time. It gave him pleasure to do so. He has no memory of being afraid of the war that surrounded them. 'When you take a poison little by little, you adapt. Everybody thought about death and war and bullets. Death was a daily matter. Something you Westerners simply don't understand.' He remembers worrying. 'You know day and night your father is in a war. The bullet kills someone randomly – you don't know who – you sleep, you eat, you are always thinking of him.' All his friends also lost their fathers, which made it a little bit easier. A year later, as the son of a martyr, Asmamaw was awarded a scholarship to study in Cuba. He stayed there twelve years completing both his high school and medical education.

The white rectangle of light at the door has shifted to a yellower, softer glow. The camp staff organise themselves to leave. Asmamaw embraces his guests, shoulder against shoulder. When the room is empty he asks if I want to go for a walk. We take the dirt road out towards the university, passing around an orthodox church. There are trees inside the high enclosing wall which make it seem enticing, but the gate is locked and there's no one around. We walk on to the wasteland that makes up the boundary of the town. Goats are grazing and three small boys are playing with the broken hub of a truck wheel. They have turned it into a rocking boat in which all three sit, shouting and gesticulating in some imaginary game.

The wind blows dust in our faces. A Somali woman walks in front of us down the track. She is carrying a heavy plastic water can on her head. Beside her a small girl who looks no more than three or four struggles along with a smaller canister on her head.

Asmamaw watches me watching the woman and asks me what I'm thinking. I am embarrassed to say. There are moments when I simply cannot get over the fairy-tale of my life. I think that one of the main reasons I am here is that it shakes me out of my feeling of entitlement. It is just luck, a simple matter of chance that I grew up in a safe country, in a middle-class family who loved me and educated me. So I end up a doctor while the woman on the track is born here and must fetch water six hours a day. I try to explain.

'You are here now.'

'Yes – with my passport, my car, my driver, my ability to leave at any moment the going gets too tough.'

I tell him a little about my own childhood. The Second World War was long past, and what I knew about conflict came from films like *Sink the Bismarck*, *Cockleshell Heroes*, *Carve Her Name with Pride* and *Reach for the Sky*. I had my own bedroom in a red-brick semi-detached house in a quiet London street. We had a cat and a dog and a menagerie of reptiles. My sister and I constructed a wigwam in our chaotic back garden, rode bicycles around the neighbourhood and walked ourselves to school.

Each Sunday was spent with our grandparents. Viennese Granny Axelrad gave us Ribena and dark Continental chocolate. We sat in the heavy armchairs in her over-full sitting room reading the comics my mother forbade us to have at home. At Granny Littlejohn's we ate lunch with the grown-ups, with lace mats on the table and two sets of forks. Afterwards they played canasta in the conservatory, while my sister and I played in the bracken in the park beyond the house, or sang along to musicals on my grandmother's gramophone. I can still sing most of *Gigi* and *My Fair Lady*. In the summer we went to the seaside. As we got older my doctor parents became more prosperous. There were summer trips to Spain and winter skiing in the Alps. Nothing very bad happened. My parents divorced and both remarried in my early teens. My new stepfather was killed in a car accident a year later. But these potentially upsetting events were muted by the continuing affection and security provided by all the family.

'Perhaps that is why you are able to immerse yourself in the tragedies of other people's lives?' Asmamaw says.

I don't think that is the explanation, or at least not the whole of it. There is something else that draws me in: not tragedy, but what accompanies it. My Bosnian friends sometimes told stories: always at night, after a glass or two in the noisiest restaurants and bars. One friend told me her main fear in 1994/95 was that if the Serbs took the town, they would not kill her 'quickly'. She was not afraid of dying. Two others talked about driving their Land Rover Defender through shelling and sniping, to collect patients, to ferry staff. Their fragmented stories came out of nowhere. They were told simply, without drama. All of them lost loved ones and risked their lives day after day as a matter of routine.

It's the same with the women at the camp. Hoden has a small daughter the same age as the child ahead of us on the track. She also has an infant who was injured when the house was bombed and they had to run. One day she told me there was another baby, burnt alive in the house. Her husband was left behind. She does not know where he is. 'The war made him mad.' Yet every day she gets up, takes care of the children, goes to work. Hoden is the best at running the mothers' groups. Everyone comes to her with their problems. When another woman had to go to the hospital, it was Hoden who took the children into her already crowded *aqal* and looked after them all.

It is not the suffering that keeps me here. It is the proximity to courage. I hope some might rub off on me.

5: FIGHT OR FLIGHT

Kosovo, 1998

The Kosovars needed courage in the autumn of 1998. The Serb police arrived at fourteen-year-old Fejza's house early on an October morning. It was a brick building in a walled yard, in a village just off the track that led up into the Drenica hills. As was common in Kosovo, two brothers had married two local sisters and the house was large enough to provide a home for both couples and their twelve children.

The police took Fejza, his father, two uncles and his twenty-year-old brother out of the yard and into a wooded area. They were all told to strip. Then they were beaten. Meanwhile, another policeman put a gun in Fejza's mother's mouth and told her to show them where the weapons were hidden. She said, 'I don't have any, so kill me if you want.' The small children were all screaming. The police searched her, pulling up her jumper and skirt. Over the children's crying she heard shots. The police stopped searching and told her to go and look for her husband. The first thing she found was some piles of clothes. Then she came to the bodies: her husband's was badly beaten and disfigured with cuts, the same with her brother-in-law. Finally she found her eldest son. Both his eyes had been gouged out. They found more corpses, but Fejza was nowhere to be seen.

It was two days before he returned to the family. 'I lost myself,' he said simply. His father had pleaded for Fejza's life and the police had let him go. He ran off and wandered, in a daze. When he recovered he could not find his family because the police had forced them out of their house and burnt part of it down. Finally he found them at a neighbour's house where they were all living in one room. For the next two weeks he clung, speechless, to his mother. She had to wash and feed him like a small baby until he became more like himself again. I first saw him three months after these events. He was going to school, 'but all I can do is write my name. I cannot put the memories away so I cannot concentrate,' he told me. He couldn't sleep much. When he did he had nightmares, about his father, about the police. He was jumpy all the time and terrified that the police would return at any moment to kill him.

Fejza's reaction to the death of his father and brothers met all the criteria for PTSD and I dutifully wrote the diagnosis in my notes. But the realities of the situation exposed both the meaninglessness of the term and my therapeutic limits.

Some of the most effective treatments for PTSD involve two things. One is talking with the patient to help them identify any irrational or distorted thoughts that have arisen as a result of the traumatic event: for example, 'It's not safe to ever drive a car,' after a car accident. Or 'I will never be able to venture out on the street at night' after an assault. Part of my job is to help my patient weigh up the evidence for and against such ideas and come to more rational conclusions. The other component is 'exposure therapy', where patients are helped to confront painful memories and slowly learn to decrease the arousal and stress they feel when thinking about particular aspects of the traumatic event, or visiting places or doing tasks associated with it.

It is one thing to use this approach when the conflict and killings are over and the terrifying places are now safe. It is quite another to attempt to reduce the distress and intrusive images caused by a tangible threat who remains present, fully armed with a machine-gun and a knife, and is visible from the bottom of the garden. Fejza's fears for his personal security were neither distorted nor irrational, nor were the traumatic events that had caused them 'post'. This was not the foggy gloom of postwar Goražde. By the winter of 1998/99 a brutal counter-insurgency campaign had raged unchecked against the

Albanian population of Kosovo for a year. Milošević's war against the non-Serb population of the former Yugoslavia had come full circle to the place where it had begun.

In 1990 Belgrade suspended Kosovo's regional parliament, imposed a state of emergency, and subjected every aspect of Albanian life to special measures. Kosovar Albanians lost the rights granted them by Tito to govern, judge and police themselves, to have their own television and radio, to state health care from doctors who spoke their language and to study their own culture and history in their own schools. Over the following years more than one hundred thousand state employees were dismissed from their jobs, depriving them of the right to social security. Arbitrary arrests, weapons searches, police interrogations, beatings and killings became routine.

In the face of this exile within their own country, the Albanians began the creation of a parallel state. In an unofficial referendum in 1991, 87 per cent voted to declare Kosovo a sovereign and independent republic. Parliamentary and presidential elections followed in 1992. The majority voted for the writer Ibrahim Rugova, supporting his ideas of Gandhian non-violent resistance. Kosovars attended school and university in garages, private houses and empty shops. They used charitable health care and developed a private economy of small businesses. Kosovo Albanians who worked abroad contributed 3 per cent of their income as tax.

But the Kosovo Albanians got a clear message from the Dayton Peace Agreement in 1995. Violence pays. If you engage in the politics of exclusion and a vicious war you get rewarded with a mini-state like Republika Srpska. Five years of non-violent struggle do not even get you a seat at the negotiating table. Years of refusing to be provoked had given the West the illusion that Kosovo was under control.

In April 1996, just after the European Union reneged on an agreement not to lift sanctions on Yugoslavia until the Kosovo crisis was resolved, the newly formed Kosovo Liberation Army launched its first hit-and-run attacks on Serbian police stations in the province. The violence escalated. When President

Clinton's special envoy Robert Gelbard identified the KLA as a 'terrorist group', Milošević had all the excuse he needed to launch a clean-up operation. Yugoslav Army tanks and bands of paramilitaries attacked Albanian communities, particularly in the mountainous regions along the Albanian border and in the central Drenica region of Kosovo, where Fejza lived. Villages were shelled, houses were burnt, cattle slaughtered, families killed. Even small children and babies could be considered as legitimate targets because, as the Serbian Rector of Prishtina University explained to me, the high birthrate of rural Albanian families constituted 'the terrorism of demographic expansionism'.

By September 1998 a quarter of a million Kosovar Albanians had taken refuge in the hills and were sleeping in the open. The UN lamented. Western powers bickered and procrastinated. Mr Holbrooke negotiated. At the end of October, NATO threatened airstrikes. Milošević promised a ceasefire and granted access to international monitors – the Kosovo Verification Mission – and humanitarian aid.

By the time I reached Kosovo in November 1998 most people had come down from the mountains. They were now camped out in plastic shelters in their skeleton homes or crammed in with neighbours, drinking contaminated water and completely dependent on humanitarian handouts. There was virtually no access to health care. In the Drenica region where we worked, most rural clinics had been destroyed and the doctors had fled. But people were too frightened to travel elsewhere. They knew that with identity cards from Drenica they risked interrogation and beating. And if they got to a hospital, without employment and social security, they had no means to pay.

I found a translator. Bini was an Albanian medical student who had been studying in Bosnia until forced to leave Sarajevo at the beginning of the Bosnian war. We rented a flat in Prishtina. We met with the handful of other agencies running mobile medical clinics and agreed who would work where in the province. We drove to Belgrade to find that our donated trucks and medications had been impounded by customs, who would not release them. We bought more medicines. Two British emergency room physicians, John and Duncan, joined us and we hired local Albanian doctors to run two teams.

We scouted the region for suitable locations for static clinics. In Fejza's village a clinic was still standing. There was a displaced family living in two of the rooms. The others had been wrecked by their former police occupants. We cleaned it up, bought plastic and wood for the windows, put in stoves, asked the displaced family to act as caretakers, and my colleagues started seeing 140 patients a day. They referred the mental health problems to me. Albanian psychiatrists still had their hospital jobs in Prishtina, but no one wanted to go there and the psychiatrists could not travel out. Space in our temporary clinics was very limited, so I saw all my patients in their homes.

After going to see Fejza, we drove back to Prishtina through what was left of his village. Only fifteen of the 170 houses remained undamaged. The white school building was gutted, as was the cultural centre. There was the usual tiny market of teenagers selling cheap biscuits, chews and cigarettes on upturned milk crates. Torched houses have a peculiar ugliness: the roofless exterior part is almost always standing. Each window has its thickened eyebrow of soot, and the chimney pots on their brick columns stand free above the eaves, like so many arms raised up in rage or despair.

The route had been off-limits to aid workers since November because a doctor working for the International Committee of the Red Cross (ICRC) had hit a mine and been killed. We passed the mangled wreck of his overturned vehicle at least three times a week. I was still nervous, and I yelled at anyone going near a grass verge on foot, or in a car. 'Being a little bit paranoid and a little bit afraid is good!' the Canadian Army officer doing mine awareness training in Prishtina told us when we first arrived. 'It will keep you alive.'

That winter of 1998, everyone in Kosovo was afraid. The Yugoslav Army continued its military actions and the KLA continued to entrench itself in the small pockets of territory it controlled.

One day John asked me to see a small boy who had been in Belgrade for three months with a badly injured leg. Quite often the ICRC was able to get child patients accepted in Belgrade hospitals. Illir had only just discovered that his father was dead, and was distraught. John and I arrived to find the front room packed with some twenty members of the extended family, all waiting for me. I had already discovered that the easiest way to begin in these situations was to get the children to help me draw a family tree on a big piece of paper. It is a common enough psychiatric practice at home, but with extended families in Kosovo I found it invaluable: the children were immediately engaged and curious, everyone got a chance to introduce themselves, while I got an approximate sense of who belonged to whom and could visibly draw attention to the bonds between those left alive. Most significantly, it allowed the family to name and identify the dead, and to say as much about what had happened as they wanted. I put all the living members present in the room onto the tree. I then asked if there were any other family members not present who needed to be included in the picture.

'My sisters,' Laura called out, 'but they are dead.'

'But we can still include them.' I drew the circles representing the sisters and added lines to connect them to their parents and to Laura and Illir. Then I put Xs through the two circles.

'And my father.' Laura explained that their father and two sisters, aged eight and thirteen, were killed by shells as he tried to load them all onto a tractor to escape. She herself was wounded and watched her little sisters die while asking for water, as they were taken to the doctor. I put an X through the square that symbolised Dad. Illir had been too badly injured to know what was going on. Now he was very angry.

When I asked if he wanted to say anything, he started to cry and an uncle rushed across the room and begged him to stop. I gently suggested that perhaps it would be good if Illir did cry for a bit. Then Illir started to rage, not so much about his dead father, but about how dangerous everything was now, how hundreds and thousands had been made homeless and how many had been killed.

'And they will lay mines and they will shell us again and they will kill old ladies and children and they do not care, and who will look after us now? There is no one and we will never be safe.' He went on and on in the same vein, curled up hot and sweaty with my arms around him on one side and his uncle holding him on the other. Bini translated fluently in a low murmur in my ear as the room pressed around us to listen. Half of them, including John, were crying as well. After Illir quietened, I said it was enough for the day and I would come again every week.

Driving home, there were small boys playing ice hockey on a frozen stream, skating on tiny blades tied onto their boots, using one rough pole to push themselves along. It looked like a Brueghel painting. But for me the landscape was mapped by the horrors of my patients' stories: the ironworks, three miles away, that figured in sixteen-year-old Dardan's nightmares because he had seen five men thrown into the furnace when he was imprisoned there; the red-brick farm where Dita's invalid non-combatant father was summarily executed with all the men of his village; the small wooded valley where Besnik's mother, aunt, grandmother and three cousins under ten were all buried, having been massacred with sixteen other members of his family.

The days blurred into each other and the stories lost their edges. Sometimes I felt as if I had been driving for ever on snow-covered roads, past small stands of oak trees, and on into the shells of former villages. I would take off my shoes at the door of a barn and be ushered over plastic and paper to a carpeted room with mattresses arranged around all four sides, smoke-blackened walls, a cast-iron stove and magazine pictures and photos tacked to the walls. The family would serve cheap soft drinks or glasses of tea, and talk to me of what had happened and who was lost and what, if anything, remained.

Fejza's mother told me that her eldest daughter often 'fainted with sadness'. Sometimes she would be 'unconscious' for twenty to thirty minutes, then she would recover and be quite all right. This pattern of fainting in teenage girls or young women was so common that I began in my own mind to call them 'Kosovar fainting girls'. A local Drenica doctor asked me to come and visit another because he could find nothing physically wrong. Sixteen-year-old Julia had been fainting every day since she lost her three sisters in another mass killing.

Again the entire extended family crowded into the room. When I asked Julia if she wanted to talk to me on her own, she looked at me in complete astonishment. No, she liked her family being present. Julia fainted at about the same time – five o'clock – each afternoon. She would lie still and apparently unconscious with closed eyes, though she responded to stimulation. Then consciousness returned and she would act perfectly normally. Julia said that she cried often over her sisters' deaths and still did not feel like eating much. She thought that she 'fainted from sadness and fear' but her family were worried that something more dangerous was going on. As they talked it became clear that everyone saw Julia as the most sensitive member of the family. She had cried most after the massacre. Her mother had never cried. She was too busy worrying and looking after her daughter. Julia wondered why her mother did not cry more.

I wondered aloud whether Julia was doing all the crying for the family. 'Perhaps it is the weight of this burden that is causing you to faint every day.' The family all thought this was a very interesting idea and that it might be possible.

'So as Julia slowly gets stronger, which I'm sure she will do, and the fainting takes less of her mother's time, do you think her mother might find she has time to cry herself?'

Systemic family therapy is a common approach in British child psychiatry. The idea is that psychological problems are located as much in the relationships between people as they are in the individuals themselves. I was suggesting that the symptom – Julia's fainting – was not so much Julia's problem as the way grief was being expressed in that family 'system' at that moment. Julia's fainting might even be useful if it was giving the other family members a way to put grief aside until they wanted to grieve themselves. As Julia recovered, this might mean her mother had space for her own feelings. The Albanian families were much more interested and accepting of this way of understanding a problem than British families had been at home. Back in England, the problem child or teenager would be dutifully dropped off at the clinic to be treated; but persuading the family to attend as well was much harder. Julia's family wanted to be in the room and she wanted them there. Kosovo Albanians believed that autonomy, individuality and privacy mattered less than family connectedness. 'If my sister or my brother have a problem,' Bini said to me one day, 'it is my problem until it is solved.'

As usual there were patients with serious psychiatric problems. One day I was asked to go to a large house in a village in the middle of Drenica. I was greeted by a middle-aged couple who walked me to the end of their yard to visit the wife's brother, who lived in a large wooden shed. A sad-looking man with stubble on his cheeks and dirty clothes was sitting on a wooden bed. He shook my hand and told me his name was Agron. The couple told me he had become so violent and aggressive thirty years ago that he had had to be shut up in a big psychiatric hospital.

'They captured me and put me away,' the man said. They had let him go after six years but he had been on medication since then. It kept him calm, otherwise he got upset and could not sleep. 'He will hear voices saying he is being attacked.' He lived out here because he preferred it. He worked in the garden a bit. He liked to talk to himself and pace up and down. They showed me a short worn pathway in the turf outside the hut. 'See, this is all done by him,' they said, 'walking and walking.' Now they were worried because they had run out of medication and had nowhere to get more. Agron told me that he liked the pills, they helped him feel better. I gave them a supply of the antipsychotic drug they were using.

But the vast majority were not psychiatrically unwell, they were simply overwhelmed by the sadness, anger and fear that follow from a massive assault. They wanted me to provide some symptomatic relief, but more importantly they saw me as a witness, someone from outside who would listen to what had happened and by listening give it validity, even if I could not offer real solutions.

The October agreement did not stop the violence. One day in mid-January I went into the pizzeria where we often ate, and found my friend Baton, one of the editors of *Koha*, the main independent newspaper, near to tears. He told me to go home and watch television. The Serbs had killed more than forty Albanians in a village called Račak. The Serbs said they were KLA soldiers. The international monitors said it was a massacre of civilians including old men and children. Pictures of tangled bodies in a shallow trench filled our TV screens. Families fled the area in panic again.

Two of the international medical agencies were travelling out to do a medical assessment. They thought I might offer psychosocial support and asked me to come. Bini and I added our old Land Rover to a three-vehicle convoy carrying food, blankets and plastic sheeting. The roads were narrow and twisting, with deep ruts carved into the frozen snow, the hardest driving we had done. But the worst thing was coming across endless small groups of people just wandering, some in outdoor clothes, some less adequately dressed. None of them had any idea which way they should go. We weren't sure either, as by this point we could hear shelling, although the direction was unclear. We told them which village we were headed for and suggested they come and pick up some supplies there.

Petrovac, three kilometres from Račak, was half destroyed and completely deserted, except for six women and girls standing crying and completely bewildered in the middle of the street. They told us there were more people sheltering in one house and a woman in labour in another. The convoy coordinator decided we should split up: he would take two cars and assess the next village. One medical team would deal with the woman in labour. I agreed to find the other people.

I was directed to a house where some twenty-seven women, children and babies and a very old man were sitting in one room, terrified, listening to the sound of shelling, which was now quite close and frequent. 'It's been going on intermittently for three days,' the house owner said. 'Most people went to the mountains but these are too old or weak to travel, so I said they could come here, but we have nothing to eat, and what everyone wants to do is leave.' A plump woman in a leather coat burst into noisy tears. Her cousin had been killed in Račak, please would I take her away.

I sat on the floor drinking the coffee that they had insisted on making me – Albanian hospitality never fails, even in such circumstances – and wondered what I was going to do. If I emptied all the materials from the car I could fit in three people. The second car would have the pregnant lady and it seemed unlikely that the other two cars would drive back into a bombardment. I said, more reassuringly than I felt, that it would be better if we all stayed inside for the moment, and that I did have some food and blankets. One fourteen-year-old girl told me she had seen her uncle killed in front of her. I put an arm around her thin shoulders and she cried and cried. The house owner said he had a more secure basement, if necessary. Then I heard someone shouting in English from the yard and went out onto the balcony to see a bespectacled man with one of the bright-orange vehicles of the Kosovo Verification Mission.

'Are you the doctor? I've come to tell you to leave, as it's getting very dangerous.'

'That's very kind of you, but there are twenty-seven women and children here and I really don't feel we can leave them behind. I can get three in my vehicle, what about you?'

The KVM man considered this for a moment.

'Probably five – look, I'll call up another vehicle, see what I can do.'

They did a great deal. We unloaded all the aid we were carrying and after about half an hour of standing in the street waiting, while the local KLA cheered us up by saying it would

be good if we could go soon as there seemed to be tanks heading in our direction, two UNHCR cars and another KVM car
turned up, just like the cavalry, and we found a place for everyone in the house. Then we drove five kilometres in convoy to
Štimlje, the nearest town. We arrived in a sunlit main street
with no sign of destruction, people shopping, my colleagues
waiting, and no evidence of war except the large number of
press fastening onto our disgorging passengers like seagulls
diving for food. The disjuncture was so great I wanted to
shake my head clear, wondering if I had imagined the whole
thing.

I actually had no idea how to do any kind of psychosocial
work in such a context. If people are terrified the only thing to
be done is to try and make them safe. No amount of empathy
or counselling can substitute for some kind of action to change
the situation. By chance that day I had been able to use my
presence as an international to improve the security of a small
group of people, though it did nothing to address the fundamental problem.

But just because I could not personally bring about a political solution to the Kosovo crisis didn't mean it was not worth
helping individuals with the physical and emotional discomfort
that they felt. I wanted to talk to my patients in a straightforward language about fear and to help them cope with it. This
meant understanding that it's a normal and useful emotion
that alerts us to danger so that we can either escape or confront it. We have natural fears that appear to be hardwired
and can protect us. Fear of strangers in infants, for example, is
likely to keep small children attached and close to those who
want to protect them. Fear of heights keeps us away from dangerous cliffs.

I drew pictures for Fejza to show how his inbuilt alarm
system worked: when he saw a policeman at the bottom of the
garden, adrenalin would zip around his bloodstream priming
his body to get ready to either fight or flee. He would breathe
faster to get more oxygen; his heart would beat faster to pump
blood to the places where it was needed, like his muscles, and

away from the places it was not, like his digestive system. His pupils would dilate to allow better vision. I made him laugh by explaining why his hair stood on end, even though humans no longer had enough fur to make themselves look as threatening as his dog did when attacked.

The trouble is that if, like Fejza, you are trapped in a situation where you cannot fight and there's nowhere safe to run, you are stuck with your body in alarm mode but not actually doing anything. This leaves you with an awareness of physical symptoms that are uncomfortable and of no use: constipation, a dry mouth, blurred vision, aching muscles, palpitations, shortness of breath. Many of the host of small bodily complaints that Kosovars brought to John and Duncan and the other doctors every day were not linked to any organic illness. They could be better understood as part of this response: a fire alarm that could not be turned off. The symptoms might be even worse if your current fears were compounded by night-time dreams or painful daytime memories of past dangers.

I found that the Kosovars, just like the soldiers in Goražde, liked these straightforward physiological explanations of their physical symptoms and the reassurance that they were neither imagining things nor crazy. Extended families were ideal natural groups in which to practise stress-reduction exercises. I hoped that taking these simple steps would make them more comfortable and more able to cope and choose the appropriate action when necessary.

Fighting or fleeing appeared to be the only choices left. After Račak, everyone who had hoped that better times might be coming was now sure they were not. In most of the villages I visited the majority of fit young adult men fought in what they called 'our army' because they saw no other way to make themselves safe. Milošević was right. There were no neutral civilians. If he wanted to eliminate the KLA he would have to remove the civilian population. Around Račak the humanitarians (meaning me) and international monitors had helped him to do just that.

*

Throughout that February and into March 1999 the international community tried to push the KLA and the Serbs into
an agreement. Kosovo Albanians were asked to give up their
demands for independence and accept autonomy; while Serbs
were asked to withdraw their military forces and police from
the province and accept a NATO-led peacekeeping force. The
KLA procrastinated. Milošević went on talking and shelling
at the same time. Albanians went on being killed in ones and
twos all over Kosovo. There were tit-for-tat grenade attacks
on Serb and Albanian bars in Prishtina. I learnt to check our
Land Rover each morning for tampering. I watched my child
patients play out their fears in therapy.

One day Laura arranged half my dolls in a box and told
me they were attending a peace conference. Illir wanted to
know 'which one is Slobodan, so I can kill him'. Laura told
him Slobo was not there, and that he should not play war all
the time, but Illir played war for the rest of the session: this
included piling up the remaining dolls, calling them Serbs and
then mowing them down with tanks, digging trenches, becoming a KLA commander, ordering the bombing of Belgrade, and
organising a funeral for dead KLA soldiers.

Not all of them played like this. Besnik was entirely constructive. An intelligent, serious five-year-old, he loved the toy
mobile phone for the different musical notes it made. He spent
many of his sessions experimenting to see at what degree of
vertical tilt he could still get the toy train to run. At our first
session he had been fascinated by drawing the family tree. The
number of dead in his family was so great that it was I who
had faltered, confused, and he who had made me cross out
relatives who were no longer alive. He and a four-year-old
sister had been at the place where the massacre occurred. No
one knew what they had seen and neither wanted to discuss
what happened. I did not push them. I have never seen my role
as 'making children talk'. Instead we frequently talked about
who was still there for Besnik, who could support him and
make him feel safe. He slept and ate well. Over the months I'd
been coming, he had started to share some of his experiences

with his father, and to look at pictures of his mother and talk about her.

By early March 1999, Serb soldiers, police and tanks were everywhere. UNHCR reported that eighty thousand Albanians had been displaced since Christmas. Fighting was going on in the north and south of the province, with continual shelling and houses set ablaze. Fejza and his family moved back into their old home but he did not improve. Whenever police passed on the main road (which was now every couple of hours) he became extremely distressed. When his family tried to calm him he shouted, 'You have not been in their hands as I have!' My techniques helped a bit but the images still filled his mind. He felt guilty for being alive when his father, uncles and brother were dead, and often thought of killing himself. Luckily he had a sensible best friend who was with him all the time. My main concern was how to help him when all the internationals might be evacuated at any moment. I decided to start him on antidepressant medication, which sometimes appeared to work for PTSD. I wanted to do it while there was still time to monitor his response.

Illir spent a lot of time playing with the toy mobile phone in his sessions, calling up John or me to come and get him as he was in danger and needed help. We worked most days with the sound of distant thunder in our ears, except it was not thunder but the near-continual shelling of villages south of Mitrovica. As in Sarajevo, one habituated. People listened, judged the distance, shrugged, and carried on with life as normal – or as normal as it could be when they had no seed and no animals. Very few fields were ploughed. Fresh grass was appearing where there should have been newly turned earth.

In mid-March, in Paris, the Albanians signed the peace accord, accepting disarmament, autonomy and no guarantee of independence. The Serbs immediately repudiated the agreement. The Deputy Prime Minister of Yugoslavia, Vojislav Šešelj, threatened the expulsion of the entire Albanian population from Kosovo if NATO came in. I told Baton I was worried about him and his family. As a prominent intellectual he was likely to be targeted. He had a small daughter. A friend rang to ask if I would take his wife Arta and their three small children with me if I was evacuated.

The trouble was I had no way to make my own patients safe. The villages in eastern Drenica were now under continual bombardment. Nine thousand fled their homes in three days. I asked Besnik how things had been in the last week.

'Fine.'

'Anything happened?'

'War, and more war,' he said in a weary way.

'Are you frightened?'

'No.'

In the last two sessions he had put various plastic animals and dolls on the railway line, taking pleasure in the train crashing into them.

'NATO will come and kill all the Serbs.'

'Do you want them killed?'

'Yes, because they are killing us.' He made a pile of all the small plastic objects.

'Look I've got ammunition – lots of ammunition.'

I told his father I was concerned about a renewed onslaught on the village. Would he let us take all the children out to Prishtina? I thought the city might be less vulnerable to attack. But he did not want them to go at the moment. He said he would ring me if he changed his mind. Knowing the children would find leaving him almost as terrifying as facing renewed shelling, I didn't push it. As always, the children helped me pack up my toys and load the boxes in the car. They solemnly shook my hand to say goodbye.

Illir had been sent to hospital in Prishtina with possible osteomyelitis. Fejza at least had a few nights' dreamless sleep after I started the medication. His cousin told me he was less preoccupied, so I left him a month's supply of drugs. When I got back into town I discovered that we were likely to be evacuated at any time; meanwhile, Illir was being discharged so I had to get him home. I spent the night unable to sleep, worrying how Illir's family would cope if they had to flee with a child on crutches.

I got to work the next day to find that the Office of United States Foreign Disaster Assistance (OFDA), who funded us, had ordered us to cancel all field operations as they felt it was too dangerous. My dilemma over Illir was solved by his consultant deciding he was not yet well enough to be discharged. Dr C. was one of Kosovo's first Albanian orthopaedic surgeons. Universally admired, he had somehow kept his job in the hospital. He promised to look after Illir. I went up to visit and found him lying on his bed staring at a battered Serbian children's book. He did not speak the language, but the ward had no Albanian books. He was very angry and fed up at not going home, so Bini and I told him about our visit to his family and I started to tell him a story. Then my mobile phone went. It was our field officer telling me I was being evacuated in an hour.

How do you tell a sick, lonely ten-year-old in a hostile hospital ward that you are leaving immediately and do not know when you will come back because there may be airstrikes? That you do not want to go at all, but have no choice because you are now simply a card in a larger game called 'Evacuate Internationals to Show Milošević We are Serious about Bombing'. And that you have absolutely no idea what is likely to happen, except that in the short term it's not going to get better. I simply said, 'Illir, I have to go right now, I am so sorry. I don't know when I'm coming back, but I promise that I will, and in the meantime Dr C. is going to look after you.' I hid some money in his trouser pocket, hugged him and left. It felt like abandonment to me, and I know that is what it felt like for him.

Then I was running across the hospital grounds, calling my friend to get his family to my house at once. By 1.30 we were in a small convoy of national and international staff on the road to Skopje. Arta's two daughters, six and four, had stopped crying at being abruptly ripped from home and school, and fallen asleep in the back of the Land Rover. Her one-year-old son dozed on her lap.

'What terrifies me is the possibility of mass killings,' she said. I did not know how to reassure her. At the border the Serbian customs officer was unusually friendly.

'Why are you leaving?' he asked Arta, smiling down at the baby. 'Nothing is going to happen.'

Somali border, Ethiopia, December 2007

You abandon home when the prospect of staying becomes more terrifying than the prospect of the unknown. But this does not mean the pull to return disappears. Sometimes it is overwhelming. When I went to see Amina today, her brother told me that she went missing for two weeks. He found her two days ago in the hills close to the Somali border. She appeared to be trying to go home. Apparently, she took the medication I had prescribed with her and continued to take the tablets intermittently, presumably because she found them helpful.

The remarkable thing is that today Amina has covered her hair, dressed in clean clothes and is able to sit and have some kind of conversation with me, albeit one still filled with the pain and misery of her experiences and still showing some confusion. 'I can't sleep, I eat very little, I feel pain,' she replies when I ask her how things are.

'Do you know where you are?' I ask. She looks round the *aqal*, at her brother holding her little son on his lap, at the unwashed pots and piles of rumpled clothes, then out of the door towards the scrubby hills.

'I don't know this place, it's a jungle, I am leaving, I don't want these mountains. I hate this life, I don't want this life. I don't want to be alive, please somebody help me.'

'Amina, I do want to help, what can I do?'

'The Somalis killed my dad and killed my husband. The family are all dead and the children are lost. I don't want Somalis any more. They killed my husband and now they want to kill me.'

Her little son crawls over, drawn by the sound of her voice.

'Do you know who this is?' I ask.

'Osman,' she replies, giving the correct name, 'but I don't know who gave birth to him.' But this time she does not push him away. Instead she picks him up and holds him against her chest, rocking and humming. I leave them, promising to return the next day.

We have started a regular weekly mental health clinic in the corrugated-iron health centre in the camp. In the afternoon

Dr Hassen, Dr Asmamaw and I see patients together. Dr Asmamaw does the consultations, Dr Hassen supervises and
teaches. I'm there to support them.

Every patient brings in the war and lays it out for us, a
gruesome, piecemeal tapestry: today there's an elderly man
with a lengthy story of multiple losses including wife, son and
daughter captured and killed in front of him, his other son
missing, his home burnt, the neighbour's six children hanged.
He has been shot in the face and leg. He would like us to
get the wounds fixed, and to help him with the troublesome
memories that plague him all the time. Then there's a boy
whose mother thinks he has 'gone mental' ever since he was
caught in shelling and knocked unconscious for two months,
but who is actually a highly intelligent and responsive teenager
who has lost his hearing. When we write down the questions,
he understands everything. He is followed by a tall, thin man
bringing his younger brother, who sits tense and staring, sometimes smiling and laughing and making one-word comments
like 'camel', 'water running'. Dr Hassen and Asmamaw diagnose psychosis, possibly schizophrenia. The problem has been
there many years, but there was nowhere to go for help in
Somalia.

The fact is that here in this dusty refugee camp, in the middle
of a desert, on the edge of a country at war, we are providing a
friendlier, more accessible mental health service than I ever did
at home in Britain.

When I worked in general practice we never gave proper
time to our mentally ill patients, we just batted them on to the
psychiatrists, who never sat in the primary health care centres.
And when I worked in psychiatric outpatients too many of
my patients never bothered to attend, in part because of the
stigma attached to the asylum, but also because we never gave
proper time to all the physical ills that plagued their lives but
for which they found it hard to get care. Just seeing patients in
an ordinary health centre close to where they live removes the
stigma in a moment, and they get treated as a whole person

whose physical and mental problems are seen as connected and equally worthy of attention.

I am also falling in love. I cannot pin down the moment. Asmamaw tells me he watched me spend my first two weeks in the camp rushing around and ignoring him completely. Now I cannot wait to see him. He is the good doctor out of the story books, everyone feels better for talking to him. Indeed, initially I assumed his warmth towards me was part of this general beneficence, but apparently not. He invites me to stay in his small, rented two-room house in the village. We sleep on cotton mattresses on the floor, read by candlelight, wash from a bucket, and use the pit latrine shared with two other homes. Nothing else is needed.

At night we sit outside to watch a sky crowded with more stars than I have ever seen. The truth is that it is easy to see beauty in a harsh environment if you have chosen to be there and have the freedom to leave. Otherwise, all the stars in a dark sky and the reds and yellows of the landscape cannot compensate for the snakes, the mosquitoes, the dirt, the lack of shade and the long trek for water.

I tell him about war in the Balkans and he tells me about returning from Cuba to Ethiopia in the midst of its own civil war at the end of 1989. He knew things were bad when he arrived at the airport in Addis and saw that almost all the soldiers were wearing torn and patched-up uniforms. The collapse of the Socialist bloc had emboldened the Tigreans and Eritreans, who knew Mengistu could no longer depend on his Superpower backer. They were engaged in a full-scale assault north of Addis.

'There were hardly any young men on the streets of the city, only wounded or elderly. The young men were at the front or in the hospital.'

One morning soldiers arrived and put up a large tent. They left without discussion or explanation. That evening at about 6 p.m., when Asmamaw was as usual the only doctor around, the ambulances started coming. There were no beds, no mattresses, not even stretchers. They lay on the floor. The hospital had no IV stands so Asmamaw hung bandages from the metal roof pole of the tent, and suspended the IVs from that. He started to triage – seven head injuries – but there was no neurosurgeon so there was nothing to be done for them. He got surgeons in for the chest and abdominal wounds, but even while he organised, people died.

'By morning five of the seven with head injuries and a quarter of the others were dead.'

The war continued for the rest of his year as an intern. In every hospital in Addis it was the same, tents full of wounded men, insufficient supplies, lice, bedbugs and death.

'Addis was full of women in black.'

'Which side did you hope would win the war?' I asked.

'Neither. I simply wanted the suffering to stop.'

6: NEUTRAL AND IMPARTIAL

Macedonia, 1999

We asked for military intervention, we got it, and the military ran the show. On 20 March 1999, the day after we arrived in Skopje, capital of the newly formed state of Macedonia, the Yugoslav Army launched a further massive offensive in Kosovo. Four days later NATO began airstrikes. Refugees started pouring into the neighbouring countries. At times four thousand an hour crossed into Kukës in northern Albania. In Macedonia there were already tensions between the resident ethnic Albanian community and the Macedonians. The government feared that a massive influx of Kosovo Albanian refugees would exacerbate the situation. So they penned thirty thousand people into muddy fields in no-man's-land until NATO built them special camps. NATO became the lead humanitarian agency and took over completely. What had we expected? This made the political partiality of the entire aid operation explicit.

All humanitarians know their founding myths: Henri Dunant's horror at the suffering of wounded and dying soldiers after the Battle of Solferino in 1859 led to the creation of the International Committee of the Red Cross. The ICRC grew over the following century to become the guardian of the Geneva Conventions, the legal framework that is supposed to regularise the conduct of war and protect both civilians and combatants. Central to its work is the commitment to three principles. Neutrality: 'In order to continue to enjoy the confidence of all, the Movement may not take sides in hostilities or engage at any time in controversies of a political, racial, religious or ideological nature.' Impartiality: people will be treated on the basis of need alone, regardless of nationality or political belief. Independence: those providing relief should have no connection to any state or body with an interest in the conflict.

The ICRC and its principles became the model for all humanitarian relief in wartime. NGOs working in emergencies claim adherence to these principles in the hope that this will protect them from being attacked by any of the belligerents and allow them access to those in need. But the nineteenth-century humanitarians I learnt about at school were immersed in political advocacy and controversy. The older idea of 'charity', whereby the fortunate had a duty to assist those less fortunate than themselves but not to better their lot, had been replaced by the radical notion that all human beings shared a common humanity and had inalienable rights to freedom, life and happiness. In this first incarnation of humanitarianism, the wish to alleviate suffering was intimately connected to the desire to improve and change the human condition.

Working to ensure that every person fulfilled their potential was necessarily a political project. Dorothea Dix endlessly petitioned the United States legislature to alleviate the conditions of the insane that she found chained and brutalised in jails and almshouses. William Wilberforce spent twenty-six years in parliament arguing for the abolition of the slave trade. This kind of humanitarianism could not be neutral because it required engagement with those who held power over the lives of others.

However, this kind of humanitarianism also provided the justification for the colonial carve-up of Africa in the name of education, enlightenment and ending slavery. The British Navy's insistence on their right to board and inspect any vessel, regardless of its flag, in order to ensure it was not carrying slaves was one of the earliest humanitarian military interventions. Nor were these early practitioners impartial. Dorothea Dix described herself as 'the advocate of helpless, forgotten, insane and idiotic men and women', yet was indifferent to the inhumane conditions of slaves in the southern United States.

Wilberforce was moved to passionate anger by the horrors of the Middle Passage and the callousness of British sugar planters in the West Indies, yet actively supported parliamentary legislation that suppressed freedom of speech and prevented working people in Britain from organising to improve their own lives.

Not taking sides is a political choice. If you want to relieve suffering, you necessarily witness the circumstances that are causing the problem. Silence about those circumstances has political consequences. In 1942 the International Committee of the Red Cross delegates voted against making any public denouncement of the genocide they knew was taking place in Nazi Germany, fearing that it might end the limited access they had to Allied prisoners-of-war and compromise Swiss neutrality. This failure continues to haunt the organisation.

It played a role in another humanitarian founding myth. In 1968 a young French doctor, Bernard Kouchner, volunteered to work for the ICRC in Biafra, which had just seceded from Nigeria. The Nigerian federal government established a blockade, which led to massive famine. Kouchner believed that the silence imposed on him and his colleagues by the ICRC made them accomplices to genocide. On his return to France he founded Médecins Sans Frontières (MSF), committed to both emergency relief and testimony on behalf of the victims. But there's a sting in the tale of this myth. Ojukwu, the Biafran leader, refused the federal government's offer of relief corridors and used the famine to manipulate global public opinion to side with his secessionists. The outpouring of concern possibly prolonged the conflict.

Neither partiality nor impartiality is a guarantee of getting it right.

I started working in the Balkans in solidarity with those being bombed and expelled. I was motivated by the same partisan sympathies that sent my uncle to Barcelona as a relief worker to help the anti-Fascist cause in 1936. As one journalist friend said, Bosnia was our generation's Spanish Civil War. There was no lack of speaking out. The Balkans were awash with journalists. During the Bosnian war, the ICRC made a public denunciation of the detention and inhumane treatment of innocent civilians and called on all parties to respect humanitarian principles. But did providing relief prolong the conflict? Aid workers bargained with the victimisers for the right to feed the victimised. Both the UNHCR and the ICRC evacuated the terrified civilians of minority populations from their homes in order to protect them. Forced to choose between being accomplices to ethnic cleansing and accomplices to murder, relief workers understandably chose the former.

The problem is that in many of the wars of the late twentieth and early twenty-first centuries, it is not a question of assisting innocent civilians trapped between enemy armies. The civilians are the object of attack and the purpose of the attack is their expulsion from a territory through terror, or their elimination. So while solidarity with the victims is definitively taking a side, failure to take it makes you a collaborator with the perpetrators.

Doctors are faced with particular conflicts because, in addition to the humanitarian mandate, there are the ethical codes that underlie the profession. The Hippocratic oath tells me to keep my patients from harm and injustice. But what if it is not disease but ethnic identity that make my patients vulnerable to harm and injustice?

Kosovo gave the old dilemmas a new twist. On a day-to-day basis you do what you can at the time. I helped a few people get out of a village in Kosovo and so assisted Milošević' with ethnic cleansing. In March 1999 I abandoned Illir and my other patients in Drenica because my departure seemed more likely to bring real relief in the long run. The agencies for which I worked were funded by the definitely partial US government. I knew we were part of the political theatre. We had already been withdrawn that February so as to push the Serbian government to the negotiating table. I hoped it would work again. I thought I would be back in a few weeks. But if the threat was not enough, I supported military intervention. I had been in Kosovo five months. I could not see how the expulsions and killings I had witnessed day after day could be stopped without it. All my Kosovar friends and patients felt the same. That meant internationals leaving, or we became the justification for inaction, just like in Bosnia. But crossing the border did not end the dilemmas.

Diary: Skopje, Macedonia, 29th March 1999

They said on Sky News that Baton has been executed. When I shut my eyes I see him lined up against a wall. My mind shies away from what happens next. I cannot stop crying. I cannot write. There is nothing to say.

Blace border crossing, Macedonia, 5th April 1999

Today's shift at the medical tent began at 4 p.m. We are situated right beside the metal gates and the cluster of offices that make up the border crossing. On the other side of the road a squalid encampment of plastic shelters stretches across the water meadows beside the railway line, as far as the eye can see. The train from Kosovo continues to shuttle into this fenced area, dropping off yet more people. The fields must contain at least 30,000.

Today the Macedonian police on the cordon have added surgical masks to their uniform of flak jacket and automatic rifle. So the Kosovars know that they are regarded as diseased as well as dangerous. Our medical tent is full. The mattresses and blankets are damp and filthy. There has been no time to dry anything out as stretcher-bearers keep running new cases in. The rest tent is completely full of paralysed people who are not sick enough for the Macedonian Red Cross to transfer to hospital. The Macedonian Red Cross tent remains empty. I spent Friday trying to persuade them to transfer three emergencies: a pregnant woman who had been bleeding for three days, a man with all the symptoms of a perforated ulcer and another with a suspected myocardial infarction. Only the intercession of the Albanian Deputy Minister of Health got them to respond.

In the evening there's the usual procession of 'Kosovar fainting girls'. No time for systemic therapy here. Clearing away the panicking crowd of attendants, checking them over and giving them a brief period of rest and explanation is all I can manage. Just before I end my shift at midnight I'm asked to see a man who is trying to bite anyone who comes near him. He is sitting tense and shoeless outside the Red Cross tent. His wife is in tears. He has never been like this before but suddenly 'went crazy'. He is too angry and incoherent to interview, but I and a colleague manage to slip our arms under his and lead him gently inside. To my relief he accepts the drugs I offer and falls into a deep sleep on one of the wet mattresses.

I don't think it's being driven from home at gunpoint that drives people over the edge, but the humiliation of suffering those experiences and then being penned into a field full of garbage and excrement, given occasional handouts of food, water, plastic and blankets, but deprived of any information or any control over what happens to you.

It is impossible to stay focused on individuals. I wake up tired old ladies after two hours' sleep to tell them their mattress is needed by someone sicker than themselves. I walk along the muddy track between the police line and the crush barriers, scanning faces for friends and trying not to hear the endless requests called out to me: 'Where are we going? What is going to happen to us?'

'I am so sorry, I don't know,' I say hopelessly.

Blace, Macedonia, 8th April 1999: My biting man is himself again today, but there's no knowing from such a short assessment whether this is the beginning of something more serious. I have never practised in this way before. One brief contact, and then I consign my patients to the void. I give his wife more medicine to administer if he becomes disturbed again and tell her to get medical help as soon as she's settled somewhere. She rummages in her bag and insists on giving me a blue silk scarf. After she leaves

I lean against the Land Rover and weep.

There are moments of grace. Baton is not dead. I found him at the other border crossing a few days ago. The queue was backed up for miles on the road through no-man's-land and very few people were being allowed through. Some friends came into the medical tent where I was working, and I immediately said how sorry I was that Baton had died.

'He's alive, Lynne! He's back there in the queue but he has no papers and cannot get across – perhaps you can help.'

At that crossing they were letting medical personnel like myself go backwards and forwards freely across the border. If we identified someone in the queue who needed medical attention, or was in trouble, we could bring them over. I had just collected four abandoned children from the line and handed them over to the Macedonian Red Cross.

I ran out of the tent, past the glass-windowed offices and the bar marking the frontier, then down the endless miserable procession of exhausted and frightened people. At some point cars were so closely parked I had to climb over them. A driver let me stand on his bonnet to stare down the whole line. I finally saw Baton with his face half hidden by a scarf, head hunched down in his jacket. I cannot describe the peculiar elation of seeing a friend whom you think has been executed, standing there alive, however miserable they look. Baton asked if I could get him across the border. He did not want to be discovered, given the terror and propaganda value his execution story had had for the Serbs. He was thinking of trying to make it through the mined fields beside the road.

'Lean on me,' I said. 'You look sick enough. Say you have very bad stomach pain.' We made our way back to the Macedonian frontier. The guards looked at us suspiciously. 'He's coming to the medical tent,' I said, far too nervously, 'he's sick.' They pulled him away from me, shouting in Macedonian.

'They are saying I paid you to bring me over here and they can see I am not sick. It's not going to work.' Baton did now look close to collapse, but we had lost our chance. But other friends were busy making calls. Albanian MPs from the Macedonian parliament turned up and walked him through. I saw him being feted in a café in Skopje this evening. He jokes that there is nothing like coming back from the dead to discover how much people care about you.

I have to admit I continue to engage in 'people smuggling'. This afternoon we found Bini's parents in the field. They have friends in Skopje so we took them to the medical tent and I backed up the Land Rover. The rear is windowless, so they were able to get in unseen and we drove them into Skopje. I have done the same for two other families that asked.

I saw another psychotic patient this evening. He is a middle-aged university professor who suddenly turned on his Albanian neighbour while they were queuing in the field and tried to kill him with the open end of a tin can. Words poured out at a fantastic rate as he sat with us explaining how his son had told him to cheer up because the red buses were coming to take them all to NATO camps. When he saw that the buses were white he 'knew' that they had come to take them to their deaths. And when he saw a policeman's head turned at a particular angle he 'knew' that his neighbour, whom he had never liked, was in a conspiracy to kill his only son. So he had to kill this neighbour first. He did not think he was ill, but was happy to take some medicine to calm down, as he had not slept for five nights.

The buses started arriving in large numbers this afternoon. When I walked into the field at 11 p.m. it was a mass of sodden blankets, torn plastic and abandoned personal possessions: shoes, wet jumpers and coats, children's toys, half-eaten food. Everyone has been moved into the calm, regimented orderliness of NATO-run camps except for the frail, elderly and paralysed, who remain in our rest tent. Somehow they got left off the list, so we will stay here until they are put back on.

Kosovo, 1999

I spent the months of the NATO airstrikes working with Kosovar refugees in northern Albania. I had strange dreams, though not about the expulsions, killings or mutilated bodies that filled my patients' stories. I dreamt repeatedly about Prishtina. There was no one there. The streets were deserted and rubbish-filled. Some buildings had been shelled. I knew for certain in the dream that we would never be able to go back. I would wake in tears, surprised at my sense of loss for a place that was not my own.

Airstrikes ended in June 1999 when Milošević agreed to withdraw all Yugoslav military, paramilitary and police forces, and accept an international peacekeeping force in Kosovo. So we did go back. German tanks and armoured personnel carriers (APCs) rolled down the main street of Kukës on their way into Kosovo on 12 June. We joined jubilant flag-waving refugees at dawn a few days later, and drove down the wooded eastern slopes of the Albanian Alps in a convoy of tractors. Nine thousand crossed with us that day, thousands more every day after that. By August almost all of the 850,000 expelled were back. It was the fastest and most complete repatriation of refugees since the end of the Second World War.

But on that mid-June morning, Prishtina was still the empty, rubbish-filled city of my dreams. The only people we encountered were journalists in the Grand Hotel and children clustered round a flower-bedecked British tank opposite the gutted pizzeria. The streets were free of traffic except for the occasional aid or military vehicle. All the shops and cafés were either boarded up or trashed. In the Dragodan area where we used to live, the gardens were full of long grass and overblown roses. Six of us camped out in Bini's parents' flat. I started looking for my old patients. I wanted to know what had happened to those who had been unable to flee.

Some of them found me. One day I heard my name shouted in the street and turned to see Illir hurtling after me on crutches. He had survived three months in the hospital. The house was wrecked, and the whole family had taken refuge in Prishtina. The families who had stayed in Drenica had a harder time. Some of them were dead. Agron, the elderly chronic schizophrenic, had refused to flee with his relatives. The Yugoslav Army found him in his bed and shot him in the head. Another of my fourteen-year-old patients was killed in the woods. Fejza's grandfather had been killed with eighteen others for refusing to say where the men in the village had gone. Fejza's mother had seen him standing stripped with the other men, in a line, with their hands against the wall.

But Fejza was better. We found the whole family living in an empty house across the road from their own, which had been destroyed yet again. There was a chair placed outside the door to indicate mourning. They poured out of the doors to hug us when we drove up. Fejza was now taller than me and very tanned. He had escaped out of a window when the tanks came into the village, then avoided one fatal selection by pretending to be disabled, putting a scarf on his head and jumping into a line of women. He escaped another by running away while a soldier was reloading his gun. Since his return home he had had no nightmares, no fear, and only occasional sadness. He thought it was thanks to my tablets, but as he had lost most of them in the first onslaught a few days after I left, I told him it might have more to do with his discovery of his own resourcefulness and strength.

Besnik was the happiest I had seen him and we played football all afternoon. The family had finally held a proper funeral for those killed the previous autumn. He took me to see the twenty-two graves. They lay in neat rows by the turn-off to the house. Each had a wooden marker and was covered in lavish cellophane-wrapped bouquets.

I kept finding patients who had recovered on their own. One boy had been so badly depressed we had started him on medication just before we left. He had run out of tablets in three weeks and escaped over the mountains to Albania. Now he was back in his own town, symptom-free and starting college. Another patient with nightmares whom I had been trying to help had survived the war in hiding and had also recovered. What had made such a difference to these young men? Certainly not individual therapy, or drugs – they had had very little of either. Rather, their recovery appeared to be intimately linked to liberation and the departure of the Serbian troops. They had coped with horrifying events and overcome them. Now they saw themselves as belonging to a political community that would build its own country. All of these things gave them a sense of self-esteem and improved their wellbeing.

Unfortunately, having bombed the Serbian administration and security forces out of the province, neither NATO nor the UN had made clear plans as to how they were going to run it. The house-burnings, evictions and revenge killings began again. This time it was Serbs and Roma who suffered. One day we found an elderly Serb couple sitting on a bench outside the priest's house in Ferizaj, bruised and crying. They had been beaten in their village, and wanted to be taken to Prishtina. The priest said he had asked for protection for his house and church, but nothing had materialised. The polite American Kosovo Force (KFOR) officer told me there was nothing to be done.

We bought soft drinks and aspirin for the couple, and as we drove to Prishtina they relaxed and told us a little about themselves. They lived in a mixed village, they were very sorry about what had happened to their neighbours but had had no part in it. They had wanted to stay. The local KLA commander had told them they could do so, but then outsiders had come and threatened them, forcing them to go. They both cried as they told the story. It was impossible not to be angry and moved by their plight. When we got to their sister's, the man would not stop kissing my hand and weeping over it, thanking us for saving their lives. I felt ashamed. The next week we went back to the town to do a clinic. The priest's house had been burnt to the ground, the priest gone, and a Kosovo Force guard now stood outside the empty church.

The UN bureaucracy was slow to organise but the NGOs were not. Before the airstrikes began, there were four medical NGOs in the country providing health services. A few weeks after the end of the airstrikes there were more than one hundred. Sixty of those offered psychosocial programmes. The agencies did not agree on how to define the terms 'psychosocial' or 'trauma' or on the methods to address it. These included debriefing, counselling, 'creative therapies for trauma healing', drama therapy in which participants were encouraged to act out their experiences, play spaces for children, sewing and coffee groups for women. Men and ex-combatants received considerably less attention than women and children. The effectiveness of any of these approaches in either improving general psychological wellbeing or preventing later psychological disorders was still generally unknown, and there were no clear guidelines as to good practice. This mattered, as by now there was some evidence that the increasingly popular 'debriefing' of everyone who had been exposed to a traumatic event appeared to make some people worse.

But never mind our ignorance, funding for 'psychosocial programmes' was abundant. After one of the endless coordination meetings in Prishtina Hospital, where I had been talking too much as usual, a man walked up to me and told me that President Clinton had made the mental health of children in Kosovo his personal priority. Would I like to submit a proposal?

'Give me ten days,' I replied.

I sat down with my Albanian psychiatric colleagues and asked them what we should do. Create a child psychiatry service. Train some of our existing residents in child psychiatry and set up clinics in the local 'health houses', they suggested. It made sense. More than 50 per cent of Kosovo's population were under the age of twenty-five. No child would ever set foot in the heavily stigmatised psychiatric unit in Prishtina hospital. Creating such a service in the local health houses would get psychiatry into the community. I wrote a proposal asking for funds to provide an immediate clinical service for 'the most traumatised children and families' in the conflict-affected rural areas, and to create a clinic in Prishtina. I knew I had to include the magic word 'trauma' to get the proposal considered, but I explained that this would be the beginning of a comprehensive child psychiatry service treating all problems. We would set it up with the trainee staff and work within the existing health system.

And that was what we did. Over the next three years the US government continued to fund the programme. We ran community-based clinics and trained the child psychiatry staff who run the service today.

A child psychiatry service was clearly needed. But I still feel uncomfortable about the ease with which we got continual funding when the United Nations Interim Administration Mission in Kosovo (UNMIK) could not pay police, judges or public-sector workers enough to avoid corruption, or keep doctors working in hospital posts. What Kosovo needed was serious investment in the institutions of law and order, the reconstruction of its infrastructure and the resolution of its political status. What it got was therapy.

Journalists rang me to ask if I thought criminality was on the rise because people were 'desensitised' to violence and in need of treatment? I could only reply that most of the people I knew, whether farmers in Drenica or intellectuals in Prishtina, made a clear moral distinction between taking up weapons to fight for a cause and using them for crime. I was astounded that, given the number of weapons floating around, the homicide rate still remained lower than in many US cities. My patients, who had suffered most, simply wanted to get on with their lives. They were disgusted both by the crime and the ethnic killings. The gun culture had developed in the vacuum created by UNMIK's failure to prioritise the rule of law.

By the spring of 2000 not much had improved. The promised International Police Force was still four thousand men down, and many of those deployed were ill-equipped to deal with armed inter-ethnic violence. Not all the local judges were impartial. Criminals were released without trial and the Mafia blossomed. Teachers and health workers left their posts to become better-paid drivers and interpreters for international NGOs. Water and power were intermittent. Prishtina roared at night to the sound of small generators.

I watched the consequences for my patients. Fejza became ill again in the winter of 2000. I found him on one visit sitting sullenly with all his female relatives chattering around him. When I saw him alone he burst into tears. He had given up school because he could not concentrate. He was restless, did not eat, and the nightmares and fear had come back. We re-started therapy but the main source of stress was clear. They were about to be made homeless. Their own house had still not been rebuilt but the owners of their current lodgings were about to return. They had nowhere to go. The family looked to him as the oldest male for a solution and he had no idea what to do. I had many patients in similar situations. They needed housing as much as psychotherapy. An Irish doctor friend of mine who had lived in Goražde under siege had given up medicine completely and concentrated on providing shelter. I was beginning to think she might be right.

It was justice that children wanted, not revenge. In 2003, five of my child patients were the key witnesses in the first trial in Serbia to prosecute a Serbian soldier for involvement in war crimes. They asked me to come with them. They each told in detail the horrifying story of a massacre in which they had witnessed nineteen members of their close families gunned down by paramilitary forces. Throughout the hours of testimony the children behaved with a courage, grace and composure that was moving and extraordinary. They were all glad that they had come to Belgrade and told the truth. It helped them feel relief and to get some sense of closure.

'I am so glad I did it,' Saranda told me afterwards. 'I stared right at him and he could not turn and look at me. I felt that I was in control. He thought he was in control, that he had killed us and it would all be quiet. But I was able to tell the world what he did, I wasn't afraid of speaking, and he could not stop me.'

The trial had changed Saranda's mind about Serbs. Much to her surprise, she had enjoyed herself in Belgrade. She had been moved by the Serbian human rights activists who had done so much to make the trial happen and by the genuine warmth of the Serb security agents who had accompanied us throughout our stay. She told me how she had liked Serbs before the conflict but afterwards all she had felt was anger and hate. Now she had decided that it didn't matter where someone was from but who they were inside. It was access to justice that had contributed to her healing.

Dire Dawa, Ethiopia, January 2008

There are three RAF airmen buried in Dire Dawa. I found their memorials by chance this morning while wandering along the airport road. I was drawn by the ruined sepulchres in an abandoned Catholic graveyard. The grass is uncut and rubble-strewn. There's a strange concrete cupola supported by four pillars housing a few of those lost to Mussolini's imperial ambitions. Next door, in immaculate condition, is a Commonwealth War Graves site: pointed stone walls enclose a small pebbled yard. The seventy or so granite gravestones stand in ranks, the names on them a reminder that Britain once summoned an army from across the globe to fight the Second World War.

Twenty-year-old Pilot Officer Paul Edwin Osborne Jago, Sergeant John Astil Wilson-Law and Corporal John Herbert Wintle died on 20 August 1940 when their Royal Air Force squadron bombed an Italian airbase in Dire Dawa. Their Blenheim was shot down in flames. The bombing raid was one small precursor to the British offensive that recaptured British Somaliland, took Mogadishu and entered Ethiopia from the north, west and south. The British Empire forces combined with Ethiopian irregulars and Orde Wingate's guerrillas to defeat the Italians. Ethiopia was the first occupied country to be liberated from Fascism in the Second World War.

I stood in the deserted graveyard, staring at all the smooth stones. Pale as a ghost, each cast its long shadow in the hot sun. The guardian who had unlocked the gate had disappeared. It was impossible not to feel the poignancy of all these deaths so far from home; impossible not to wonder what if? What if those fifty-two members of the League of Nations had lived up to the commitment they gave Haile Selassie in October 1935 that an attack upon a member state was an attack upon all, and that the offending partner should be stopped?

The history of the ineffective interventions taken by the League to halt the Italian aggression against Ethiopia reads like a primer for the delayed interventions in Bosnia, Kosovo, Rwanda and many other places, more than half a century later.

There are the back-room deals by the 'Great Powers' (Britain and France) that allowed Mussolini to believe he had 'a free hand' to invade and occupy the country. There are the ineffective sanctions that left out the oil and metals necessary to the functioning of a modern mechanised Italian army. There are the secret partition plans to dismember the country, leaving a tiny unoccupied rump state. There is the arms embargo imposed (at Italian prompting) on *both* sides of the conflict, thus depriving the Ethiopians of any means to defend themselves beyond the spears and rifles already in their position. There is the unexpected resistance from the Ethiopians, who held out for more than seven months, even though they were so poorly equipped and were bombarded with mustard gas. There is the ill-thought-out lifting of sanctions when the conflict was over, permitting the aggressor to continue to act with impunity; and finally a public outcry on behalf of the victims, along with 'neutral' humanitarian assistance.

This was the first conflict to which the ICRC sent its own delegates. Dr Marcel Junod witnessed the Italian bombing of Red Cross hospitals and the use of poison gas. He described 'an Italian plane spraying the area with an oily liquid which fell like fine rain and covered a vast area with thousands of tiny droplets. Each one that fell on the *tégument* caused a small burn which developed into a blister a few hours later.'

Yet when the League of Nations asked for access to such reports the ICRC refused, arguing that the duty 'to alleviate the sufferings of the victims of war' meant not departing from apolitical principle. Well and good, except that the then President of the ICRC, Max Huber, was an adviser to the Swiss Foreign Office, which believed Ethiopia could only benefit from Italian colonisation and advocated a policy of appeasement within the League. Like the Swiss, French and British governments, Huber believed a close alliance with Fascist Italy was the best protection against both Nazi Germany and the Soviet Union.

No one knows for sure how many Ethiopians were killed in what the League chose to call the 'the Dispute' between Italy and Ethiopia. The numbers are estimated at many tens of thousands. The Italians sacked Addis in early May 1936. Mussolini declared his *Impero Romano* on the ninth of that month. At the end of June the exiled Emperor Haile Selassie addressed the League of Nations with a speech of extraordinary prescience. 'I thought it to be impossible that fifty-two nations, including the most powerful in the world, should be successfully opposed by a single aggressor.' He requested the League not to lift sanctions and abandon Ethiopia to her occupiers, asking if states were 'going to set up the terrible precedent of bowing before force? . . . What undertakings can have any value if the will to keep them is lacking? . . . It is collective security: it is the very existence of the League of Nations . . . It is international morality which is at stake.'

Sanctions were lifted on 4 July. Franco began his attack on the Republican government of Spain two weeks later. Hitler had already used the opportunity of a distracted and impotent League to annex the Rhineland the previous March. In October Mussolini and Hitler signed the first Italo-German agreement: the Axis was born.

Italy continued to use poison gas in Ethiopia until March 1939 in its attempt to pacify the country. Ethiopian resistance to the Italian occupation cost thousands more lives. Luckily these did not include Asmamaw's young grandparents, who were both part of the rebellion in the east. Asmamaw's grandmother and great-aunt – with extraordinary courage, or extraordinary foolishness – broke into an Italian camp on their own and made off with two large metal boxes of what they hoped was ammunition. When they opened the boxes at home they were found to contain condoms. Asmamaw has a photograph of his grandmother in the customary baggy trousers, an ammunition belt round her waist and a rifle on her shoulder.

After the Allied forces liberated Ethiopia, they occupied it. Ethiopia was recognised as independent, but until 1944 the British ran the police force and had the right to place their military wherever they liked. It sounds very familiar. They stayed even longer in the Ogaden region – that large eastern area of

Ethiopia just to the south of Dire Dawa and Jijiga – hoping to create a Greater Somalia under their protection. That did not happen. But the Ogaden has never settled. The continuing unrest provided the excuse for the war that killed Asmamaw's father, and is one of the reasons justifying Ethiopia's intervention in Somalia today.

Ethiopia invaded Somalia in 2006 with United States blessing and a few supportive airstrikes. The stated aim was to assist the transitional government in its fight with the Islamic Courts Union, who then controlled Somalia. Ethiopian intervention involved indiscriminate carpet-bombing of sections of Mogadishu, killing no one knows how many and causing almost half a million to flee.

Ironically, some ten thousand of those refugees are now guests of the Ethiopian government in our camp. Ethiopia is on the front line in the fight against 'Islamic terrorism', so there's little complaint from the current 'Great Powers'. The trouble is that this 'intervention' has done absolutely nothing to improve things in Somalia. Far from liberating Somalis, it has just further radicalised some of them. If people thought the Islamic Courts Union was unpleasant, they should see what is emerging from the shattered pieces.

I was invited to a coffee ceremony in a shop yesterday. While we sat drinking from the tiny cups, a young Somali man told me he admired Al Shabab, the radical Islamist group that is now fighting the remnants of the Somali government over the border. He dreamed of a caliphate across East Africa, it was only a matter of time.

'These would be the same people who think it appropriate to stone thirteen-year-old girls to death after they report a rape to the police?' I wanted to ask. I am ashamed to say I chickened out, not wanting to cause a scene as a foreign guest.

The violence is unending and unbearable. Oddly, with war to the south and east, our destitute refugee camp seems like a haven of calm. But no one thinks of going home.

In the afternoon we drive back to Jijiga. Just after Babile, before you climb the Karamara Mountains, there are wide-open pasturelands that stretch south-east towards the Ogaden. As-mamaw tells me this is Kore, where his father died. There has never been a way to find the body. The area is still mined. We cannot even stop the car for long as it's a high-security area. At his request I sit in the front beside the driver and take quick furtive photographs. I look back and see that he is crying si-lently, through closed eyes. We drive on.

7: INTERVENTIONS

Doctors are inclined to be interventionist. You see that some-one is sick or hurt and you want to do something to stop the pain. The urge to act is compelling even when the outcomes are uncertain. We all learn the injunction, 'First, do no harm', but needless to say this has not stopped us. Our attempts at curing disease have included bleeding patients to death to remove poisonous humours, blistering and ulcerating the skin to rid them of mysterious internal inflammations, and poisoning them with mercury for almost every complaint. Dr Guillotin believed developing a more humane method of killing was a first step to abolishing the death penalty altogether.

Psychiatrists have come up with particularly imaginative interventions to cure insanity. We have whirled patients in ro-tatory chairs in order to dislodge delusions; infected them with malaria – this won its inventor a Nobel Prize; sent them into diabetic comas, and severed the connections between the fron-tal lobes and the rest of the brain. When such interventions didn't work, the patient was blamed.

Therapeutic failures in the nineteenth century led to grow-ing interest in 'degenerationist' theories and a preoccupation with heredity. Psychiatrists warned of the growing dangers of a toxic combination of mental imbecility, criminality and poverty. You could not shut all these people away. There were too many. 'Would it not be better to weed out and extermi-nate the diseased and otherwise unfit in every grade of natural life?' asked A. K. Strahan, writing in the *Journal of Mental Science* in 1890. The United States pioneered a more humane intervention: compulsory sterilisation. After all, it was 'better for all the world if instead of waiting to execute degenerate offspring for crime, or to let them starve for their imbecility, society can prevent those who are manifestly unfit from continuing their kind'. In his Supreme Court judgment Oliver Wendell Holmes spoke for many racial hygienists of the day. The compulsory sterilisation programme of the mentally unfit continued in some US states into the 1960s.

The Nazis saw US eugenic policies as a model and an inspiration. German psychiatrists enraged by 'the therapeutic inaccessibility of so many mental patients, psychopaths and habitual criminals [that is, Jews] moved from treating the individual to treating the national body, the *Volkskörper*'. The necessary intervention was extermination. Robert Jay Lifton meticulously documented what followed.

'I am a doctor and I want to preserve life. I would remove a gangrenous appendix from a diseased body. The Jew is the gangrenous appendix in the body of mankind,' explained Fritz Klein, one of the Nazi doctors who worked in Auschwitz, when Lifton asked how he could reconcile the gas ovens with his Hippocratic oath. It is salutary for me to remember that psychiatrists were on the selection ramps at Auschwitz.

Health interventions that sacrificed the individual for the greater good did not end with Nuremberg. The United States Department of Public Health actively denied treatment for syphilis to black Alabama sharecroppers in order to understand the progress of the untreated disease. The study was closed only in response to a public outcry in the seventies. In the name of a better understanding of disease processes, doctors have, among other things, given developmentally delayed children hepatitis and injected live cancer cells into people with dementia.

This history of the harms done by well-meaning medics trying to serve the common good should have made me wary of abandoning my pacifist principles to advocate 'humanitarian' military intervention. Yet the pacifist pastor Dietrich Bonhoeffer, faced with Fascism in Nazi Germany, argued that

'abstract principle' can get in the way of 'concrete responsibility'. He went on to engage in the plot to assassinate Hitler
and died in a concentration camp. I cannot imagine having
his courage. But it was partly because of his writings that I
put pacifist principles aside. Once the simplicity of 'principle'
is lost, though, all choices become questions of judgement.
How can one predict the consequences yet to come? If but-
terfly wings in Hong Kong set off tempests in the Atlantic,
how do we ever know what may happen? In Bosnia I thought
the choice was between using violence to end violence, and
allowing genocide to continue. I still believe we were right
to intervene there and in Kosovo, wrong in our failure to
protect the Rwandan Tutsis from genocide, and right to intervene in Sierra Leone and East Timor. I did not anticipate
how these choices would lead to the dreadful consequences
seen in Afghanistan and Iraq, or Ethiopian intervention in
Somalia.

Like Emperor Haile Selassie, I wanted a world where small
states – including new ones – had the right to self-defence and
to call for assistance when subject to aggression, as laid down
in Article 51 of the UN Charter. 'If we tear up the rules of a
game in which we ourselves are participants, what protection
is there for us in the future?' I wrote in 1993. 'It is now open
season for anyone with enough Kalashnikovs, howitzers, SAM
missiles, nuclear or chemical weapons, take your pick, to intervene wherever and whenever they like and commit the crime
of genocide with impunity.'

The tragedy was that military successes were followed by
political cowardice. On the brink of complete military defeat,
the Serbs were rewarded with an ethnically partitioned Bosnia.
After NATO airstrikes reinstated the Kosovar Albanians in
Kosovo, the UN administration that followed was unable to
protect Serbs and other minorities from revenge attacks and
expulsions. One thousand were killed and maybe one hundred
thousand fled. Today in Kosovo there is rampant corruption,
organised crime, organ-trafficking, a dysfunctional government, unemployment is at 50 per cent and infant mortality is

still the highest in Europe at 35–49 per 1,000 births. Members of the KLA leadership who fought in the war have been indicted for war crimes. Baton was tried and fined at The Hague for exposing the identities of protected witnesses. The state declared independence in 2008, but still has no seat at the UN. My Kosovar friends are enraged by KLA corruption and incompetence but are sure that without NATO's intervention all Kosovar Albanians would have been exiled or killed in 1999.

The Rwandan genocide brought home to humanitarians the true cost of non-intervention. Between April and July 1994, eight hundred thousand Tutsis were killed. It was the largest genocide of modern times. At the height of the slaughter, additional Western troops arrived in Kigali. Their mission? To protect and evacuate their own citizens and soldiers. MSF France actively campaigned for the use of force, declaring, 'You cannot halt a massacre with medicines . . . the genocide must stop and those responsible must be brought to justice!' The US government labelled the killings a 'humanitarian crime' so as to avoid invoking the Genocide Convention, which would have committed them to action. But yet again the presence of humanitarians on the ground allowed the international community to procrastinate. In the end it was only the military intervention of the Rwandan Patriotic Front that saved the Tutsi population from being entirely annihilated.

In August 1999, 98.6 per cent of the East Timorese voted for independence. I was happy when the deployment of Australian peacekeepers stopped Dili from being burnt to the ground by an angry Indonesian military. I was also glad when the British Army finally intervened in 2000 and ended the two-decades-long conflict in Sierra Leone. Then the World Trade Center was bombed in New York and everything changed. As the 'Osama Wanted Alive or Dead' rhetoric echoed around the world, I wrote to a friend:

> . . . the odd and alarming thing is that my 'anti-bombing in the Balkans' friends are mostly pro-bombing now, although no one has succeeded in explaining to me how this

will catch Osama or end world terror or stop anthrax in its tracks, while it quite obviously will kill millions of Afghans through starvation this winter, which confirms yet again that the only important lives and bodies are Western ones . . .

The Bosnians, Albanian Kosovars, people of Sierra Leone and the Timorese had all asked for military intervention to end killing and displacement. The Afghans made no such request. Bombing them to get rid of Osama Bin Laden seemed like stamping on mercury. It would do nothing to end their years of misery and starvation under the Taliban. But by October of 2001, 74 per cent of the British public supported the idea.

I went on a peace demonstration in Trafalgar Square, the same place where I had stood and made a speech in favour of military intervention in Bosnia six years earlier. Inconsistency, according to Gandhi, is a sign of growth, an ability to see the truth as it appears at that moment in time. Perhaps I was becoming clear-sighted. The US and British governments dropped food parcels as well as cluster bombs, which unfortunately looked rather similar, and scattered leaflets asking illiterate Afghan mothers to consider how they would feel if they had lost a baby in the World Trade Center attack.

I felt the same about military intervention in Iraq. I joined another peace demonstration in autumn 2002. But the simplicity of the Stop the War Coalition bothered me. In the peace movement of the eighties, a group of us had tried to articulate the complex connections between peace and freedom and advocated campaigning for both at the same time. That meant protesting against human rights abuses and the lack of democracy in Eastern Europe, as well as against the new generations of nuclear missiles in the West. Each justified the other. A similar analysis seemed obvious here. The peace movement had to challenge and oppose Saddam Hussein's human rights abuses – otherwise, that agenda was left to Blair and Bush and the pro-war lobby. I could not find this argument among the 'No Blood for Oil', 'Stop the War' and 'Star of David = Swastika' posters on the march. I did not go on the next peace march in February 2003. I wrote a letter to the press.

> I cannot get round the fact that Iraq would not have let the inspectors back in nor be making any changes without the coercive pressure and the threat of military action initiated by George Bush. On the other hand without the pressure of the anti-war movement it is likely that there would have been dangerous and precipitate military action weeks ago ... So perhaps both need to keep on doing what they are doing!
>
> Personally I have been in favour of regime change since 1991 when we first abandoned Kurd and Marsh Arabs to Saddam's mercies – it would have been nice to see a million marching on their behalf then. Or if we had all marched in protest at Saddam's use of chemical weapons in 1988, there might not need to be any marching or bombing today.
>
> The problem is that the anti-war movement is very good at saying 'No war' and very poor at coming up with the non-violent options for the democratic changes that are so desperately needed in so many places. This is why it always appears to support a very ugly status quo, and leaves the field wide open to aggressive imperialism ... 'No' is no longer enough, we have to say what we want instead.

The letter never got published. Not surprisingly, my ambiguous position succeeded in alienating all my friends and family. The consensus most of us had shared over military intervention in the Balkans had shattered, and the debates played themselves out in the press. The 'liberal hawks' who had advocated intervention in Bosnia now argued that this was the moment to overthrow tyranny in the Middle East. Ends justified means.

I had been on a brief assignment in Afghanistan which had made me question my earlier opposition to military intervention in that country. The women I had met there all welcomed the fall of the Taliban, although they asked me repeatedly:

'Where is the promised international assistance?' If we were going to intervene, did we not have an obligation to follow through and help them rebuild? On the other hand, David Rieff, a writer on human rights and humanitarian issues that I admired, argued that human rights advocates and humanitarians had gone too far in their pursuit of a liberal and just world order. There was nothing humanitarian about war, and democracy and justice could not be imposed by force.

The historian Brendan Simms took me to lunch in the oak-panelled dining room of Peterhouse College, Cambridge. We had campaigned together for intervention in Bosnia. He asked if I now wanted to live in a world where no one intervened on anyone else's behalf, governed only by national self-interest? Where Russia and China had the veto on right action? 'An interventionist US is much better for the world than an isolationist one.'

A Foreign Office friend whom I trusted assured me that there was definitive evidence of weapons of mass destruction, and they had to be found or we were all at risk. There was an imminent threat. Meanwhile, my anti-war friends saw my silence as shameful and wondered why I was not sitting down in protest in Whitehall. But like Michael Walzer, I did not want to be part of 'an anti-war movement that strengthened the hand of Saddam'.

The arguments that made most sense to me came from Faleh Jabar, an exiled Iraqi Communist and research fellow at Birkbeck College. He argued that Saddam's Baathist Iraq was

> a menace to its own people, the region, and the world at large. Leaving the monster in its place is an invitation to future catastrophe. This may sound like an endorsement of the war camp. Not at all. Warmongering is as short-sighted as philanthropic pacifism. The former deliberately neglects the possibilities of a political solution to the problem; the latter does not recognise the existence of the problem. Both are locked in an ideological cage.

He warned against the attempted 'surgical' removal of Saddam as likely to

> unleash latent, uncontrollable, institutional and social forces beside which fantasy will pale. A civil war may begin nobody knows where and end up in nobody knows what ... War is as pernicious as totalitarianism. Both breed violence and mayhem. Opposing the war in itself is good but not good enough. Letting the Leviathan off the hook is a grave mistake for which we will pay sooner rather than later.

Jabar argued for non-violent, coercive, political measures rather than waging an illegal pre-emptive war: Saddam should be threatened with indictment for his previous illegal use of chemical and biological weapons and offered safe passage along with his elite. The remaining clan elites should be supported in transforming the regime through a mini-Marshall Plan. This should be backed by the threat of force. This kind of supportive pressure would embolden people to take matters into their own hands. 'An invasion, on the other hand,' he said, 'would wrench matters out of Iraqi hands and would risk untold consequences.'

But no one was listening. And ambivalence, like silence, has a moral price. If you refuse to join a side, then by default you share the position of the prevailing one. On 18 March 2003 I wrote to a friend:

> So now we are all on the front line and bombs will fall and tanks roll and more people die than have died already and this war whether won or lost will provide the blueprint for the next and the next. To fight in this way at this time is wrong ... I cannot concentrate. I am filled with foreboding. I endlessly watch the news and learn nothing. I see no point in lying on some pavement or cutting the fences of missile bases as I would have done ten years ago. That kind of action is to convert the public mind

through symbolism, but the public already know what they think. If anything there is too much action and too little thought. How to recreate the democratic connection between people and government and a working international order that CAN provide security? These are the questions that should trouble us now.

I felt complicit. Miserable, perplexed and confused, I retreated back into the asylum.

That April I got a short-term position standing in for a consultant on an acute adult inpatient ward in a large city. The nineteenth-century buildings were mostly closed, waiting to be turned into luxury flats. The wards were in self-contained units set up in the hospital grounds. My sad, bothered and agitated patients never mentioned the war. Their own pains took up all their energy. Most of them were confined to the hospital because they posed a danger to themselves or others. So our dramas and conflicts centred on the degree to which I might intervene to limit their personal freedom, for their own good.

What to do for Angie, who didn't know whether she wanted to be alive or dead? She had been cutting herself since the age of seventeen. On my first day she ran away and then brought herself back late in the afternoon. She sat whey-faced and miserable, whispering that she had gone to the local park with a packet of pills to kill herself, because she was having flashbacks of abusive experiences as a child. The tablets made her gag so she gave up and called the hospital on her mobile. She still wanted to be dead and still felt hopeless. As she spoke, her thumb twitched in the characteristic way of someone on neuroleptics. At least I could fix that. Fixing how unloved and unwanted she felt would take much longer. I promised we would talk in the morning. The nurse sitting in with me told me this was all a 'put-on' for the new psychiatrist. Angie's notes began with two paragraphs by a junior doctor calling her a sociopath, making no reference to her history or the likelihood that she had PTSD, or any recommendations for her care. She was now in her thirties, half that time spent in hospitals. I put her on constant observations.

And there was Jim, whom the nurses wanted me to discharge. He had been admitted with hallucinations by the duty doctor. The nurses knew him well. They said he was making up his symptoms to get a bed. He sold drugs to the other patients. Painfully thin, in a grubby purple sweatshirt and torn jeans, he was homeless and had been sleeping on the street. He admitted he took drugs, but not recently as he had no money. He could talk coherently but still had the anxious, distracted look of someone hearing voices. 'They go on and on,' he said, 'talking about me, telling me I'm shit, I should walk under a car.' Occasionally he blanked out, sometimes he muttered. If it was an act, it was a good one. Could we make a deal? I asked the charge nurse. Strict rules about behaviour, no taking or selling drugs and we would keep him in until his social worker had sorted out temporary accommodation and the addiction team got involved. Otherwise, he would be out and in again as an emergency in a few more days – only more hostile and less cooperative, and what was the point of that? Could we try trusting him?

In the evenings I watched the war with friends. It became the permanent backdrop to our lives, our senses numbed by the media's love affair with split-screen reporting: a talking head accompanied by continuous repetitions of undated and untitled 'highlights': oil wells burning, soldiers running or shooting or putting their gas masks on and off, Iraqis being arrested and searched, helicopter wreckage. Along the bottom of the screen the ticker summarised events, interrupted by flashes of meaningless and often inaccurate 'breaking news'. How does one provide the whole picture when broadcasting live from under a tank in a sandstorm? I was sickened, and yet it was addictive. In a newly liberated port, the 'liberated' Shia grabbed their rations and cursed us, yelling for our defeat.

Lilac bloomed outside the dark brick asylum walls, astonishing in its loveliness. Sticky buds appeared on the chestnut trees. The amazing spring days seemed inappropriate. I felt the weather should match the mood: cloud, rain and an early darkening, not such florid beauty.

Angie said she was feeling more positive and asked me to stop the constant observations. We did. I hoped she now had enough structured attention to tell us rather than show us when she was distressed. The next day she walked up and down outside the office with a plastic bag in her hands, then retreated to her room and pulled it ostentatiously over her head. I pulled it off and sat at the foot of the bed.

'What do you want, Angie?'

'A magic wand to take the pain and thoughts away.'

'I haven't got one,' I said, 'there are no quick fixes.'

I knew she did not really want to die, but she didn't want to take the drugs or engage in the psychotherapy we offered, either. In one breath she told me to put her in a secure unit as she could not be responsible for herself – in the next, to lift her section and allow her the freedom to go home. I wanted to bang my head against the wall in frustration. She sat rocking and crying, face distorted and miserable. I asked what she would do if Ronnie, her small nephew who sometimes visited, stuck his hand in the fire.

'Pull it out!'

'Even if Ronnie protested?'

'Of course.'

'Well, if you behave like a child, which is perhaps how this illness makes you feel, we have to intervene to protect you, until you feel well enough to be an adult.'

I felt like a jailer. But on my last afternoon Jim went off to see a new flat with his social worker. He told me all about it. He was signing up to the drug rehabilitation that was part of the deal. I got up to go, relieved that at least one intervention had worked.

'Dr Jones, wait a minute.' Oh no, there's a glitch, I thought. 'I just want to say thanks very much for giving me a chance. No one else has bothered. I really appreciate it and I won't mess it up.'

President Bush promised the Iraqi people that war would be

'directed against the lawless men who rule your country and not against you. As our coalition takes away their power, we will deliver the food and medicine you need. We will tear down the apparatus of terror and we will help you to build a new Iraq that is prosperous and free.' An estimated 3,000 to 4,000 Iraqi civilians lost their lives between 20 March and 20 April 2003, along with some 7,000 to 8,000 Iraqi combatants. Many more were wounded. 'The Iraqis are sick people and we are the chemotherapy,' Corporal Ryan Dupre told a journalist outside Nasiriyah that March. Soldiers engaged in 'humanitarian' military intervention now used medical metaphors. The Marines had just killed twelve civilians as they tried to escape the city. 'I am starting to hate this country,' the corporal continued. 'Wait till I get hold of a friggin' Iraqi. No, I won't get hold of one. I'll just kill him.'

Neither US nor British forces could provide sufficient security in the 'liberated areas' to prevent widespread looting. The public health service collapsed. Health centres and hospitals were stripped of beds and medication. 'There is no serious looting,' a British officer in newly liberated Basra said on television, as the same news item showed food stores and banks being gutted. When a young British soldier brusquely turned away a group of Iraqi doctors who had come to discuss security with his commander, I felt ashamed.

The humanitarian community was divided in the run-up to the war. European agencies and donors were reluctant to either prepare for or put aside funds for the humanitarian consequences of a war that many saw as illegal and which was deeply unpopular. US NGOs were more pragmatic. Used to being funded by the US government, most of them saw preparation as a responsibility and cooperation as a necessary evil. They argued that it gave them a chance to remind the government of its obligations to the Iraqis under international humanitarian law. They thought that once the conflict was over the military would confine itself to the necessary role of providing access and security, and that leadership of humanitarian affairs would return to the UN, as in other conflicts.

This would allow them to maintain a fig leaf of independence from US government policy and to deliver aid securely.

Except that Colin Powell had already said in Afghanistan that US NGOs were 'force multipliers' and 'such an important part of our combat team. [We are] all committed to the same, singular purpose to help every man and woman in the world who is in need, who is hungry, who is without hope, to help every one of them fill a belly, get a roof over their heads, educate their children, have hope.' Andrew Natsios, head of the United States Agency for International Development (USAID) made it even clearer in a speech in May 2003. US NGOs who received US government money for their activities, he said, were in effect 'an arm of the US government'. If they did not make the US government origin of their funding explicit to beneficiaries, as private contractors did, he would personally tear up their contracts and find new partners.

In the Balkans I had worked both for agencies who only took voluntary private contributions and for those that were government-funded. I had no ethical objection to the latter. I preferred my taxes going to aid rather than to weapons, and someone had to implement the aid programmes. I wanted to go to Iraq. I had failed to clearly oppose the war and I wanted to contribute whatever I could to clearing up the mess. Half of my friends were there already. I thought that if the UN took charge, humanitarians would soon be able to work with Iraqis to improve things. I took the first job that was offered: to do a mental health assessment for a US-funded agency.

Diary: Baghdad, 23rd July 2003

I now have a room in the maze of small apartments in which the agency is housed. The power and air-conditioning are on two hours a day. According to the World Service the two hottest places in the world at the moment are Death Valley in California and Baghdad. I also have a radio – my call sign is 'India 83' – and four bits of plastic hanging around my neck with other call signs, phone numbers and two forms of ID. It's quiet today but Ken our security guy is full of gloomy prognostications of it getting worse before it gets better. If the house is attacked, we all have to make our way to a sandbagged position on the roof. What happens next is rather unclear. Perhaps the cavalry will arrive (in Black Hawks, not on horses) and it will be like a John Ford movie. The idea is to give the intruders free run of the house and come downstairs when they have gone off with the computers, or whatever they wanted.

There is some risk to any journey outside, but there's a risk to staying indoors, not least from going bonkers and getting exceedingly fat. Everyone is trying out disguises. The UN stopped being white because the Coalition were shooting at white vehicles belonging to the fedayeen. So they've painted themselves blue with fluorescent orange letters, making a lovely target that can be seen by all at 100 metres. We drive in unmarked battered-up old cars, keep away from the military, and hope we go unnoticed.

Baghdad, 25th July

The UN has said that attacks on humanitarian workers can no longer be considered random and something should be done to protect us. An ICRC worker was killed outside the city, as was someone from IOM [the International Organisation for Migration]. Two car-jackings outside the UN in the last 24 hours, with a driver killed in one; a bomb thrown into an NGO compound last night. The odd thing is that as the situation deteriorates I have adapted. It took a few days, but just like in Sarajevo, your idea of what is normal radically alters and you acquire the useful sense of denial that lets you get in the car to go to a meeting, and the dangerous sense of being bullet-proof.

Strange how I feel about the tanks: when I first got to Bosnia I regarded the SFOR [NATO-led Stabilisation Force] guys as basically friendly and on our side. (They pulled my Volvo out of a ditch once.) I had to adjust in Kosovo. All the tanks and APCs were Serb so we would give them a wide berth. Then NATO came into Kosovo and I began regarding convoys as friendly once more. Here, any Coalition hardware needs to be avoided. The drivers are good at it, even parking completely to allow a convoy to pass rather than getting caught up.

I met an elderly doctor at WHO this morning who told me his house was bombed by the Coalition but he still thought they did a great job. There were a lot of fedayeen in his garden, so he thought the bombing was justified.

Baghdad, 26th July

Driving in Baghdad is the most dangerous thing I do. There are no rules. This morning we drove briefly down the wrong side of a four-lane highway with the oncoming traffic barrelling towards us, then across the rough ground that made up the divide, ducking into the fastest stream going the correct way. Most traffic lights don't work. Those that do are ignored. My driver told me 'it's dangerous to stop at a red light or you'll get hit from behind'.

I was late for my meeting because it takes 20 minutes to get onto the bulging elevators at the Ministry of Health. The building was entirely gutted during the looting and is now being restored by WHO. Dr J. is the WHO point person for mental health. His vision is to put psychiatry into primary health care and get teachers trained in mental health. Over the last two years he ran small courses for teachers and GPs. He gave me the manual he wrote, then nervously took it back and started to pull out the glossy picture of Saddam in the back.

'Please don't,' I said, 'I'm happy to keep it as a souvenir.'

He gave an embarrassed laugh. 'I thought you might be offended.'

'Of course not.'

'And he is very good-looking,' he added.

I and my driver drove out to Al Rashad, the large mental institution for chronic patients on the edge of Baghdad. Dr J. thought I was foolish to go. 'They will just ask you for things.'

The city disintegrates at its edges. The larger villas and apartment blocks give way to walled compounds, mud-brick houses and wasteland. Bedraggled palms struggle up between piles of rubbish and toxic-looking streams. There are also pools of vivid blue water, reed-fringed, a ghostly hint of beauty, although rubbish floats in these as well. In one, a dozen white egrets swoop and fish, along with diving terns and other small waders I cannot recognise. But never mind the beauty of the birds, the road was increasingly empty. Areas are divided into three grades: 'OK', 'Uncertain' and 'Hostile'. This felt 'uncertain', if not actively 'hostile'.

'Is this a safe area?' I asked my driver.

'It's good and the hospital is five minutes away.'

That at least was correct, although my unease increased when I saw two Coalition vehicles pulling into a compound. We pulled back to give them space.

During the hotter phase of this war (I am no longer going to talk about it as if it is over), Al Rashad mental hospital was on the front line between advancing US and Iraqi forces. Marines smashed in the front gate. After they had gone, looters rushed in. The patients and most staff fled in terror. Dr G. who remained at his post tried to negotiate with the looters, explaining that this was a public facility and nothing to do with Saddam. They stuck a knife against his ribs so he gave up. He had no means to go home so he spent the night locked in his office. The anarchy lasted two days, and the looters took everything.

Dr G. then left the now deserted hospital and went to town to try and tell 'the government'. He discovered there was no government, so he went to the ICRC, who had supported the hospital in the past. They have put it back together, cleaning and refurbishing wards, putting in fans and air-conditioning. Six hundred of the former 1,200 patients have come back or been returned by their families. Six hundred are still missing, including the 160 mad, bad and dangerous, deliberately released from the maximum-security wing, adding to the hazards of the city.

I found Dr G. writing ICRC a letter of condolence because of the death of one of their staff in the rocket attack
two days ago. He wanted to know if I and Dr B. (an
English-speaking psychiatrist who joined us) thought he
should mention God in the letter. He was worried it might
offend the ICRC.

'Of course not!' We both agreed. 'If you want to mention God, you do so. They will be touched by whatever
you say.' He also wanted to know why I had a scarf round
my shoulders.

'I sometimes put it over my head, depending where we
are. Should I do so in the hospital?'

'No, no, you should not! Don't! It is not necessary, and
you should always refuse!'

'Well, I don't want to give offence, especially in such
insecure times.'

Dr G. shook his head. I saw I had disappointed him
as a potential warrior in the battle for female emancipa-
tion and modernisation. We discussed the attacks on aid
workers.

'The trouble is there are a lot of rumours about international organisations,' Dr B. said. Iraqi people believe
they are supporting the reintegration of Jews back into
Iraq. Some people think most of the foreigners are Jewish
and are here to reclaim their property.'

'What happened to the Jewish community in Iraq?'

'A quarter of Baghdad was Jewish before 1948. They
were the elite, they ran many things. But after the Arabs
lost the war, there were massive deportations, killings and
burnings. What are you doing here?'

'Learning as much as possible at the moment,' I replied,
and asked what the long-term plans for the hospital were:
'Deinstitutionalisation?'

Dr B. laughed. 'That is for the West. Here we institu-
tionalise as much as possible. This society believes the
mentally ill should be in an institution. We have no plans
to put them in the community. Not here. A long time ago

there was talk of halfway houses and day hospitals, but with all the wars nothing came of it.' I mentioned Dr J.'s ideas about increasing primary health care involvement.

'Dr J. is a dreamer. Maybe too close to the government. He held a lot of workshops for GPs but I think it was futile. If you want to change things you must change society first. Ordinary people don't want chronic patients back home. No one wants a mentally ill person in their home. They want them here. They are "the untouchables", the neglected; this is the dark side of humanity. As health workers we have to respond to this and take care of these people. I'm not talking about neurotic illnesses. Some things can change there, but not with schizophrenia or mania.'

'But what about when people have recovered?'

'In the Iraqi mind a mentally ill person is ill for life.'

'Do they seek other forms of treatment?'

'In the countryside, ignorant people go to faith and folk healers. They keep going until they realise it does not work. Then they come to us. That's part of the problem. We always see patients so late, when the problem has become chronic.'

'What sort of treatments do they get?'

'Prayer, exorcism. It may work for some problems such as conversion or somatic symptoms, but not for serious illnesses.'

'Perhaps even there, it might be calming?'

'Not Muslim treatments, they are too exciting,' Dr G. broke in. 'We use things such as flogging, bloodletting, chaining. Muslim clergy will beat the patient into recovery if they can. Sometimes people arrive with bruises and head injuries and we ask the family, "What did you do?" "Nothing, it was the healer," they say.'

'Perhaps we could quickly rehabilitate some of the inpatient psychiatric wards in district hospitals? They must be even more neglected than here?'

'It's a very good idea but this is the wrong time for

such programmes, the wrong time for any of you to be here. You Westerners don't get it. The fedayeen are not the problem. The fundamentalists are. You are part of the game. They hoped to draw you into a war to get rid of Saddam and the fedayeen, and they succeeded. Now with just a few terror attacks they will get rid of you all, and they will be in control.'

'Is that what you want?'

'Of course not, but it will happen. It is not safe for a British person to work here at this time. People will smile at you but they have a knife behind the back.'

He walked me around the hospital in the hot sun. From the outside it wasn't so bad. Freshly painted blocks divided by gardens of palm trees. All the wards were barred and locked. There is no legislation, but all mental in-patients are involuntary in Iraq by default. The high wall of the empty maximum-security unit dominated one side of the garden. Then we went into a ward: a rectangular courtyard with six small bedded rooms. It was clean, the beds had mattresses, and there were fans. One woman stood naked in the hot sun while another, very modestly dressed, yelled and expostulated with her to dress herself. The one nurse on duty took no notice. The other patients sat around listlessly or walked and muttered to themselves. It was the asylum of my medical student days – food, bed, medication and neglect. The patients were on their own.

'We don't have enough nurses and they have no train-ing, so mostly they stay in the staff room and avoid the patients except to give them medicine.'

'To be honest, I am pessimistic,' he continued. 'I feel we are in a tunnel without an end in sight. The Coalition will pull out and then there will be fighting between the Sunni and Shia extremists, each certain he knows the best way to govern.'

'You're not hopeful about the new Iraqi authority?'

'Exiles from abroad. They don't understand us.'

'They are not all exiles.'

'All the politically astute ones are.'

As we left the hospital I saw a couple of Coalition APCs finishing a house search. A disgruntled group of men and boys stood, arms folded, outside the gate as they pulled away. We drove back past the egrets and the rubbish piles. Back at the office Ken told me I had been in a 'hostile area'.

Baghdad, 29th July

Pick a war, any war with sufficient media coverage, and after it has officially declared itself over, there you will find the humanitarian community: international, multi-ethnic, well-meaning, naive, rich, or at least phenomenally well resourced. The larger the community, the greater the dis-organisation, and the more time we spend in meetings coordinating. The psychosocial meeting is as good a place as any to see it in action.

UNICEF is coordinating and today they invited every-one engaged in 'psychosocial activities' to come along. 'Psychosocial' is one of those wonderful words that can mean anything you want, so almost every agency does some of it. Some 50 aid workers stuffed themselves into a tiny office. There was the usual scatter of Italians over here to play with children; a young woman with a pony-tail explained that 'Bridges to Baghdad' is organising summer camps. There were Iraqi schoolteachers planning to reform the entire teacher-training system. An intelligent friendly woman called Jill Clark is trying to organise a na-tional child protection assessment. The French Enfants du Monde, who have been here for years, are trying to help children in institutions. And UNICEF intends to assess traumatic reactions in all 11 million Iraqi children.

The UNICEF representative was in full flow when two more Iraqi gentlemen arrived. Both smartly dressed, they squashed themselves into a corner and looked bemusedly at the rather scruffy crowd, as if they had expected some-thing else. Professor D. introduced himself. He has been appointed by the acting Coalition Provisional Authority

Minister of Health, to be in charge of mental health at the ministry. I asked Professor D. if he knew Dr J.

'Who is he?' Professor D. replied.

After the rep finished, and cooed her enthusiasm at all the wonderful work we would do together, two more Iraqi psychiatrists wanted to discuss their project to set up a child guidance clinic. Professor D. bristled. 'Have you got funding?' he asked.

'Not yet,' said one of the doctors nervously.

Money is power in this country. If you are funded you can act. There is very little to stop you. However, the Coalition Provisional Authority [CPA], who as occupiers are the de facto government, are trying to control things. They have announced that they will vet all proposals. So before you can dream of asking OFDA [the Office of US Foreign Disaster Assistance], DFID [the UK Department for International Development] or anyone else for any money, you have to check with them. This won't bother MSF and other independently funded NGOs. But the CPA is determined to stamp its authority. It has already told WHO and the World Bank that their planned massive needs assessment has to be done through them. The CPA knows best what is needed; although to date it hasn't done its own assessment. I should be pleased, as they have prioritised 'mental health'. Four million dollars has been allocated to PTSD. Dr K., whom I met the other day and who is here with Professor D., will have a leading role.

Dr B. told me that Dr K. used to be a military psychiatrist. 'The military psychiatric unit closed along with all military facilities. And all those staff are hanging around the MoH wanting to be redeployed. Of course, now they are the biggest Saddam opponents. They changed very fast.'

Baghdad, 31st July

I and a colleague met Professor D. for coffee. He is an Iraqi child psychiatrist who left some 35 years ago but continues to travel back and forth. He shares at least some of my scepticism about the PTSD bandwagon. He intends to turn the planned 'trauma clinics' into a comprehensive service for children.

As for training GPs in mental health: 'I have plans for that problem. What we will do is invite the drug companies in. They will offer gifts and incentives, so all the GPs will come. Then they will train them in the treatment of anxiety and depression, which is all GPs really need to know about.'

'So shortly we can expect everyone in Iraq to be on Valium and Seroxat?'

'This is a long way off. It is not a priority.'

He could see the horror on my face. 'That is the way things are going in psychiatry, unfortunately.'

And so in mental health we have all the elements for conflict that exist in the country at large: the locals who view each other with suspicion, depending on what they thought each other was doing before the war, and who are all competing for money; the foreign exile, brought back by the US to run things; the NGOs, WHO and UNICEF and the occupying forces, all with their own agendas. But money talks. The Coalition in its wisdom has decided that, having starved and then bombed everybody in the name of freedom, what Iraqis need now is stress counselling, to the tune of 4 million dollars.

Northern Iraq, 2003

The trouble with doing a 'needs assessment' for a particular agency is that you rarely get the opportunity to focus on the neediest. If NGOs prioritised according to need we would all have been in Burundi or the Democratic Republic of Congo, dealing with a catastrophe on the scale of the First World War. Instead we were in Iraq because that is where the politicians, the media and the public funds that followed wanted us to be.

NGOs are prostitutes: 'project' appeal matters just as much as country appeal. Children and trauma are sexy, mental hospitals and chronic schizophrenics are not. My boss wanted me to go north and follow up on an earlier US government emergency assessment. This had identified needs among the internally displaced people (IDPs) in the three governorates that made up Kurdistan.

The good side of this less than impartial means of selection is that sometimes quite forgotten groups of people are suddenly remembered. The north was awash with displaced Kurds: 850,000 or more. Some had been displaced more than five times, beginning in the seventies when Saddam burnt villages on the Iranian and Turkish borders and forcibly relocated Kurds into military-run collective towns. This was followed by the Arabisation campaigns that drove them out of Kirkuk, Mosul and Baghdad; the Anfal campaign of 1988 when Saddam used chemical weapons and probably killed 100,000; then by the First Gulf War when, betrayed by us, they fled to the mountains, and finally by the internal fights between different Kurdish factions in the mid-nineties. I'm exhausted simply writing the list. Approximately one in six people in Kurdistan lived in a displaced collective community of some kind, and a fifth of the population lived in destitution.

After the heat and chaos of Baghdad, I found the north beautiful. Five of us shared a staff house in Ankawa, the Assyrian suburb on the edge of Erbil where most international organisations had their offices. In the pasturelands beyond the town storks nested on telegraph poles, fields full of wheat stubble rolled away towards parched hills and flocks of sheep grazed in the white light. Driving through mountains to get from Erbil to Sulaymaniyah was like crossing a rough sea. Sharp-edged limestone ridges and softer folds of clays and shale all flowed towards the west. The rocks were the colour of sunset.

This was the one part of Iraq where the notion of 'shock and awe' was popular. In Sulaymaniyah multicoloured banners praised Bush and Blair for victory, and admonished the population to remember Saddam's Iraqi victims. Almost every

IDP family I visited had photos of George Bush stuck up on their walls and told me with delight how much they admired Tony Blair. But although Blair had trumpeted the human rights of the Kurds as an argument for getting rid of Saddam, 'liberation' had been a disaster for Kurdish IDPs. The UN, who had administered the area since 1991, had made plans to improve IDP living conditions. Funded by the 'Oil for Food' programme, they planned rehousing, water and sewage systems, income regeneration and improved schools. After the 2003 war, such plans were suspended indefinitely.

The Kurdish local authorities were determined that the IDPs should not be made too comfortable, as this would be a disincentive to going home. The obvious misery in which these IDPs currently lived justified the political demand for the right to return to contested oil-rich Kirkuk. But the authorities provided no assistance for going home. The UN was on its way out, the Coalition Provisional Authority had not arrived. Both had voiced concerns about destabilisation if large numbers of Kurds returned to Kirkuk and Mosul too rapidly. Everyone bickered about what should happen right now.

Hana, my translator, and I travelled around making site visits in two cars. One was back-up and security in case the other broke down. I became sick and spent my nights lying feverishly in stuffy hotel rooms, wondering whether it was worse living for three years in a barren wasteland in a boiling-hot tent provided by DFID, or spending fifteen years in the Police Machinery building. In the former the children got nosebleeds from the dust and their biggest fears were scorpions and snakes. In the latter families slept on concrete floors, twelve to a room, in the small cells where Saddam's victims had been tortured. Outside, raw sewage mixed with unexploded ordnance.

Such places were hardly conducive to good childcare. All the children I met told me they were regularly beaten, or burnt with hot knives or scorched with the ends of cigarettes. One father banged his son's head against a wall because the boy failed sixth grade. Another beat his six-year-old daughter whenever she went outside. A fifteen-year-old who collected garbage three hours a day for 2.50 dollars a month said quite simply, 'I would like to die.' He hated his life and saw no reason for living except that his parents needed him.

Meanwhile, the international and government agencies played their favourite game of blaming the victims. UNICEF's child protection officer, a well-dressed local woman, told me the families stayed in the shelters 'because they want an easy life'. She had never visited these places herself, but assured me that IDP children had access to all the same services as everyone else in town. The children told me that IDPs were turned away from the youth club, and stoned by town children on their way to school.

'They say things like, "We will put a pole up your ass",' one girl told me.

'People look at us like scum and it makes me feel like scum,' said a boy.

In the shelters, all of them were scared.

'The Islamic army said they were coming to butcher people; I did not sleep all night.'

'They have knives.'

'They have long beards . . . my cousin saw them.'

'This is inhuman and it has gone on for thirteen years. We are stuck between the earth and the sky and no one cares,' said the head man at the Police Machinery building.

'The trouble is people don't want to give up their comfortable lives in town,' the minister responsible for the displaced people in Erbil explained. 'Here they can earn money, go to school, they have TV and satellite dishes. They don't want to return to the relative hardship of the village.'

We were sitting in his large office. There were tasteful contemporary oils on the wall, hinting at historic Kurdish events. He was elegantly dressed, wore a bright-orange silk tie and spoke English with a thick German accent, a result of his ten-year struggle on his people's behalf as their political representative in Germany. I felt the familiar tide of anger rising.

'Have you visited the Police Machinery building?'

'Where is that?'

I explained how he could reach the IDP shelter closest to his office, and asked if he could recommend other sites to visit or give me some overall figures. He looked anxious and embarrassed. He went to his desk and flicked through papers. He called his assistant. They did not know.

Driving back to the agency house that Tuesday night, Hana caught a line of radio news and muttered that something had happened at the UN. The Canal Hotel in Baghdad, which housed the UN headquarters, had been bombed. I opened my email to discover that Sérgio Vieira de Mello, the Special Representative of the Secretary General in Iraq, was dead after being trapped in the rubble for hours. There was a flood of kind enquiries about myself. One of those Tuesday-night emails was from Jill Clark. She wanted some child mental health material, and asked after my health. The following day I discovered she was one of the twenty-two who had been killed. Death reaches out and touches us all. I was just lucky. What else can be said?

I kept the World Service on all the time. Kofi Annan said responsibility lay squarely with the occupying powers whose job it was to make us all secure. Donald Rumsfeld said no changes of any kind were needed. Japan said it was certainly not safe enough to send any of their elite troops to Iraq. Holbrooke called for the Coalition Provisional Authority to hand over to UN leadership.

Al-Qaeda circulated a letter claiming responsibility for the Canal Hotel bombing. Lengthy and articulate, the letter made it clear that it regarded the UN and the humanitarian enterprise as just as illegitimate as the US occupation. It accused the UN of an anti-Muslim bias and listed all the failures to act on its own Resolutions, from Kashmir to Srebrenica to Palestine to Chechnya. Innocent Iraqis killed in error could be sure of a place in heaven. Occupiers, humanitarians and collaborators were wished an 'unhappy trip to hell, damn them'.

None of this was surprising. The Coalition in its wisdom had dissolved the Iraqi Army and sent its mostly Sunni soldiers home without salaries but with their guns, as part of its programme of de-Baathification. There was no organised programme of demilitarisation or retraining, and most were now unemployed, angry and easily recruited by Al-Qaeda.

The UN presence downsized by 90 per cent. This was a message to the Coalition that it was not doing its job as an occupying power in providing security. The Coalition's official response was 'great disappointment and regret that the UN was withdrawing and a sincere hope that it would come back soon'. Posters went up in Mosul calling on locals to attack any foreigner, or any Iraqi who worked for them. Rumours circulated: there were plots to blow up the Kurdish parliament (false), Islamists had kidnapped a local politician (true), UN Habitat vehicles packed with explosives were circulating in the area (who knew? but I closed the office anyway and sent everyone home).

My agency offered voluntary evacuation. I really did not want to go. I did not want to sit around with bored NGO workers in Kuwait, eating buffalo wings and gossiping. I was still discovering hellish shelters where forgotten IDP children lived in squalor. I wanted to finish my report. I still had to arrange the medical evacuation of a nine-year-old who had lost both eyes and an arm, playing with one of the bright-yellow cluster bombs we had so carelessly dropped.

It was hard to make a judgement. It was not like the Balkans, where the risk was visible, audible and palpable. Everything in our quiet Ankawa suburb felt quite safe. The only difference was that there were fewer internationals and far more concrete bollards. Perhaps the former had been turned into the latter? I was reading too much *Harry Potter*.

I spent the evenings in the garden at a friend's house and swam in his tiny deserted pool. Then I sat on a swing seat among the pomegranate and fig trees and watched the light change, as flycatchers and martins gave way to bats. In the morning I walked to the office along quiet, sunlit suburban streets. There was the fruit seller pushing his wheeled trolley with figs and grapes covered in sacking. Here was a perfectly groomed small boy and girl sitting in front of their gate. The boy had the blond hair common in Assyrians and wore knee-length shorts. The girl wore a small pink straw hat. They looked like the cover of a *Janet and John* book and always said good morning in perfect English. At work, the drivers hung around in the kitchen drinking tea, bored because we didn't go to many places these days. Rouham was doing the finances, Nasir the morning radio check. Adrian was talking to Baghdad. It was quite impossible to imagine something cutting through the middle of this – glass shattering, limbs smashed, the fruit scattered, the children killed. I could not picture it. So it could not happen.

And if I did leave, when would I come back? Humanitarian workers could be kidnapped or blown up anywhere, not just in Iraq. Actions are as infectious as ideas. So either one had to find a way of working as best one could, or do something else. But most important, just as in Bosnia and Kosovo, I had made local friends and did not want to abandon them.

It didn't help that those who were supposed to advise us on security had their own agendas and conflicting views about what was going on. The CPA always told us 'the environment is permissive'. After a car bomb exploded in Erbil, Master Sergeant P. from the Civil-Military Operations Center told us that northern Iraq was 'calm and stable' but that 'the threat is out there and it's real'. Elegant Colonel Q., former Indian Army and now head of UN security, thought it was 'reasonably stable but very sensitive'. To be precise, Mosul (mortars and IEDs every day) was 'very sensitive', Kirkuk (three drums of TNT on a bridge) was 'quite sensitive', and Erbil (one car bomb) was 'slightly sensitive'. The colonel suggested digging a moat around Ankawa. It was not clear, even with added stakes and boiling oil to hand, how this would protect us as we drove around the three governorates. And how would it protect our neighbours?

The car bomb had been destined for a safe house where US Department of Defense men lived. It had blown up short of its target, killing one child, blinding another and injuring forty-five Iraqi adults. In the past I had worked in situations where the presence of internationals was sometimes protective.

Now I had to face the possibility that our presence was contaminating. We were like the plague. It was dangerous to get too close.

In the end an infected root canal decided me. I could not find a dentist I trusted in Erbil. After some days of lying on the sofa clutching a vodka bottle from the icebox to my cheek, Adrian told me to go to Amman and get it fixed. While I was in Jordan the Canal Hotel was bombed for a second time, as was a bus, as was another hotel and a pornographic cinema. In October ICRC headquarters were bombed, killing two of the staff. Thirty-five Iraqis were killed at the same time in coordinated attacks across the city.

By now almost all the NGOs had international staff working long-distance from Amman. As I was leaving one of the endless humanitarian coordination meetings one morning, a donor from OFDA came up to me. He wanted to thank my agency for the wonderful job we were doing in Iraq, 'flying the flag'. But he also wanted to make clear that there was absolutely no pressure from donors for staff to stay. Why, though, I wondered, were the big donors from the US and the UK not ordering compulsory evacuation, as they had done in Kosovo? It was now clearly more dangerous in Baghdad than it had ever been in Prishtina.

The answer was that this was a different political game. The evacuation of humanitarians from Kosovo signalled the intent to bomb. Humanitarians on the ground in Iraq signalled 'mission accomplished', the environment is 'permissive', reconstruction in Iraq is 'going well'. No one mentioned that 596 Iraqi civilians had died that June, 648 in July, 793 in August.

At the beginning of September, a close friend of mine in the Baghdad office of our agency wrote to headquarters:

I have reached the point where I cannot, in good conscience, continue working on a humanitarian project that I feel is more politically driven rather than being politically informed. I'll drop the jargon. I feel that we have lost a great degree of autonomy as a humanitarian NGO and

that we are actively contributing to the American occupation of Iraq which right now is doing more harm than
good.

She asked to be redeployed. It had taken me rather longer to
realise she was right. Not only had I failed to protest strongly enough against the war, but my attempts to address the
damage done were probably making it worse. In Bosnia I had
complained that the military had become relief workers and
had failed to do their job in ending an unjust war. Here in
Iraq relief workers like myself had been recruited into a failing
military occupation. There was no independent humanitarian space. If that was the case, I wanted to work in a country
where at least I could be on the side of the angels. I too asked
to be sent elsewhere.

Somali border, Ethiopia, April 2008

There's a new woman in the mother and baby group this week. Unlike the others in their multicoloured shifts and vivid knotted headscarves, she is dressed in plain brown cotton with a nun-like cowl, the full head covering that tightly frames the face and covers the upper half of the body. She sits staring solemnly at us all, holding her two-year-old daughter tightly on her lap. At first the child appears equally solemn and shy, but as the other children roll around and play with each other and the toys on the mat she starts wriggling to join in.

The mother releases her and lets her slide down onto the floor where the little girl immediately grabs a soft cloth-covered brick. To her complete delight, it makes a squeaky noise when squeezed. She keeps squeezing and shaking the toy and holding it up towards her mother, to join in the fun. But her mother just stares back, her face impassive, until the child turns away, lower lip trembling, at which point another mother leans forward and holds out her hand for the brick, beginning a game of catch.

After the group ends, Hoden explains that the woman, Ashraf, was raped by a neighbour last week. Hoden brought her to the group to try and make her feel better. This is a change from when I first got here. Then, the women told me of a woman who'd been gang-raped and made pregnant. She had been completely ostracised and committed suicide. These women in the group are being supportive. Hoden promises to persuade Ashraf to come to the clinic.

Ashraf is at the clinic the next day. However, she has brought her daughter with her and only wants to discuss the girl's cough. I go and get Hoden, who comes and takes the girl and persuades Ashraf to tell us about her own problems. Ashraf sits, head down, twisting a bracelet round and round her wrist, while whispering the details of what happened. Her husband is still in Somalia. Normally she lives with a sister and her daughter but her sister has gone to Addis. So she was alone and her daughter was sleeping when the man came in the middle of the night. He covered her mouth with his hand and forced himself on her. She closed her eyes but she cannot get the smells or the sensations out of her head. She cannot sleep or eat. She feels her life is over.

The man has been arrested and is in jail. But no one has done a formal medical examination or started her on anti-retrovirals to prevent HIV. Dr Asmamaw goes off to sort these things out and Dr Hassen continues to talk gently with the woman. She explains that the man's family have told everyone she wanted intercourse with him. Now people come up to her and say they heard the man was her boyfriend and that she invited him in. She wishes she was dead and prays to God to finish her off. It is only the presence of her daughter that stops her killing herself.

'The gossips are liars. You are the victim here, you have done nothing wrong,' Dr Hassen says firmly and quietly. 'God knows this, as do you and I and all the people that matter. We trust you and respect you and you can come to us at any time. We are here to support and protect you.'

The woman nods and for the first time looks up, saying, 'I thank God I am here. If I was in Mogadishu I would have been beaten and killed already.'

Non-believer that I am, I'm thanking some God for Dr Hassen's presence. It is not just his calm, gentle, unintrusive manner that's so encouraging. It's the fact that he is a Muslim himself, a doctor from this region who can speak with genuine authority. As a white foreign woman, I can sympathise and be angered by Ashraf's situation but do little to make her feel re-assured. We arrange with Hoden for the other women to keep her company overnight. UNHCR have arranged to transfer her tomorrow to the safety of the hospital in Jijiga and we will see her regularly to support her.

I endlessly puzzle over how to walk the line between respect for cultural practice and protecting those who are abused in the name of culture. Like so many humanitarians, when confront-ed with someone like Ashraf I swing between angry messianic zeal, my wish to uphold what I regard as universal human values, and embarrassment at my own arrogance. Some argue that we shouldn't be there at all, as we lack proper cultural un-derstanding and impose our own values. But this would mean

I could work only with white Western middle-class women, because age, gender, work and class – never mind ethnicity – all create their own microcultures within society. Dr Hassen laughs when I raise the issue with him.

'And where should Dr Asmamaw and I work? He is from an orthodox family, I am Muslim. We both come from Harar. There are more than eighty ethnic groups in Ethiopia. All my work is cross-cultural.'

In fact what I admire in both is that they are deeply rooted in their own cultures, having been born and brought up locally, but their education abroad allows them to see things from both inside and outside. They know how to be respectfully critical.

By now I have worked out that the simplest way is not to 'teach' on these subjects, but to have conversations where we share our personal opinions as to the best way of understanding or doing things. On one occasion I was talking with the mothers about child-rearing and I asked them if they would like to change anything about the way Somali children are raised. To my surprise, everyone brought up female genital mutilation, without prompting. In this area they remove the prepuce of the clitoris; or do the full works: the pharaonic, which is the removal of everything. Afterwards the girl is stitched up with a thorn to leave her almost impenetrable.

This is all done when the child is five years old or younger. The women gave me a host of reasons for it. All were based around the fear that if women enjoy sex they will be uncontrollable and go out and have a great time with one and all. There were a few contamination fears thrown in, such as the belief that the clitoris has the power to kill the first-born if the baby's head touches it. Others seemed to think that women are just downright dirty and smelly and this is a way to clean them up.

All the mothers deplore it, saying it hurts the girl and endangers her life because of the risk of HIV from reused instruments or clumsy surgery. It is now illegal in Ethiopia. But all except two of them had had their daughters circumcised. One told me it was essential, or her daughters would be seen as prostitutes and never get a husband. Another said her own mother had kidnapped all her daughters in order to perform the operation. The women also brought up a host of other cultural medical practices that are still used on small children. These included putting a sharp stick up the child's nose till it bleeds to cure sinusitis, or up their bum to cure worms, and cutting the uvula to prevent tonsillitis.

At least in these instances we could agree that modernity and Western medical practice had something better to offer.

When it comes to cultural understandings of distress I am not so sure. I have discovered that Somalis make clear distinctions between different kinds of sadness. There is *murugaysan*, sadness which responds to encouragement and does not require a doctor; *barooranaya*, the grief that comes with the loss of a loved one; and *quusasho*, severe deep sadness where a person is hopeless, suicidal, has no appetite, can't sleep, thinks all the time, has no energy, and speaks and walks very slowly. This person won't get better just with encouragement.

So the Somalis make the distinction between normal and abnormal sadness, a concept that has existed in Western medical thought since classical times. Aristotle described 'groundless despondency', where the misery was too intense and went on too long to be regarded as normal. In the seventeenth century, Robert Burton distinguished 'sorrow without any cause' from the 'transitory melancholy' from which 'no living man is free'. In the twentieth century, psychiatrists as different as Kraepelin and Freud made a similar distinction between pathological and non-pathological sadness.

Unfortunately, this common-sense approach was abandoned in the new symptom-based classifications that started in 1980. Now, unless you are bereaved, you can be diagnosed as having a 'depressive disorder' purely on the basis of having, for the past two weeks, experienced particular symptoms such as low mood, loss of interest in normal activities, insomnia, loss of appetite and loss of energy, regardless of any underlying causes or your current life circumstances. Perhaps it's not so surprising that increasing numbers of people in the West are diagnosed as 'depressed'. And this despite increasing levels of material comfort beyond the wildest dreams of most of the refugees here in the camp.

When such symptom checklists for depression are used in non-Western contexts the results can be problematic. A study of 160 women in Afghanistan, conducted in 1998 by Physicians for Human Rights after four years of Taliban rule, found that 97 per cent demonstrated evidence of major depression, and 86 per cent had significant anxiety symptoms. But what did that mean in a context where women were denied their most basic rights – to education, to work and to autonomy?

I was sent to Afghanistan in 2002 to assess mental health needs. I found one ward of the General Hospital in Kabul full of gaunt, sad-eyed women, some as young as seventeen, being treated with antidepressants and benzodiazepines for anxiety and depression. After thirty days or so they were sent home: to the confinement of purdah, unhappy marriages, bossy first wives or mothers-in-law, and the stressed and sometimes violent husbands that had made them ill in the first place. Everyone I talked to told me self-harm was a major problem among young girls. Opium, self-burning or shotguns were the common methods, all easily available, and no one was shy about discussing the reasons:

'Because they are forced to marry young, because they are unhappy, because most men in this area have more than one wife, because they are poor, because they cannot go out, because they don't have boy children, because they are always working, because there is no escape,' one doctor told me. I asked him what he did to help.

'What can we do? We inject water, a little placebo, we give phenobarbitone, and we send them home. This is the culture.'

If expressing psychological distress was a response to stressful living conditions, my worry was that a mental health programme that was not properly thought through could contribute to that quick transit from home to hospital and back again, helping husbands to define their unhappy wives as mentally unbalanced and in need of medication to calm them, thus legitimising seclusion and confinement when they themselves were the cause of the problem.

Purdah long predates the Taliban. It is a cultural tradition, albeit not one I wanted to reinforce. But there were changes I did think would help: programmes to educate, empower and provide employment for girls and women. But I knew these would have to come from the Afghan women themselves. They could not be imposed by outsiders.

And here on the Somali border neither Dr Hassen nor I want to train health workers to recognise 'mild, moderate and severe depressive disorder' on the basis of symptom checklists that can be administered in less than thirty minutes, taking no account of the culture, the life experiences or the meaning people give to their symptoms. What's striking is that even when people tell you they are sad much of the time, they are still coping: setting up small market stalls, building better shelters, getting their children to school. I have three volunteers working with me who are so friendly and energetic that it's easy to forget what they have been through and what it takes to get here.

They have all grown up knowing nothing but war. In the last few months their homes have been bombarded, their families injured or killed; they fled to avoid recruitment, then spent months in the hellhole of a registration camp before getting permission to live in this 'proper camp'. Now they are here in the dust and heat and the freezing nights. Last week when teaching on grief and loss, I asked one volunteer to draw a map of all the connections he had at home. A spider's web filled the page: school, work, family, friends, the village, the neighbourhood, the mosque. Then we took a new sheet to draw what he has here. He drew one line and two dots. He lives alone. There is one uncle. He did not know any of his neighbours when he arrived. But still he volunteers.

If people are *murugaysan*, we need to help them encourage each other, not tell them they are sick and hand out antidepressants. I have begun to believe that pathologising sadness is as big a problem as pathologising fear and traumatic responses.

8: HEALERS

Sierra Leone, 2003

In Sierra Leone the Krio word for sadness is 'poil-heart'. The literal translation is 'heavy-hearted'. A teenage girl explained it to me.

'Someone who is poil-heart is in a group but she's withdrawn from it, she suffers from something and does not pay attention. If she has a baby she is confused and can neglect the baby. When she or he imagines what happened, she cries all day and cannot sleep or eat. She tries to work but it's no good. When she is at school her concentration is poor.'

I met this girl with a group of teenagers in a half-rebuilt national school in the remote town of Kailahun, in Eastern Sierra Leone. Her country had been at war for the previous decade. It began when disaffected army officers and youths formed the Revolutionary United Front (RUF). Backed by the notorious Charles Taylor, President of neighbouring Liberia, the RUF had engaged in a 'war against poverty and injustice' that was financed by exporting diamonds and included raping women and cutting off arms and legs in order to terrorise the local population. Most of the health facilities and schools in the countryside were destroyed. Two million people, half the population, abandoned their homes.

Kailahun province was an RUF stronghold and had been under rebel control until they were disarmed in 2002. When I arrived in 2003, half the town were registered as ex-combatants. Many of the children in the group had spent the last few years in the bush fighting. The others had spent their war in refugee camps in neighbouring Guinea or Liberia, and had only just come home. Families lived in the ruins of their former houses. Life expectancy was less than thirty-five years. Almost every child in the group had lost at least one parent. Many lived Cinderella-like existences with foster-carers who made them work and beat them.

But none regarded feeling poil-heart, because of these experiences, as an 'illness'. It was a matter for friends or family, whose job it was to 'encourage' you.

The eloquent girl continued her explanation: 'If my friend was poil-heart I would go to her and talk with her to encourage her. If there was a football game I would encourage her to go. If lonely, I would ask her about her problems and exchange ideas. If she told me she could not sleep or was afraid, I would take her to my bed and share it. One should hear the problem, explain it and solve it.'

Nor did they confine themselves to individual solutions. The children were writing a play to educate people about the problems they faced. It was about a child who lived with foster-parents and was neglected, beaten, overworked and not allowed to go to school, while the foster-parents' natural child was treated beautifully. Later, this foster-child was married off early and died in childbirth. The drama was called *All Is Not Lost*.

Everyone recognised that there was also something called 'severe poil-heart'. The teenagers told me about a boy who was so severely poil-heart that the previous week he had gone down a well, stood in the water up to his neck and refused to come out because he did not want to live. The police had eventually talked him out. The children explained that in this case the boy was 'out-of-head', the evocative Krio word for madness, an all-encompassing term for anyone who acts strangely – equivalent to our 'crazy', 'loony' or 'bonkers'.

In fact, the Mende-speaking health workers with whom I worked in Kailahun had a more detailed way of classifying madness. The Mende word for 'out-of-head' was *kpowa* and it came in two quite distinct forms. People with *kpowa pom pom* were 'very, very crazy, they eat their own shit, talk rubbish, stop taking care of themselves so that their clothes turn to rags, stop washing'. Such people might go off into the bush by themselves, or behave strangely. They might be aggressive and abusive; but, significantly, they might recover. In a second form, called simply *kpowa*, they were still 'out-of-head' but it came and went, mostly in keeping with the cycles of the moon. This *kpowa* had two states: in one, the person might wear strange clothes or rip them all off and run naked in the street, or steal and act without shame. They might talk and talk without stopping, or cry all the time, or be aggressive, angry and abusive. In the other state they might stay silent, sitting without speaking or moving for long periods. Or they might appear completely well for a time, but unlike *kpowa pom pom*, this *kpowa* was lifelong.

So Mende people recognised the two forms of madness that Emil Kraepelin had identified at the beginning of the twentieth century and that I had learnt about in my training at the Allinton. There was a lifelong relapsing illness related to mood, that could either disinhibit or silence you; and another in which bizarre speech and behaviour and self-neglect were the predominant features. Bipolar disorder and schizophrenia, or *kpowa* and *kpowa pom pom* – take your pick.

When it came to causes, I was on less familiar ground. Everyone believed that both witchcraft and malign spirits (djinns) in the trees, water and rocks could trigger either illness. However, *kpowa* might also result from someone being severely poil-heart, while *kpowa pom pom* could be caused by jealousy in your family, or by wrongdoing. And both illnesses could be 'in the blood', that is, inherited.

Were these multiple explanations so very different from our own? At home, researchers have known for years that upsetting life events and troubled relationships can trigger episodes of severe mental illness and that genetic inheritance plays a role. We also know that sending young schizophrenics back into families who are overly emotional and critical can result in relapse. Were our causative 'biopsychosocial' models so different from those of the language of blood, bewitchment, jealousy and complex family relationships through which the people in Kailahun constructed their problems?

I was discussing sadness and madness in Kailahun because I wanted to discover how people defined their problems and what kind of help they needed. My agency was already rebuilding the local hospital and training the local district medical officer in emergency surgery and obstetrics. They were also reconstructing primary health care centres across the province, and training staff. After I left Iraq, they sent me there to find out if more could be done in mental health. There was one run-down psychiatric hospital in the capital city, Freetown, where most of the patients were chained to their beds and dependent on relatives – if they had any – for food. A WHO report had recommended decentralising mental health services to local communities. But I had learnt by now that if I wanted to avoid medicalising distress I had to ask the people themselves what they saw as mental health problems and where they went for help. I started in Freetown, with Sierra Leone's single psychiatrist.

Dr Nahim was a remarkable man. He had trained at the Maudsley Hospital in Britain and, unlike so many of his contemporaries, decided to return home in 1980. Since then he had been trying to address the needs of four million people with the help of two psychiatric nurses. Young doctors did not want to do psychiatry: 'Because no one likes the subject, because it does not pay much, because the patients are all poor, they don't have families and they don't come back,' he told me gloomily.

Dr Nahim had made clear how aggravating he found international NGOs the moment I staggered into his office, in the crowded heart of the city. I say 'staggered' because I had just put my back out and so had to stand propped against the wall, while listening to him telling me about the problems people like me caused when we failed to understand that *he* was the government's focal point and responsible for the ministry strategy for mental health in Sierra Leone.

His aggravation was completely justified. Freetown was awash with international psychosocial programmes of various kinds, offering counselling to amputees and child soldiers, but few of them had asked him what he actually needed. Recently he had found an Islamic foundation to help him renovate the hospital and train more nurses. I slid into junior doctor mode – easy to do, as he reminded me of my professors at the Allinton. I assured him we always collaborated with government authorities and followed government strategy. That was why I was here, to learn what it was. I explained our ideas for community-based services in Kailahun. There was a slight warming. Was this because he liked the idea, or was it because I was going a long way away? I was not entirely clear. Could he recommend who else I should talk to?

'Traditional healers,' Dr Nahim told me caustically. 'Of course there *is* a mental health system in this country. Traditional healers provide all the care in remote areas. You must work with them.'

He wrote me a formal note saying that I was working under his authority and supervision. He told me I was welcome to consult him and refer to him at any time. He would try and visit when he had time.

That was that.

After the meeting I lay flat on my back on the empty veranda of the agency house. I watched a small bird with a bright-orange head hop about the glossy, wet mass of palms and shrubs that stretched down to a wide lagoon. Beyond that were more palms, a line of shacks along the beach and then the surf. Egrets commuted home in low-flying formation, the sun turning their white backs mauve. I was in agony but I didn't care. I was just delighted I had official permission to stay. I had fallen completely in love with Sierra Leone. I couldn't get over the brightness and immodesty of the women's clothing: short skirts and skimpy tops, or longer ones wrapped tightly to reveal incredibly sexy figures of all sizes.

I loved everything: the crowds swirling in the streets making it impossible to drive; the hand-painted signs on every shop, offering things like 'self sufficiency, efficiency and godliness' along with a haircut; the crumbling, mouldy, stone or wooden villas that lined the cobbled roads running along the low hills around the bay; the strangely familiar street names like Liverpool Crescent, Angus Road or Sir Samuel Drive; the schoolchildren walking home in immaculate, rather British-looking uniforms – neat shirts, shorts or pinafore dresses. After the parched landscapes and hidden terrors of Iraq, Sierra Leone felt like paradise.

In the winter of 2003 it still took fourteen hours by road to get from Freetown to Kailahun. After Kenema, where we stopped the night, 'road' was no longer an accurate description. Think ribbon of mud through dense forest. Kailahun must once have been a substantial town. Elegant stone buildings edged the marketplace. The paramount chief's house was three storeys tall with windows that would have graced a Georgian villa in London. But it was pockmarked, gutted and empty. Most people now lived in mud and plaster one-room huts roofed with plastic, either clustered near the stream that ran through the centre of the town, or spreading out along the main road. My agency had patched up the local bank. I was given a small cell-like office with bed, chair and table, mosquito net and fan. We ate and worked together in the cool, open central room.

Our neighbour on one side was a small, newly built evangelical chapel, from which noisy singing and clapping issued forth most of the day and night. 'This is one of our main forms of psychotherapy,' Dr Nahim had told me. 'Muslims and Christians alike attend. They get reborn and feel much better.' On our other side stood the four-towered mosque, freshly plastered and repainted by the Pakistani battalion from UNAMSIL (the UN Mission in Sierra Leone). The mainly Mende population of Kailahun was at least 60 per cent Muslim, but there was no religious animosity. At the start of almost every meeting, large or small, including the hospital management ones, everyone sat with palms turned up and open while a Muslim blessing was followed by the Lord's Prayer.

Kailahun had two traditional healers, or *Karra Mokos*, as they were called in Krio. I found Sheku Bangura sitting on the floor in his mud hut on the edge of the town. He was a Muslim religious healer, *Kaar Moi Sia* in Mende. His father had been the *Kaar Moi Sia* before him and sent him to Guinea to be apprenticed when he was six years old. He had studied and worked for twenty-five years with a very famous *Kaar Moi Sia* before returning to Kailahun.

Sheku Bangura told me he treated almost everything: impotence, headaches, fever and all forms of being 'out-of-head'. The treatments were complex and lengthy. Recently he had treated a young man who had begun dancing and shouting immediately after having a fever. First he talked at length with the family, and then he consulted the spirits, who could be seen in a special shaving mirror. They guided him as to diagnosis and treatment. He then wrote a special prayer in special ink on a special board. It had to be written out two thousand times. Each time the board was full, he washed off the ink into a bowl and saved it. This process took two days, after which the inky drink was given to the young man to take every day for two weeks. He was literally drinking the word of God. And he recovered.

'The most important thing is the Book,' Bangura told me, holding out his large, old and battered Koran for me to see. Although on some occasions the spirits would guide him to use particular herbs to make infusions, which should be inhaled or drunk. Some problems were simple. Fear could be treated by writing a prayer on the door to prevent the devil from entering. Or if my husband went off to Freetown and I wanted him back, Bangura would give me a special paper with his name on it, wrapped in white cotton. If I hung this above the fire, my husband would feel uncomfortable and come home. As we talked, he kept glancing at the mirror lying at his feet. It had a pattern traced upon it. He sprayed it with some liquid.

'The spirits are asking who you are and why you are here.' He smiled at me: 'I have told them you are a friend and they should go away.'

I felt touched and honoured. Here was an elderly man who had spent far longer than I in the training and practice of his profession, and was now explaining its intricacies to this completely strange white Western woman who had turned up unannounced at his door. I tried to imagine how Sheku Bangura would have been received if he'd arrived unannounced at the Allinton and asked to discuss mental disorders and their treatments with one of the consultants. It did not bear thinking about. I asked him if he was ever unsuccessful. Not often, he said, although there were cases where the mental disorder came directly from Almighty God and could not be removed. Nor could he use treatments to cause harm. He had not been taught how to do this. His job was to treat the ill-effects of harm caused by others. 'Suppose you have a garden,' he explained. 'Someone steals something from it so you go to the herbalist and get him to make something that makes the thief go off his head. So the thief may come to me for help to recover.'

Mr Ibrahim, the local herbalist, or *Haegbah Haaleey Blaa Sia* as such a person is called in Mende, also assured me he never used treatments to cause harm. Unlike Sheku Bangura he had not inherited his position, and had had no formal training. But one night twenty years ago he had had a dream in which he'd been offered books and leaves and told to become a teacher and healer. In the morning he woke to find the Book and leaves were there. He converted to Islam and Almighty God had taught him which leaves worked for which patients, through dreams. In one dream he had been instructed that a particular tree would cure people with mental illnesses.

'My treatments are based more on leaves, and the *Kaar Moi Sia* uses the Book. Although I may sometimes use the Book and he may use leaves,' Mr Ibrahim explained. He had only recently returned from Guinea where he'd been living as a refugee. Now he was seeing at least twenty adults and perhaps ten children a week. The children's problems were numerous: for example, if witches captured them at night it would stop them sleeping and cause them to lose weight; or they might reject the breast; or they might still have a fever after being in hospital; or one child might shake and talk senselessly. All of these problems could be treated with leaves in various ways. He invited me to come and meet one of his patients. The young man had been with him for a week and was just finishing his treatment.

We walked down the hill behind his house to a simple shelter made of tarpaulin stretched over wood. Outside, a large iron pot containing water and leaves boiled on a fire. Inside, a young man named Thomas was sitting on the ground with an old blanket round his shoulders, waiting. Mr Ibrahim took the pot off the fire and put some of the liquid in a jug. When it had cooled a bit, he took some soap and used the liquid to wash the man's head. Then he rinsed it and placed the still-steaming pot on the ground between the man's legs, pushing his head down towards the vapour and telling him to inhale, while pulling the blanket over him. 'We do this twice a day,' Ibrahim explained. A week ago the man had abandoned his family and gone to live in a ruined house on the edge of the town. He made small piles of sticks, cried, spoke rubbish in answer to any questions and shouted accusations at all who came near. So his family had brought him to Mr Ibrahim, who had tied him to a log so he could be treated.

Thomas was not tied down any more. He cooperated with the treatment and afterwards was happy to talk to me. It was not the first time he'd been sick. In the mid-nineties he had been a trader in a neighbouring village but had fled to Guinea. When he got there he started believing all his friends and family intended to harm him. He couldn't sleep and destroyed his possessions, so his family had taken him to a herbalist who had cured him using the same treatment.

Then he got married and had a small son. They had come back to the village where his father lived with his wives. Thomas had started another small business that was going well until he became ill again. He was afraid of his friends. He could not pay attention. He felt angry and irritable and would argue and become aggressive with people. He was sure he was being poisoned so he would only eat food prepared by his wife. He was unable to sleep for more than a few moments and had palpitations. Finally the fear was so great that he moved into the ruined house. He'd been frightened to come to Mr Ibrahim, but now he was glad his family had captured him and brought him here. After a week of treatment he felt completely well.

It was impressive. But as I listened I could not resist trying to fit the story into my own diagnostic frameworks. A little voice in my head was murmuring: 'Acute paranoid psychotic episodes? Or perhaps hypomanic? No doubt the immediate precipitant was stress: first through leaving home in the war and then on return. The treatment works because he's removed from the stress and the herbs are sedative . . . or perhaps they have an antipsychotic component . . . Perhaps there's an underlying condition?'

'Were you ill as a child?' I asked.

'Actually I did have problems. I went to school but it was difficult to study because I saw something evil coming. It is hard to explain. My mother had me treated by a herbalist and it stopped.'

Mr Ibrahim's explanation was completely different. Thomas's last attack of illness was due to a spell. Someone had recognised his business skills and had bewitched him out of jealousy. Thomas's father had many wives and Thomas had at least five older stepbrothers, who would ask him for money. 'If you don't give the money they are offended. This is a common problem for small brothers,' Thomas explained. He agreed with Mr Ibrahim. He planned to move with his wife and son into Kailahun town to be nearer his mother's relatives. Ibrahim assured him that the illness would not return. Thomas trusted that God would protect him.

There was a conventional health system in Kailahun, headed by Dr H., a dynamic district health officer who had decided to train the rebel combatant 'medics' who had been running the clinics during the fighting as vaccinators. In this way he had pushed vaccination coverage up from o to 55 per cent in a couple of years. There was also Dr Y., the district medical officer, who ran the half-destroyed district hospital that my agency was rebuilding. And across the province a network of dispensers, midwives and community health officers (CHOs) worked out of small health posts and dispensaries in the remote rural areas. In many ways these were the most impressive of all the healers I met.

Isaac was one such community health officer who had come back to the area six months previously. He had a small house and a bright, freshly painted government health post from which he took care of the health needs of thirty-eight thousand people with the help of one midwife. The ministry had yet to pay either of their salaries. But Isaac loved the work. Community health officers trained for three years at a college in nearby Bo. They were the heart of the primary health care system in the country. Isaac knew much more than me about the diagnosis, treatment and prevention of malaria, Lassa fever and tuberculosis. I watched him do a three-hour clinic where he addressed sensibly a range of ills from vaginal discharge to liver disease.

In between times he put a very dehydrated elderly lady with fever on a drip, and saved a baby in acute respiratory distress by hijacking a food distribution truck as an ambulance, and sending him to Kailahun. 'The baby was ill for days but the mother went to the false doctor. She only came today because he was not getting better,' Isaac complained to me. 'So I only get to see people when it is almost too late.'

By 'false doctor' Isaac meant a traditional healer. However, if a relative was mentally ill, Isaac told me, he too would send them to a traditional healer first. Almost all his government health-worker colleagues felt the same: Kissy Hospital in Freetown was too far away and too frightening to contemplate. 'Doctors cannot treat mental illness,' I was told repeatedly. 'They do not know how . . . They don't understand it and they don't have the power to treat sickness caused by witchcraft or djinns.'

As my health-worker colleagues saw it, Western doctors

took an entirely biological, mechanistic approach to mental illness. They gave pills and did nothing to treat the underlying complex web of causes including family jealousies and the upsets in the physical and spiritual worlds. Traditional healers took a much more holistic approach. This was similar to the arguments my friends made back in Britain when they took themselves to various complementary therapists, be it acupuncture, homeopathy or herbal medicine. Ordinary doctors just wrote a prescription and paid no attention to the whole person.

The district medical officer, Dr Y., had no patience with such views. He often came round to our house to watch television after work. We would sit on our colonnaded balcony off the main room and watch the sun set over the tin roofs of the marketplace. When I told him I was considering how to collaborate with the traditional healers, he became quite upset. 'People are dying and mutilated because of their care.' He reminded me of Josephina, a beautiful fourteen-year-old girl who had fallen and fractured both legs and gone to a local bone-setter. Infection and gangrene had set in and the legs could not be saved, so he and our Ethiopian surgeon, Dr T., had amputated both. He could show me many such cases, and anyway it was government policy to stop people going to these 'false doctors'.

Outside the main hospital in Bo there was a large hand-painted poster. It showed a woman in a bright-red dress and a child with stick-like limbs and a swollen stomach. The child was being offered an evil-looking black drink by a man waving a horsehair fly-whisk. He was dressed in a loincloth with arm and wrist bracelets and an odd little pixie hat. In front of him was a skull and crossbones. But the woman was waving him away and had turned towards a friendly nurse in Western dress, complete with bib and small hat, sitting at a desk with a stethoscope. The nurse pointed to another building adorned with the word 'hospital'. 'Kam Ospitu en pay Smal Korpo for you wel bodi', said the slogan. Even I could understand the message.

I thought banning would simply drive harmful practices underground. I told him about Isaac's healer friend Emmanuel, who had brought his own son to the clinic that afternoon after the child had fallen and grazed his head. Like Ibrahim and Sheku Bangura, he was modestly dressed in plain trousers and shirt. There was no pixie hat or fly-whisk in sight. He told me of two patients he had treated in the last month with the holy ink drink and herbal infusions: a man who had started beating his wife after a bad dream, and a woman who kept undressing herself in the marketplace. Apparently the man was now good to his wife, and the woman was a model mum, breast-feeding her baby.

Emmanuel had begged us to accompany him on a home visit to another patient. We found a rake-thin eighteen-year-old girl lying on a bed in a darkened hut. She had a puffy face, swollen belly, and grossly swollen ankles that pitted deeply when I pressed my thumbs into them. She had been like this for a month and ill for a year before that, after a miscarriage. Her kidneys were tender. It did not look like a mental illness to me. Emmanuel thought it was 'worms'. He had been treating her for a week but there had been no improvement.

'The thing is,' I explained, after examining her, 'whether she has worms or not, Isaac and I think there may be something wrong with her kidneys. Do you know what they are?' He shook his head. 'Well, they're a bit like drains in your body. All the water that you drink goes through them and they clean out the stuff you don't need. But they can get damaged and then they won't work properly, and so all the water goes into other parts of her body, here and here' – I touched her ankle and face. 'We need to get her kidneys working again or she will become much, much sicker.' I could not imagine any of my physiology lecturers being at all comfortable with this gross oversimplification of renal function, but hoped it would do for now.

'Of course, you are the doctor and this is your case, but with your permission we would like to send her to the hospital for some tests. If we are wrong she can come back to you.'

'We have been to the hospital!' the woman's sister said. 'It was no good, they did not help.'

'You mean the pharmacy,' Isaac cut in. 'You have been to the pharmacy and they gave you medicine.' The woman nodded, looking cross.

'The local pharmacies are another big problem, they just give patients anything and don't send them to me,' Isaac said, addressing me.

He turned back to the family: 'Look, the hospital is different. They are ex-pats, they are good doctors, they are free, and they will help your sister.'

Emmanuel was delighted. It struck me that his eagerness to show me the case was actually a face-saving way of getting help with a problem he couldn't solve.

'If Isaac and Emmanuel collaborated they might be able to change bad practice.'

Dr Y. shook his head. 'Good practice on *our* part is the best advertisement. People will see that we offer better medicine than the alternatives.'

I didn't think it was that simple with the mentally ill. Some of their patients did recover, but I could hardly claim 100 per cent success for Western psychiatry.

Humanitarians, the third group of healers, were here in full force just as we had been in the Balkans and Iraq. There were community rehabilitation programmes providing training in tailoring, carpentry and hairdressing; educational support NGOs were setting up schools and children's clubs; there were child protection and gender-based violence projects, and at least two separate trauma counselling programmes. In health, my own agency supported primary health care and surgery, while another medical agency had set up a field hospital providing obstetrics, medicine and paediatrics. The idea was that when the district hospital was complete, both agencies would work together providing training and support until the local staff could work on their own.

So was I needed? Dr H. suggested there was an easy way to

find out. I was working with the government primary health care staff. He would announce my availability to treat mental health problems on the radio and we would see who turned up. Within ten days I had accumulated a caseload of some twenty-five patients with severe mental illnesses. Whenever I went to an outlying clinic I found more waiting for me even though I hadn't told anyone I was coming. The majority of them were psychotic. Many had been sick for years and had already been to traditional healers at some point, but it hadn't worked. Many were ex-combatants, self-medicating with palm wine and marijuana.

Not all. Paula, a paediatrician at the field hospital, wanted me to see Rosina, a ten-year-old girl who was unable to walk properly. Paula could find no organic cause. The weakness had begun a week earlier after Rosina was raped by a neighbour who had found her alone at home. Her mother noticed her walking oddly when she returned and took her to the hospital. Paula put the child on a cocktail of antiretrovirals to prevent HIV, but staff could not get her out of bed. When I came to visit, Rosina was walking very slowly and painfully with crutches, her legs held rigid and wide apart. She complained that her arms hurt. She had repeated nightmares about the rape. She was terrified because she knew her neighbour was not in jail, but free pending a court appearance. Wonky legs at least kept her safe in hospital.

As a trainee psychiatrist in England, I had once been given a patient that no one else wanted: a woman on a medical ward who had lost the use of her lower limbs after being dismissed from work. The physicians had told her there was nothing wrong. The nurses hated her. They saw her ills as imaginary and time-consuming when they had other 'genuinely' sick people to care for. They would try to trick her into walking by ignoring her bell when she rang for help to go to the toilet.

'If she really wants to walk, she will walk,' one of them said. The woman wet her bed, causing more aggravation. Certainly, the symptoms were fascinatingly inconsistent with any known organic pathologies. She had full movement and sensation in her feet, but nothing in her leaden legs.

This was what used to be called 'hysterical paralysis' and is now called 'conversion disorder'. In simple terms, an unresolvable psychological conflict or inescapable stress is 'converted' into a physical symptom. Such symptoms tend not to improve in the face of proof that there's nothing wrong – because, of course, there is. What sometimes works is accepting the language in which the person is signalling distress and offering treatment in the same tongue. The woman's paralysis responded well to physiotherapy and graded swimming exercises in the hospital pool. As she recovered the use of her limbs, she started talking to me about the people who had 'stabbed her in the back' at work.

I took the same approach with Rosina. We talked about her aches and pains and how brave and strong she was, and how the bruises inside and out would take time to heal. I explained that in order to help her walk again, she would need to do very gentle exercises, every day. Eventually the pain would lessen and she would get stronger. We did some gentle walking and arm raises that first afternoon and I asked the nursing staff to encourage her with small exercises every day. By the second visit she had begun walking without assistance, so we all clapped and cheered.

Then we started on the nightmares. I asked Rosina: if she could change just one thing in the frightening dream to make it safer, what would that be?

'I would dream that my dog came in and barked at the man and scared him and then he ran away before he did anything.'

'So tonight, before you fall asleep, just tell yourself that good-dream story, picture the whole thing in your head like a movie, and you will dream that one instead.'

I sounded much more confident than I felt. Rosina was distracted and not paying full attention, and dream-scripting like this usually takes practice. I kept visiting. We started doing *Monty Python*-style 'silly' walks and playing with puppets. Then one afternoon Rosina suddenly announced, out of the blue, that the previous night she had dreamt that her dog had bitten the man and he ran away. She thought it was magic. I told her that if it was magic, it was her doing, and she should keep practising it. Rosina's case reminded me again how much my own capacity to heal rested on the same kind of 'magical' authority, and the same power to suggest, as the *Karra Mokos* possessed.

Kailahun began to feel like home. In the evening I would sit on the balcony and play with our mother cat and her kittens. Salonians thought ex-pats were out-of-head about pets; they usually put cats in the pot, to eat. Ours kept me sane. It was almost Christmas. Small boys banged sticks, while straw-covered demons danced and jumped around in your compound until you paid them to go away. It was impossible to sleep at night with a brass band practising on one side, loud prayers and music on the other, and all the usual chatter from the market area. And just when I finally drifted off, the call to prayer from the mosque next door would jerk me awake at five.

So I started running. It was a forty-minute jog along a hilly dirt road past the school and the Catholic church, through the bird-filled forest to the river. I was never lonely. Small children would shout 'Hey Pumoy!' ('white person' in Mende) and I would shout 'Hey Nulele!' ('black person'). Others would run after me, laughing, to slap my hands. I had two personal trainers: Dr T., who simply cruised up and down the hills as if they were not there, then patiently jogged on the spot as he waited for me to catch up. The other was a six-year-old girl in flip-flops carrying a water bottle, who would regularly run with me the whole way without taking breath. Then I would walk across the market area to the office or the field hospital to see patients.

One day Mr Ibrahim asked me to come and see Peter, a new patient who had just arrived. He was around twenty and had been ill for a few years: there were repeated episodes when he started talking rubbish and then ran out of the house. The family had a real struggle tying him up and he'd got a few cuts and bruises, but after two herbal treatments he was calmer. Mr Ibrahim explained that he had divined the problem through the 'Book' and talking to the family. Peter had witnessed a violent fight between two men when he was a refugee in Guinea. One of the men in the fight had bewitched him to stop him making trouble. That spell had caused these episodes.

Peter was chained by one leg to a log, under the small thatched roof. He sat rigid, propping himself upright, uncomfortably twisted. As I walked up he said in clear English, 'Thanks be to God.' Then he turned his head away and refused to speak. He kept spitting quantities of saliva. His eyes were bloodshot and his skin hot and dry. A fly grazed undisturbed on a cut on his abdomen. His food was uneaten. I wondered if he was catatonic, but didn't feel able to interfere. He was not my patient, and this was what the family wanted. I told Mr Ibrahim I could bring disinfectant for the cuts, and he agreed.

I returned with the disinfectant and with Dr T. that evening. Mr Ibrahim was not there but Peter's father was visiting his son. Dr T. had treated the father's infected leg wound in the past, so he was really pleased to see us. He told us more about the strange episodes.

They were always the same: Peter would suddenly go rigid and blank; although his eyes were open and he was not sleeping, you could not communicate with him. He would spit repeatedly. Sometimes he would shout, other times he would actually run out of the house but he wouldn't know where he was. If you tried to interfere he would become very violent. Then after a short while he would recover and be himself again, with no memory of what had happened. Listening to the story I suddenly thought: complex partial seizures, not psychosis, perhaps the boy has a form of epilepsy? It would make sense of his state earlier that day.

There was more. The father was unhappy with the treatment that his son was getting. I asked why he had brought him here rather than to us, given that he'd been happy with Dr T.'s treatment of his own leg.

'I know, I know, but my wife was crying and insisted, but now today he has a terrible burn between his legs.' Peter was now unchained, moaning softly and lying back on the straw mat, covered with a blanket which, on this occasion, I pulled back. I wished I'd done so before. The boy had deep, ugly third-degree burns on both inner thighs. He lay there uncomplaining while we examined him. Dr T. looked horrified.

'Can you fix this?' I asked.

'Of course,' he said, 'but not here, he needs a graft.'

'How much are you paying Mr Ibrahim?' I asked the father.

'Well, it depends if he is successful, but maybe fifty thousand leones.'

Mr Ibrahim arrived. He too looked at the burn. He shook his head, clucking. 'It's terrible. The children did the treatment yesterday and they did not take care with the pot.'

'Mr Ibrahim, I know you are in the middle of a treatment and that's important, but this burn is very bad. Perhaps you would let us take him to the field hospital to get the burn treated, and then if he still needs your help we could bring him back. I could reimburse you now for your trouble so far. Would twenty thousand leones be all right?'

Mr Ibrahim nodded happily. Just like Emmanuel, he seemed relieved to have a problem beyond his care off his hands without losing face. I hoped so, because I knew that any mental health programme we created here would depend on his goodwill. It was my first experience of buying a patient.

Dr T., the father and I lifted Peter into the vehicle. He lay propped in his father's lap, and we drove him over to the ward. We started him on an anti-epileptic drug and Dr T. treated the wound over the following days. By the end of the week he was transformed. Mr Ibrahim came to visit and I explained my thoughts about epilepsy, how in my own country it had in the past been treated as a form of madness, but was actually disordered electrical activity in the brain. He was fascinated.

'If I get the funding to come back, perhaps we could do some joint clinics where we learn from each other?'

He agreed.

But not all patients were so lucky. A few nights later the ambulance brought in a woman who had been in obstructed labour for three days in a remote village. She had been treated by a local healer, with no effect. Dr Y. was away and Dr T. asked me to assist in theatre.

When we got there the woman was already in the small pre-op room with no palpable blood pressure and two nurses trying to find veins. Dr T. inserted a gloved hand into her vagina and shook his head.

'Gas gangrene.' He made me feel the edge of the womb: spongy and bubbly from the gas and the hard edge of the baby's collarbone that told him it was a shoulder presentation.

'Gram-negative septicaemia and almost certainly multiple organ failure already. It is very bad, very bad. But we must get the baby out and do the best we can.' The nurses had got a nasogastric tube in and were drawing up what looked like coffee granules. They were shaking their heads and muttering about 'false doctors' and the herbal remedies the woman had been taking for the last two days. Even with the nasogastric tube in and Dr T. doing a cut down on her ankle to get a drip in, the woman was chatting away to me in Mende, in a slightly confused manner. The nurses translated bits. She was in her mid-twenties at most. She had already given birth to six children. Three had died.

'And I don't want any more!' she said emphatically.

The nurses succeeded in getting another drip into her arm and prepared the theatre. For theatre, think tiny concrete room with a suction machine, oxygen for the patient, and lit by generator-powered lamps. The scrub nurse had come in so Dr T. asked me to help Luke, the anaesthetist. Sterile gowns were in very short supply, and that way I wouldn't need one. Meanwhile, I sat at the woman's head, holding her hand as she talked feverishly. I knew these might be the last conscious moments of her life; someone had to hold her hand and talk comfortingly, even if she could not understand a word I was saying. Voice and expression must count for something.

We pushed her into theatre while Dr T. and the nurse scrubbed up. Luke was looking at the woman's terrible teeth pointing in every direction. He took her down with ketamine and got an endotracheal tube inserted with amazing speed. Dr T. was still worried about air entry and asked me to check it, while Luke ventilated her with one hand and fiddled with the drip with the other. As I listened to the air filling her lungs, I suddenly heard the heart stop. Actually, I don't know how to describe the sensation of hearing a silence. And for a few seconds I refused to believe it, pushing the stethoscope around her chest wall: silence.

'Heart's stopped,' I said.

'Are you sure?'

'I am sure!' I replied, starting to push with both hands.

Dr T. already had the abdomen open, but put the knife down and came round and took over, while Luke put adrenalin in the drip. We took turns for seven minutes, and after injecting adrenalin directly into the heart, it restarted. She had been ventilated throughout, so perhaps it would be all right. Dr T. went back to work, asking me to sit with the stethoscope strapped to the chest wall. So I listened to her heart for the next hour: the beat strengthened and quickened with the operation, as Dr T. removed the very dead baby and then the womb itself. Then it began to fall away again as he closed her up. She arrested again just after he finished, and he was now listening himself. This time we got her heart pumping again in two minutes, but two hours after the end of the operation, during which time Dr T. had successfully removed a retained placenta from another woman, we were still giving her oxygen; she showed no signs of recovering consciousness. She died an hour later. There was no more to be done.

Kailahun, Sierra Leone, 2004

It didn't end there. I went home and wrote reports and submitted proposals, and finally a donor gave us money to train a community health officer who would run mental health clinics at the hospital and outlying health centres.

In the autumn of 2004 I returned to Sierra Leone to set up the mental nealth programme. Kailahun was bigger and noisier. There were more people in the town, more goods in the market, more metal roofs, more young men on motorbikes and far fewer trees on my old running route to the river. Dr Y. gave me an office in the newly refurbished district hospital and I found a good translator: Dan. Finding a trainee was more difficult. I was suffering from Dr Nahim's problem. Despite the offer of an NGO salary, no one wanted to work in a remote area with patients that no one liked and thought were bewitched.

'If you do that work they will think you are out-of-head as well,' one of our nurses said. The stigma of mental illness was infectious, but the patients turned up anyway.

'One for you, Doctor Lynne,' a nurse called out, while I was fighting with a new photocopier. I looked over the balcony at a skinny young woman in a torn green dress, shouting and gesticulating in the street. The nurses were all laughing at her. To my surprise she accepted my invitation to come up, sat herself down heavily on the office sofa, then started peeling oranges and stuffing them into her mouth. Her words poured out:

'My name is Annie. I am a doctor from London. I have a son in London, he treats mad people. You can find out if I am lying you can find out . . . my name is around the world, I have worked all over when you hear about Sierra Rutile and Sulongo, I did all criminology, I did police, I did CID, I worked as military police, after an MP, I was a cadet, I went upriver with Marda Bio, I told him I am born again and he told me he was Jesus . . .'

Without prompting, Dan was simultaneously translating in the first person, giving me all the incoherence as it came, as well as explaining her references to diamond mines and one of Sierra Leone's military presidents. She continued loud, fast, jumping from one idea to another. Sometimes the only connection between sentences was that they contained words with similar sounds. Faced with someone this agitated, I always let them talk and listen intently. They can see I am not dismissing them, and I can learn what's bothering them and the way their thoughts are working. Annie clearly had grandiose ideas, as she was not a doctor in London, not world-famous, nor was she in control of any of the diamond mines, as far as I could see. Finally, after about fifteen minutes she wound down and sat there slightly breathless, staring at me wide-eyed.

'How do you feel right now, Annie?'

'I don't feel well. When I am on the street people provoke me and stone me and say I am crazy. See, I am wounded all over.' She pointed to the visible cuts and bruises on her legs and arms; some were bleeding, fresh and dirty. Her clothes had ash and mud on them and were torn. 'See, my hair, its cut like a man's!' It was shaved close to her head. This, in a society where women either have complex plaits or buy elaborate wigs ready-braided.

'Annie – may I call you Annie?'

'Call me dirt bag.'

'I'm sorry?'

'Call me dustbin, everyone does.'

She was close to tears. She told us she had been in the psychiatric hospital in Guinea 'because I went off'. They had given her medicine but she had run out. She had come to Kailahun to live with family, but they had quarrelled and she had moved into the local spiritual church next to our office. Dan found the pastor. Annie had turned up on his doorstep and joined in the praying, and they'd agreed to give her a place to stay. Possibly, non-stop singing, dancing, praying and clapping made an overstimulating environment for someone on the edge of a manic episode. She had become more and more demanding, shouting, and refusing to stay indoors. When she'd gone out dancing in town the night before, the pastor had refused to let her back. However, when we promised medication and support, he agreed to look after her while we searched for her family.

The arrangement broke down in a week. We found Annie dishevelled and dirty in the marketplace again, shouting at a trader. We still hadn't located her aunt. I went round to the maternity ward in the field hospital. They had an extraordinary nurse called Alice, who had taken my patients in before. To my relief she agreed again.

By now Gabriel had joined us, a well-trained, highly intelligent community health officer who genuinely wanted to learn about mental health. We started running clinics in the hospital, and in outlying health centres. Mr Ibrahim joined us in the weekly hospital clinic. It was very useful. We saw a boy who fought with his mother, accused her of poisoning him, and wiggled his eyebrows in a strange way. He said it kept the witches away. Mr Ibrahim told him this was complete rubbish and he should take the medicine we prescribed. This was more valuable than anything I could have said.

A few days later, I found Annie in the hospital pharmacy shouting at the dispenser, who was telling her to go away. She agreed to come and talk with Gabriel and myself. She was calmer and more coherent than before, but still loud and irritable. She had left the maternity ward because the night nurse had said, 'Who is this crazy woman on my ward? I won't have her near my mothers.' She had come here for a skin cream because her skin itched so much. It did look horribly red and infected. I went in search of Dr Y.

'Is she the lady who abused me this morning? She was very rude!'

'Dr Y., she is not well, she's hypomanic, we are treating her but it takes time, she is really not to blame!'

'I have done psychiatry! She was very unpleasant. We could not calm her.'

'Well, please can you see her with me? She's much calmer now and I don't know what to do for her skin.'

He agreed. When we returned with Annie, the nurse at his door stopped us and tried to push Annie away.

'Excuse me,' I said, 'she is seeing Dr Y. with me.'

'But she's out-of-head!'

'Does that mean she cannot see a doctor?' I asked.

The nurse pulled a face and shrugged, letting us by. Dr Y. was kind and courteous and Annie was a model patient, submitting to a skin snip to check for the microfilariae that make you itch and cause river blindness. Dr Y. gave her a note saying she was a 'vulnerable' patient so she could get free medication, and the dispenser politely dispensed.

We finally located her aunt. She had been away at a wedding and was back in town. We all agreed to meet at our hospital consulting room. Annie arrived first. She pulled out a plastic bag full of different medicines: antibiotics, painkillers, worm pills, anti-cold remedies and sleeping pills.

'Who prescribed all of these?' I asked in amazement.

'It was a CHO.'

Annie had obviously decided to take advantage of her new 'vulnerable' status.

'I had a pain here,' she pointed to her shoulder.

'Did he ask you any questions or examine you?'

'No.'

There is now solid evidence that patients with mental disorders die up to twenty years earlier than the general population, both because it is harder to live a healthy life when you are mentally ill and because their physical ills are neglected. Neglect can include prescribing inappropriately to get a patient you don't like out through the door as fast as possible. I restrained the urge to go and talk to the CHO, whoever he was; I knew I would end up shouting.

We went through the medications. She was rubbing the powder from one of the capsules into one of her ugly skin sores, a common local approach – with some effect if the pill is an antibiotic, but none at all if it's an anti-parasitic medication as in Annie's case.

'Annie, they won't work like that. You have to clean those sores. I will help you but you really don't need all these, believe me. I will keep them for you. And you can take these. They are for worms.' I caught myself sounding like a senior prefect at my public school: bossy, firm but kind. I really didn't like this voice, but Annie didn't seem to mind. Perhaps she was just relieved to have someone else take control and help ward off some of the chaos inside her head.

'All right, doctor, please can I have a glass of water?'

I gave her one.

'I don't want to go to my aunt's house, she will beat me!'

This was new information. I laid my forehead on the table, then turned sideways for a moment so I could stare out through the mesh-covered window at the green trees and the piled-up storm clouds. It was a very hot afternoon. It had been a very long week. We were seeing at least two new, acutely psychotic patients a day. We had spent all the previous day doing a workshop with health and community workers. I had begun with a poll on people's beliefs about mental illness. Everyone, community and health workers alike, thought that most mentally ill people were 'bad, violent, abusive and aggressive, stupid, lacked initiative, did what they liked, were unreliable, could not be controlled, hurt themselves and others, did not obey the law, and were unable to learn'. Not surprisingly, it followed that the mentally ill 'should neither marry, nor vote', but 'be locked up, restrained or beaten'.

The aunt arrived. I pulled myself together and sat up.

She told us more about Annie. Her mother had died in childbirth and her father had disappeared, leaving the daughter in the care of the aunt, who had no children of her own so she loved Annie like a daughter. But she was very poor. Annie had been married to a rich man in Freetown at a very young age. He had used her as a maid, abused her and beaten her and refused to let her go to school. She had run back to her aunt on a number of occasions but the man had always found her, tied her up and taken her back. When the war came she had escaped to Guinea as a refugee, and in the camp there she had been happy for the first time in her life. But then Annie had obtained a good luck charm from a medicine man and had not paid for it. The aunt was sure that the man had bewitched Annie in revenge. She'd been hospitalised for six months until her aunt brought her home to Kailahun. She had then had two months of treatment from a local healer and got better. But the healer had told Annie never to drink. She had got very drunk on palm wine at a local celebration and had been out-of-head ever since.

'My aunt would rather I was dead than alive. Even now she sets demons on me. I had a dream and saw my aunt with a red dog. I told her to put it down, she refused and told me she would kill me.'

'Annie, you are like my own daughter! I expect you to take care of me when I am old,' the aunt said. 'After all the money I have spent on you, how can you say that I don't care?'

'You have to understand, when she was sick she would shout in the village,' the aunt went on. 'People insulted me, I cried all night wishing I was dead.'

'She beats me and chains me up!' Annie jumped in.

'Because you are abusive and steal things.' The aunt turned to me. 'If you send her back to the village now, people will abuse her, and torment her, it will be too hard.'

'I don't want to go there!'

I could see that this was likely to be true.

What to do? How to protect Annie and those like her from the abuses and torments of the crowd in the marketplace, in a country that had just crawled out of a twelve-year civil war?

It had become clear to both Gabriel and me that what mattered in recovery was not the severity of the illness but whether there was anyone to care. Matthew, for example, had been sick for a year. He had developed the idea that many of his school mates were witches and could read his mind. He could also hear them talking about him on the radio. He was terrified, and wanted the shutters to the clinic closed because witches were trying to get in and harm him. His mother had walked seven miles to bring him to the clinic, accepted the medication we prescribed, listened to our explanations and promised to do all she could to care for him. When we saw him again a few weeks later he was much less frightened.

I always kept Vikram Patel's brilliant, simple, understandable textbook *Where There Is No Psychiatrist* to hand. It was the bible for my training programmes, and lay on my desk. Matthew took it away to read and came back the next visit having helpfully ticked all the symptoms that he had. He was very bright and wanted to sit his exams and go to college. Having a caring mother made it possible.

Ahmed was a different matter. He brought himself in to see us because his friends had told him to come. He had filthy torn clothes and dirty matted hair and beard. After spending a little time with him we knew he had a chronic psychosis as well as an ugly ulcerating sore on his foot. I found his family living close to the marketplace, but they could not manage to care for him – they had eight other children. It was too difficult for them to keep him at home or get his foot dressed or give him medication. So he went back to wandering round the market again, laughed at, stoned and neglected. Whenever I bumped into him I would beg him to come and see me again. He was always polite but always had somewhere else to go at that moment.

I longed for access to a small asylum. Luckily, the pastor stepped in again. Annie could stay with them as long as her aunt came to feed and take care of her there – which she promised to do. But then Annie disappeared. We searched the town, no one knew where she was – perhaps in Guinea. There was nothing I could do. I hoped she had taken the tablets with her. New patients kept coming. We had to start waiting lists in the outlying clinics. There was more and more epilepsy. Word had got round that we could treat it, and people with 'fits' now outnumbered those with psychosis.

Dan found Annie drinking palm wine and sitting like a queen on the riverbank, amidst the purple flowers and the orange and white butterflies, watching the waders spin up from the rocks in the river. He persuaded her to come and see us again. She told us she had crossed to Guinea to look for an old boyfriend, but she got lost and decided to come back. She was quite coherent; she had been taking her tablets because they helped.

'But the drink does not help you, Annie, you know that.' Annie pulled a face. Mr Ibrahim was with us. He turned towards her and looked at her sternly over half-moon glasses. In his robes, he reminded me of a Methodist minister from Wales. He gave Annie a lengthy lecture on the iniquities of drink and the importance of family. She was to go home and stop drinking.

It was just what was needed. Annie managed to look both astonished and meek at the same time. She promised to stop, and return to her aunt. We promised to check she was not beaten. The Annie that came to see us two weeks later was a woman I had not seen before: soft-spoken, her face relaxed and pretty, hair elaborately plaited; talking about how nice it was that people could see she wasn't crazy, and how the hospital dispenser had been polite to her when she had gone there with her prescription. She wanted to start cooking and selling baked goods in the marketplace. Her aunt was all smiles.

Meanwhile the boy with the wiggling eyebrows was getting on with his mum again. She said he was unrecognisable. Annie came to tell me clients were buying her food. There is nothing as de-stigmatising as recovery.

Jijiga, Ethiopia, November 2008

'If you are unfortunate enough to be the victim of a disaster, here are some dos and don'ts for gaining maximum attention and assistance:

'Timing is very important. Don't have your disaster just after one in a very rich First World country. Don't have it just before Christmas: people are too busy shopping. Have it on Christmas Day – Boxing Day is even better if you can manage it, when everyone is exhausted by present-giving, feeling overfed, watching TV and wishing they could do something constructive, especially if it does not involve physical effort.

'Location: it is best to have your disaster close to a beach. This ensures attractive locations for both media and aid workers looking for a nice place to work. Avoid chilly mountainous regions with severe deforestation, bad urban planning and poor Internet connections.

'Victimhood: avoid being black. Try not to be old, any age under ten is excellent. Do not live in a state with Sharia law or any association with terrorism. Nice Muslims in lacy white headgear are acceptable, but Buddhists and other religions that have monks and flowers are preferred.

'Nature of disaster: do pick something catastrophic and unusual, preferably something that has not happened before. Tsunamis are good, although they might be passé now. Earthquakes – it depends. Floods, sinking ferries, long-running wars, forget it.

'Numbers of dead: this is much less important than you might think. More may sometimes be better, but will always be trumped by the other factors listed above.'

I am reading Asmamaw my opening to an article about the Pakistan earthquake in 2005, written for a glossy American women's magazine. My editor loved it and it was included in the page proofs. The editor-in-chief did not. She cut the section from the article. She sent a message to us both: 'Our women readers will not appreciate the irony and will feel insulted.' There was no argument. She was on a yoga retreat in Colorado, and not taking incoming calls or messages from anyone.

'I think perhaps she was right,' Asmamaw says.

'Yes, maybe, I was feeling particularly jaded at the time.'

I wrote it while I was living in the North-West Frontier Province of Pakistan in December 2005. An earthquake of magnitude 7.6 had just killed seventy-eight thousand people, and I was a very long way from a beach. Balakot had been reduced to rubble along with hundreds of remote surrounding communities. Winter had begun in earnest and 1.9 million people were still living in three hundred thousand canvas tents. In the hills and mountains around us, houses that had withstood the earthquake collapsed under the weight of fifty centimetres of snow, landslides occurred and helicopters stopped flying.

Some of the small roads that wound up the sheer faces of the Karakoram Mountains became impassable. In the camps in the valleys below, UNHCR and the Pakistani Army argued over whether to provide heating by means of individual stoves or communal gender-segregated tents, while families came up with homemade options that caused respiratory infections and lethal burns. Then when the army and UNHCR finally agreed on covered stoves, the government insisted that families who had lost everything and had no compensation had to pay for the kerosene, because aid agencies were creating 'dependency'.

I remained mystified as to what people should pay with when their houses had fallen down, they had no jobs and no possessions, and still had not received their compensation cheques. (If no one had died in the family or you did not own your house, there was no compensation.)

I tell Asmamaw these stories sitting over coffee on the back porch of the agency house in Jijiga, eating breakfast with him and the office staff. I am back on the Somali border after five months away. The kitchen hut now has a stove inside and we have a wonderful cook called Bizu. I have dragged an old cane sofa out here so we can look at the blossom over our neighbour's fence, admire a single tree that's struggling up in our own yard and watch the eagles circle above us on the updraft. It takes very little to make a home, easier still if you are loved. Asmamaw and I plan to get married. We are just sorting out the paperwork. We don't know where we will live. There is work for both of us here right now.

'Are we creating dependency here in the camps?'

Asmamaw smiles and shakes his head. We both know that what all the Somalis want to do is get out of the camp and get a job, any job, and make a life. All everyone dreams of is 'resettlement', and just like last year, wherever I move a crowd hover around me trying to thrust various scraps of paper into my hands: letters of appeal, official documentation of war in-juries, of rape cases, about relatives abroad – never mind my protests of complete powerlessness and my inability to move anyone anywhere. There is some resettlement going on from camps further south, where people have been living at least twelve years. One year is nothing.

I spend my daytimes talking to the most vulnerable families in the camp. They all tell me the same story. They are cold: UNHCR issues one blanket to two people, and it's freezing at night. Yesterday I met a family of fifteen who had only six blankets. Sometimes they use them as extra cloth on the door or roof of the *aqal* to keep draughts out, which leaves them lying on plastic on the floor. They are hungry: World Food Pro-gramme (WFP) rations are a minimum 2,000 calories in wheat flour and beans, but the Somalis hate this food so they sell it, get short-changed and have even less.

They don't have enough medicines. The new clinic is almost finished but it doesn't have the capacity to address the chron-ic problems like old gunshot wounds, or illnesses like asthma and diabetes that have gone neglected for years in their dys-functional homeland. These are referred to Addis, but because there's a long waiting list it takes months.

They don't have shoes, or clothes. One family of ten chil-dren lined up for me: they were all in the torn garments in which they had left Somalia three months earlier and between them had eight pairs of shoes, six of which were broken. No agency or generous public is donating these 'non-food-items', as they are called, which is another reason the poorest families sell their food rations and go hungry. They were all scratching themselves and complaining of fleas keeping them awake at night. UNHCR issues one bar of soap per person per month, so skin infections are the number-one complaint at the clinic. And there's not enough water so there's fighting at the communal taps, where usually the 'minority' clans, like the Somali Bantu, come off worse.

'We fled Somalia because we were discriminated against and it's just as bad here. They call us "big nose" and "curly hair",' one father told me.

Another six and a half thousand refugees arrived from Somalia this summer, a small-scale disaster unrecorded by the Western media. They've been placed in a new camp on a hillside in a constant, biting, dusty wind and their needs are even greater. Asmamaw has been shuttling back and forth, doing clinics in both camps all summer.

In the new camp I can say things like: 'It will take time.' In the old one, some things are getting worse. Although some families are obviously doing well because they have money sent by relatives abroad. Their shelters have grown in size and comfort and are now five-roomed 'buses' round a yard with satellite dishes outside. They charge camp children one birr a time to watch TV. And there's now a proper school, boys are doing sport, and there's some informal education for adults.

'But they don't give us eye-glasses, so we cannot read,' one middle-aged woman told me.

At least Amina is getting better. I went to see her on my first day back. She was sleeping, but her brother insisted on waking her. She got up bleary-eyed and took my hand in greeting – an astounding change in itself – before sitting back down in the darkness.

'Hello,' I say, 'I'm Doctor Lynne, I work with Dr Hassen and Dr Asmamaw. We met a few months ago, do you remember me?'

She stares at me and nods. 'I do.'

'And how are you feeling these days? When I saw you before you were very upset.'

She shakes her head. 'Not good, I ache here and here, my headaches, I cannot sleep . . .'

I'm actually delighted to hear this catalogue of physical woes. She sounds like a normal Somali woman, we are having a coherent conversation about aches and pains, her son is cuddled up in her lap and her daughter is going to the new school. An enormous change. Her brother agrees.

In the evenings, Asmamaw and I go for a walk. We have found a flat, shallow lake surrounded by cracked mud just outside the town. Mengistu never completed his plans for a reservoir here. We take the dirt track along what was once intended as the dam so that we can watch the sun set behind the mountains to the west, and the lake and pasturelands turn gold to the east. Today we have the whole place to ourselves except for one family walking their cattle home. There's a great mass of birds: mostly moorhen and grebes, sacred ibises, Egyptian geese, but also avocets, stilts, and one fish eagle making its leisurely way around the margin, stopping every now and then to drink. As we pass each cluster of birds they startle up briefly, their feet beating water, then air, and their wings catching the light.

'It's almost a beach,' says Asmamaw.

9: AFTER THE WAVE

Lamno, Aceh, 2005

The story my landlord told me was that the river suddenly drained dry. When it came back it was full of bodies. He knew who some of them were. After the Balkans, Iraq and Sierra Leone, I thought I knew something about death and destruction, about lives abruptly ripped apart and buildings destroyed. But none of that had prepared me for standing on a devastated muddy plain on the west coast of Sumatra in early 2005 to be faced with . . . nothing. I looked out over a river estuary where thirty thousand people had once lived. All that remained was mud, rocks, shattered tree stumps and the indecipherable remains of clustered dwellings.

I was staying in Lamno, once a sprawling community of twelve thousand on the west coast of Aceh, now reduced to a village with a main street. The street ended in a bridge across a river. On one side were smiling people, open cafés and small shops. There was a market selling fruit, vegetables, clothes, dried goods. On the other was desolation, a landscape scoured clean of every sign of life, stretching for three kilometres down to an unfamiliar sea. In the early evenings we drove to the new shoreline, edging the car cautiously over wide fissures in the road. My driver peopled the space with brief sentences.

'Eight thousand lived there. They are all gone.'

'No one on that side of the river survived.'

'Two hundred people lived in that village.'

'The flags tell you where a body has been found and still needs to be collected.'

'Those tents are where they put the bodies.'

'That was a house, it does not belong here. It was a kilo-metre downstream.'

'This was my house,' he pointed to a bare patch of mud. 'This was my shop,' he pointed at a concrete foundation, 'and I had a bus. All gone.' In relative terms, he knew he was lucky: his wife and child survived and only his brother died, but all his neighbours were killed.

So were the five hundred boys and hundred or so girls in the Islamic boarding school. The substantial three-storey building was one of the few in the entire flood plain to remain standing. The boys on the topmost storey survived, but had the agony of watching their friends and classmates below swept away. Their young teacher had been outside the school drinking a coffee. He saw the wave coming, ran to slightly higher ground half a mile away and watched his students drown. He walked around the empty classrooms in quiet fury, telling us, 'My heart has turned to stone. I cannot stop seeing it.' A few upturned desks remained inside against the downstream wall. The silence was full of ghosts.

The Indian Ocean tsunami on Boxing Day 2004 was caused by an underwater earthquake of magnitude 9.1, which shifted a twelve-hundred-kilometre section of the earth's crust and re-leased energy equivalent to more than twenty-three thousand Hiroshima bombs. In Aceh some three hundred miles of coast-line were hit by towering waves of water within the first thirty minutes of the disaster. In some places the tsunami was more than twenty metres high. Salty debris-filled water raced six miles inland, drowning entire communities. At least one hun-dred and thirty thousand people died in that province alone, and more than a quarter of a million across fourteen countries.

The catastrophe was up there in the world's top ten worst natural disasters and generated an unprecedented outpour-ing of generosity. Humanitarian agencies of every description flocked in. Coordination meetings in Banda Aceh, the pro-vincial capital, were standing room only. There were at least thirty-three local and international agencies offering some kind of 'trauma counselling': many offered stress debriefing, while Scientologists offered 'therapeutic massage'. But we were seemingly incapable of addressing the fact that some communities were getting nothing at all while just down the road six agencies jostled for space.

In Lamno there had previously been two doctors serving the population of thirty thousand. One had died, along with most of the town's educated elite, who lived in the larger houses closer to the shore. The other had left. Now there was a Pakistani field hospital with a staff of fifteen in the local primary health care clinic, and three other medical NGOs, including my own, running mobile clinics in the surrounding area. My first feeling on arrival was bewilderment at the arbitrary perversity of human generosity. I thought of poor Dr Y., single-handed in the Kailahun government hospital, back in Sierra Leone. My second was to wonder whether I should ask to be posted back there.

But as I daily crossed that bridge between life and death, I changed my mind. The individual needs were vast, everyone I met had been stripped bare of absolutely everything: their possessions, their livelihoods, their homes, their landscape and most of those they loved. The fact that the public had still not understood the intensity of suffering in Sierra Leone or Darfur did not make the people of Aceh less deserving of help.

And something else was going on. Aceh had been struggling for independence for thirty years. Martial law was declared in 2003 because of fighting between the Free Aceh Movement (Gerakan Aceh Merdeka, or GAM) and the Indonesian National Army (Tentara Nasional Indonesia, or TNI), and the area had been closed to outside agencies. Now suddenly the world was invited in, and for all our flag-waving, our quarrelsome competitiveness, our clumsiness, our cultural ignorance and lack of coordination, this massive international presence was having a benign effect. Local NGOs blossomed as internationals scurried around looking for local partners with whom to share the world's largesse. Human rights activists welcomed us as possible brakes on any abuses. Never mind what we thought we were doing, the sheer mass of agencies all following their own agendas, independently funded and to a degree 'out of control', made it difficult for the Indonesian government to push through any particular 'political' agenda.

For example, in those first months the main plan for rehousing the surviving population was relocation into barracks. In Lamno survivors had initially found accommodation with friends or relatives, or lived scattered in small clusters of homemade tents in school yards, around mosques, in the university grounds. Then we were told the twelve little camps would be concentrated into three big camps. It's simpler to deliver water, food and medical care to displaced people all lined up in neat rows of tents or barracks. But it was not lost on the locals that if services were concentrated in large camps, it was easier for the TNI to control a potentially subversive population.

I went to visit one of the relocation sites, five kilometres inland from town in an isolated position in a narrow valley next to the river. Large wooden barracks were crowded close together around squares. Each section had its own row of latrines and was labelled with a large sign: Blok 1, Blok 2, Blok 3. There didn't seem to be any space to grow anything or to play.

'How will we live here?' my driver asked me. 'How will we find food? How will the children go to school? And people wonder why all this wood is being used to build temporary relocation camps rather than help us rebuild permanent homes?' Good questions. I had no answers.

'See that hill,' he pointed at a cliff overhanging the road back into town. 'That's a GAM gun position. The GAM and the TNI were fighting the night of the tsunami. Even before the tsunami came our hearts were racing because of the guns: boom, boom, boom. People are afraid.' He felt it was a no-win situation. With TNI 'protection' the camp population would be more vulnerable to attacks from GAM. 'Before the internationals came we were beaten up all the time and accused of being GAM. It has stopped now that you are here. And when you distribute food, everyone eats.'

We walked back to the car.

'Please tell all the internationals,' he continued. 'Don't go! We love you being here.'

On one of our evening drives we came across a group of men sitting on plastic chairs not far from the shore of a newly formed lagoon. They waved and beckoned us over. A cardboard sign with the name of the village, 'Ujung Muluh', was tacked to a post, a large fishing net was stretched across a bare concrete area they said was the mosque, and there were two tents. I was surprised to find them so close to the sea.

'We are fishermen, we don't know how to farm,' one man said.

The others nodded.

He went on: 'This is our home, this is the land where we were born, and it is hard to leave. But we have nothing, everything is gone, some boats disappeared out to sea, the others are destroyed.' He pointed across the road. 'There were trees with large oranges, they were famous. We played soccer in that field. There were twelve hundred of us, only four hundred are left. We sleep in the camps at night and come here every day. We want to come back here and be right next to the sea. Can you help us?'

'Aren't you afraid?' I asked.

'No, no, no,' said one.

'We are all afraid but it is up to fate,' another said quietly, 'but all of us who survived want to live here – one hundred per cent.'

'I want to be here,' said a thin man. He had lost his entire family: wife, mother, father, parents-in-law, sister, nephew and his own daughters aged twelve and nine. 'This is where I feel closest to them.'

'They told us we are not allowed to live here for at least three years. But we don't want to go elsewhere,' the first man said. 'We have made a pact among ourselves. If they build for us elsewhere we will refuse to go. We have told everyone. Please, my sister, if you want to help us, please help us to stay here.'

All the men had tears in their eyes.

It was the same everywhere. In the camp next to our clinic,

two hundred and seventy people remained from a village of two thousand. They were all related and wanted to stay together, next to what remained of their village and their property, in what remained of their family groups.

'I prefer to be where I can remember,' I was told all the time. I was glad my own agency understood this and insisted on providing services in the places where people wanted to live.

And as I wandered about I realised we were needed for another reason.

'Indonesians love to talk,' a medical student explained at a lecture I was giving in Banda Aceh, 'and we are all talking and talking and talking about what happened, but none of us can listen or pay attention.' Just as I had first discovered in Sarajevo, there was a need for unscathed outsiders who could take time to listen. This was particularly important in Aceh where there were so few remaining survivors, and where to smile and look happy in spite of pain suffered is an essential part of social relations. The capacity to listen doesn't require a degree in counselling, or a seat in a traumatic-stress clinic. The main requirement is empathy. The man from Thames Water who was setting up a purification process could do it while he taught his Acehnese counterpart to filter water. World Food Programme staff could listen while giving out rice. So when passing journalists asked if I was 'counselling', my answer was always, 'No, I am just paying attention.'

In fact, to say that I was unscathed was not strictly true. In the first week of the year, just before I had flown out to Aceh, one of my closest friends had died unexpectedly. Paul and I had gone to medical school together, trained together, and he had become a talented child psychiatrist. He had accompanied me through many of the ups and downs of my disorganised life, inviting me to take up a training post with him after my first marriage had broken down, supporting my international work and coming out to Kosovo himself to teach.

As a happily married father in what he had hoped was the middle of his life, his death had the arbitrary unfairness that all unexpected deaths do. Not surprisingly, the funeral service in the tiny country church was packed. Wife and children were surrounded with love, support, friendship, people wanting to help in every way they could. All of us who mourned the man could both express and alleviate the pain of losing a friend, relative or neighbour in this way. One man in one community was gone, but his possessions – the photos, his jukebox and collection of discs, the garden on which he had spent so much time, the village in which he had lived – all remained. These were painful to contemplate in the immediate aftermath of loss, but would be comforting tangible reminders over the years to come.

I was to learn the same lessons all over again six months later when my father died after a short illness. I was away at the time and could not stop weeping. I dreamt every night that he was alive and it was all a mistake. It was only when I slept in his house, surrounded by his things and the reality of his absence, that the dreams stopped.

'So what do you do if every single thing is swept away: house, furniture, photos, clothes, every single thing?' another medical student asked me at the next lecture in Banda Aceh. 'And all the neighbours and family who should come to mourn, help out and share their memories with you,' I could have added, 'and the places you walked and played.' So much of what makes a person is what we remember. What happens when all the markers are gone?

'I'm learning this myself,' I replied. Find the good memories inside yourself, put them down on paper, share them with others, find some way, any way, to memorialise and treasure the past. This was why going home was so important. Even in this strange, bare, stripped-clean landscape, being close to the familiar overrode the fear. It was a place to begin. So no wonder people clung to the foundations of their homes and wanted to rebuild in places they knew well. Better to live with familiar ghosts than with strangers. The survivors won the argument. A minister announced at the end of March that people could go back to their own homes. After that, return was unstoppable.

Another source of continuing pain was what had happened

to the bodies. No one had been able to follow the traditional custom of burial within twenty-four hours. Either the body was completely absent, or it had been scooped up by a road digger and shovelled unceremoniously into one of the mass graves that had been constructed in the immediate aftermath of the disaster. At my father's funeral in Wales, I could speak about his life, standing next to his coffin, watch it be put into the ground, and listen to the stories all his friends and relatives told at the wake. Every society in the world has some form of ritual to help us accept a death, honour the person, and say goodbye.

But months after the tsunami many had not been able to hold a funeral of any kind. Many of the young men who came to my clinics were working in clean-up programmes run by organisations like Oxfam to get 'cash for work'. In May and June they were still finding the bones of two or three bodies a day.

'We all know these could be our mothers and sisters, so we treat them with care. We only clean our own villages. So they are not strangers,' one man told me. The bones were given to experts for identification. He had not found the bodies of his own family. One of the reasons he did the job was in order to keep looking.

Another problem was the numbers. The fact that two hundred and twenty-five thousand had died in a matter of hours might have captured global attention and brought aid workers and journalists en masse to South East Asia; but if your loved ones are just a fragment of this enormous number, it actually diminishes their significance. We want strangers to know that someone we loved and lost mattered. After 9/11 the *New York Times* ran 'Portraits of Grief' of every person killed: small stories that brought people whom I had never met to life. Like Kirsten Santiago, a twenty-six-year-old insurance broker who took her dog Sailor to play with Alzheimer patients every Sunday. Other therapy dogs attended her memorial service. Such details stuck in my mind. But here in Aceh the lives and stories of the dead had drowned with them. Each individual was lost in a sea of numbers.

The importance of this acknowledgement by strangers was brought home to me vividly in Sri Lanka when I travelled there from Aceh that April. I was walking down the street of a former fishing village. All that remained of the houses were skeletal fragments of walls. The street was deserted, so I decided to take some photographs. Suddenly I saw a man running towards me from the far end, waving and shouting. I put my camera back in my bag and waited until he came up to me, breathless.

'I am so, so sorry,' I started to say, 'I had no intention to cause offence, please excuse me, I'm not a tourist. I work here and these pictures will help me explain what has happened to others at home.' I was babbling in my embarrassment.

'No no no!' the man said (like many from the area he spoke excellent English). 'Please take more pictures. Please take a picture of *this* house.' He pointed to the one beside me. 'My mother lived here!'

I took the picture with him in front of the house. Then we sat on the roadside looking at it on the camera viewer, while he told me all about his mother. I suddenly understood. What mattered to him was that his mother was not lost among the fifty thousand who had died along that coast, but was an individual with a life that counted, a story worth telling, whose home was worth photographing. I told him that she sounded like a wonderful mother and I would always remember her. And I do.

The tsunami was a discriminating killer. Women and children at home were killed while their fishermen husbands and sons out at sea survived. But there were also surviving children, and teachers at the Islamic elementary school asked me to help them make sense of what had happened. They explained that normally when someone died, children under ten were told that that person had gone to study and they would see him at the end of life. If the child was more than ten, everything was explained. But as all the children had seen so many bodies, they wanted to know how to talk about death with them.

Children in Kosovo had already taught me that when there's

mass killing there's little point in lying about death, even to the smallest child. They know that someone they love is inexplicably absent and the lie confuses rather than comforts. By now I had developed some simple rules: make sure the child has as much continuity with their previous life as possible and is cared for by someone loving and familiar. Never push a child to talk about what has happened if they don't want to, but listen if they do. Answer all their questions simply and honestly, including ones like 'Where is my mother?', and in a language the child understands. Find a way to help them make sense of what has happened. Find simple ways to make memorials. Find normal activities to distract them from the pain.

On one occasion some villagers asked me to see a little girl who had not spoken for the six weeks since the tsunami. She and her mother had both been swept away by the Wave. She ended up in the top of a palm tree, alone above the flood water, crying for her mother and unable to get down. She was there for two days before she was rescued. There were snakes and a crocodile in the water but somehow she survived, although her mother had drowned. She was happy to sit with me, nodding and shaking her head in answer to my questions. She did not want to tell me what had happened, and having obtained the story from a relative, I did not ask her to do so.

Instead I got out my finger puppets and asked her to choose one. She chose the most brightly coloured bird, and I asked if she would like a story.

She nodded, so I told her about some birds that lived in a forest. When a strong wind came and blew all the nests away, one small bird lost her mother. But she was incredibly brave and managed to hold on to a branch and to stay there, even when other forest animals came and tried to frighten her. The little bird hung on and hung on until a kind monkey came to rescue her. He took her to some other birds in her family who told her she could live with them. But the little bird was still so sad, she did not sing any more. Nobody minded, though, because sometimes birds just don't feel like singing. But little by little, as school began and the little bird saw her friends and they told her how brave she was, she felt a little less sad. And even though she thought about her mother all the time, the frightening memories grew less, and the happy ones, of times they played together and her mother kissed and sang to her, came back. Then one day when the sun was shining and everything in the forest looked so pretty, she did feel a bit like singing again.

It was just a start. All I was trying to do was create a story that acknowledged her loss, confirmed her strength and bravery, let her know that she was talented and loved, and that the pain would lessen over time. When I'd finished I asked if she wanted to keep the bird. She nodded. When I returned the following week she had brought her elder sister and her cousin to see me. Both wanted to tell me what had happened to them. I had brought all my animal puppets this time, explaining that they had heard of the bravery of the children and wanted to meet them. So I placed them in a circle with me, and we listened as the two explained how they had clung to branches as the wave swept by. Both children then wanted me to repeat the story I'd told the previous week. So the strong wind came again, and this time it all ended as happily as possible in a small safe clearing in the forest.

In Aceh my puppets became my co-therapists, helping children to talk about their symptoms and have brief conversations about what death was, because many small children don't understand that it is permanent; and about responsibility, because they are the magical centres of their own worlds and often blame themselves for such events. This indirect method of dealing with these hard subjects seemed to work much better than direct questions and held the children completely.

One afternoon we were asked to visit a woman and her only surviving grandson. The plump, very elderly lady welcomed us into her tent, clutching my hand and taking it to her forehead in the traditional gesture. Then we sat cross-legged on the raised platform with a few boxes piled around us, and she burst into tears. Every time we asked the boy a question, the grandmother answered for him, weeping, while he smiled and said nothing. So Dian our psychologist took her aside to talk with her alone, and I got out my puppets. The boy chose the cat and I took the rabbit and we had a conversation.

'Rabbit and Cat are friends,' I said, 'and Rabbit has come to visit. "Hello Mr Cat, how are you?"'

'I'm fine,' said Mr Cat. It was the first word the boy had spoken to me.

'I heard you lost your mummy in the tsunami.'

'Yes, I did.'

'I am so sorry! How do you feel?'

'Very sad.'

'Did you lose anyone else?'

'Yes I did,' said Cat, 'my two sisters and my grandpa. We were at the market and they were at the beach.' Now that I knew the boy was using the cat to talk about himself, we could discuss everything. Cat told Rabbit that he could not sleep at night because he always remembered how his mummy used to help him with his schoolwork and tell him a story. Rabbit learnt that Cat was not afraid and liked fishing; he had just caught some shrimp that morning. Cat liked school and had lots of friends.

'What's your favourite subject?' asked Rabbit.

'Catching mice!' said Cat.

We continued to visit these children and support them through play, and they all did well. In fact most of the children I met were doing well: eating, sleeping with few nightmares, enjoying school, playing sport. I saw no signs of the 'epidemic of PTSD' predicted by more than one newspaper. On the contrary it was the stoicism, combined with the courtesy, charm and hospitality of the Acehnese people, that was most striking. In the midst of disaster, we were all their welcome guests.

Nonetheless, there was some evidence of PTSD. Meurah thought about his two lost sons every time he saw a child in the street. When I first met him he talked for almost thirty minutes without a break, hunched forward, not smiling, telling in vivid detail how some half a dozen of his neighbours all ran into his house near the sea after they heard the sound of the wave coming, because they thought it would be safer inside. The water crushed the house. He had his infant son in his arms and the older five-year-old clutching his shirt. His wife was swept away and he smashed into a tree and lost the older boy. Later, as the water filled with sharp objects, he could not hold on to the infant and he let him go as well.

'At the last moment my son did not look like my son and it was easy to let him go. Now I remember him all the time. How could I not have recognised my own son? He was alive in my arms.' Meurah's memories had a different quality from many others I had listened to. They were agonising, vivid and intrusive. He wanted to be rid of the images and his feelings of guilt, as well as the irritability and jumpiness, the aches and pains, that he had felt since the tsunami. He wanted to go back to his village and rebuild his house but if he went near the place he felt completely overwhelmed.

Those who were actually physically immersed in the water and fighting for their lives appeared more likely to have classic post-traumatic stress disorder than those who suffered losses but escaped the Wave.

Grief trumped fear, however. When people came to our clinics their commonest symptoms were sadness, sleeplessness and 'remembering'. Usually these were not intrusive memories of frightening or upsetting experiences, they were sought-after memories of beloved lost companions. I called it 'Tsunami distress'. One woman saw her daughter's face every time she opened her Koran. She didn't want to lose the image, she wanted to hold on to it, but it also gave her pain. The question was how to find comfort from it rather than distress.

Even a single object could help. Another man who had lost his home, his canoe, his parents, his wife and three sons found a hat belonging to one of the sons: a torn remnant of a red and white baseball cap that he kept turning over in his hands as he talked with us about the boy and his life. It clearly put him more at ease. Mementoes appear to help focus grief because there's something solid to touch, around which to tell a story.

With nothing left at all, one remains immersed in a swirling mass of incoherent longing.

Meurah came back three weeks after our first appointment, completely transformed. He looked a different man, smiling, smartly dressed, relaxed, saying he felt much better. He slept, he ate, the aches, pains and jumpiness had gone, he no longer felt guilty and although he dreamt of his family often, they were no longer drowning. It was in the early evenings, coming home from work, that he missed his sons most.

'What has made so much difference?' I asked, rather bewildered at such rapid change. I had planned to start cognitive therapy but we hadn't begun, and I'd started him on a small amount of antidepressant, but it was too low a dose and too soon to have had such an effect.

'Talking to you, your suggestions, prayer, the medication. I sleep and eat better. I don't blame myself now – this is destiny. God chose my sons and I tried to do my best. He has work for me and if I am alive it is important to be a good Muslim. I won't forget, but I don't want the memories to make me sick.'

There was more to it. He had plans to help his brother replant trees back in their village, and intended to marry a new girlfriend he had met.

'She won't be the same, but I realise I can have another wife and children.' Although we both agreed he should stay on the medication for a while, I thought it likely he could have done without. The essential treatments appeared to be love, faith, reconnection and work. I had little control over the first two, but I thought we could do more to provide the latter.

Everyone who came to see me complained of having nothing to do all day but think, and no means to restart their lives. 'Cash for work', through clearing debris, could not go on for ever. The tsunami had swept away almost everyone's livelihoods, filling the rice fields with salt water, wiping out orchards and plantations, smashing up fishing boats and destroying small businesses. One day I came across a thin, tearful man sitting with two infants on his lap. He had lost twenty family members and all his knife-making equipment. Then there was a woman who had lost the stove on which she cooked snacks for the local shops; a village headman who spent sleepless nights worrying about how to get things going for the twenty survivors in his village. He wanted agricultural equipment.

And it was not just work. The boys in Teumareum wanted a football field. Apparently the one they had lost was one of the best in the area and people had come from Banda to play there. The young men in Gle Jong wanted a volleyball court. Some of the other agencies who dealt with livelihoods had set up a council where requests like this could be submitted for funding. But my agency also had funds to use for this purpose. For the first time in my career as an aid worker, I did not necessarily have to direct my patients elsewhere. I could set up these programmes myself.

Gle Jong was a seashore village a few kilometres from Lamno where everyone under five, and most of the women, had been killed. One hundred and two of the original six hundred survived. Asiyah and her sister lived in a shack built out of salvaged wood. Their coconut trees had been washed away, and they had lost their sewing machine. They wept and worried all day long. In May 2005 I began to work with them both and the other twelve surviving women, all of whom were grieving. I told the women I had some funds to help with livelihoods and asked them to decide what they wanted to do with it. An animated three-week discussion led to an agreement on a tailoring project. Oxfam promised the sewing machines, our construction people promised to put up a workshop, and our livelihoods manager said he would get the project up and running. I left happily for Sri Lanka.

When I came back in November, Dian our psychologist and Eddy our community psychiatric nurse sighed when I asked them what had happened.

'The sewing machines were donated by Oxfam, but the workshop is still not finished.'

'The women are not happy with the workshop.'

'Why ever not?' I asked.

'They don't think it is big enough.'

'But they gave us the measurements they wanted.'

'Yes, but now they want something bigger.'

'Well, they can't keep changing their minds,' I replied somewhat irritably, momentarily forgetting that this was a group of women who had lost every single thing they possessed, including all the children in their village. Dignity, and the right to change their minds, or to be as stroppy and demanding as the rest of us, were all they had left.

'And there is Teumareum . . .'

'Yes, I know, we promised to redo their football field.'

'That's not finished either.'

'But we thought it would take a week!'

'We began, but the previous site manager insisted on trenches and he built them too big. When the monsoon came the field collapsed into them and the flooding made it harder to build and it needed more and more trucks of stones.'

'And the community is very angry with us for being so slow.'

'But we're not gods. We can't stop the rain,' I complained.

'It's not just the rain. It's the shoes.'

'Shoes?' By now I was a bit bewildered.

'We promised all six villages football shoes, but the brand they wanted was not available, so they agreed to compromise and accept something else. We got that, but after wearing them for fifteen minutes those shoes fell apart.'

'But they *must* be guaranteed! Can't we change them?'

'Yes, but the guarantee lasts a week from purchase, and our logistics department was slow, it took two weeks to get the shoes to Lamno, so we cannot return them.'

'The boys are mad at us. Poor Eddy was threatened with a machete a few weeks ago.'

There are times when I hate the giving business. In this disastrous year I had seen unwanted donated clothing lie rotting on the beaches at Aceh, and outside churches in post-Katrina Louisiana. I had had a lengthy correspondence, via our public relations department, with a very important federal bureaucrat in the United States. His office insisted on 'giving something' from the children of the United States to the children of Aceh.

I suggested money, so that Acehnese children could choose for themselves. They refused. Eventually, after talking with local teachers and children, I came up with schoolbags with art materials inside. The very important bureaucrat visited without the bags: dignitaries, handshakes and promises, photos and press coverage all round. Eventually the bags, books and crayons were all sent separately by DHL. Our Indonesian staff spent hours packing them up, but were upset because the bags were of such poor quality they felt embarrassed to give them. The children could buy far nicer, cheaper bags in the local market. The crayons, sent from the United States at such great expense, were all in boxes labelled 'Made in Indonesia'.

Here's the thing: givers choose to give because they want to feel good about giving, but receivers never choose to receive – they are usually forced into this position. Why, when people have lost everything, should they reward us with gratitude? And why should they be fobbed off with cast-off clothing, expired drugs, surplus grain, cheap football boots or anything else we would not want ourselves?

I set off for Gle Jong, anxious to learn how all my best-laid plans had gone so wrong. I didn't recognise the road out to the shore any more. The empty, wrecked tarmac was now a highway pulsating with traffic: pushbikes, motorcycles and trucks. The tideline marking the divide between devastated flooded and unflooded land had completely disappeared under the vivid green of a new rice harvest. Homemade shacks of driftwood and canvas had been replaced by new houses. The tsunami was a great leveller in more ways than one. Even though some had elaborate two- or three-storey villas before the Wave, everyone now had a one-storey tin-roofed house of some description. Whether wooden, breeze-block or concrete appeared to depend on the lottery of which agency was rebuilding your patch: the Turkish Red Crescent did wooden cabins; Terre des Hommes were building concrete villas in Teumareum across the river. Out in Rumpet, next to Gle Jong, someone had built the stilted houses with individually roofed porches that create the layered, overlapping effect so beloved in this country.

The shelter agencies had not yet reached Gle Jong, but the ramshackle cabins had acquired potted plants and small yards which, in the bright sunlight and with a breeze blowing off the sea, had an air of homeliness. In the middle, though, was an ugly concrete building painted in our agency colours. Thick pillars on low walls supported a tin roof. It looked like an oversized municipal bus shelter. Motorbikes were parked inside. This was the sewing-machine house. It was not the simple, airy, elevated wooden structure I had imagined. No wonder the women were unhappy. Dian gathered them all together. They told me the full story. The workshop was quite big enough and they didn't mind the concrete. They had not started work because other things they needed hadn't been supplied. We ran through them: lino for the floor, tables, chairs, cupboard, materials and some shutters to rainproof and lock the building. It was our own ex-site manager who had frozen all these requests because he thought the building too small.

Meanwhile, our livelihoods programme manager, fresh from microcredit work in India, had told the women they had to start a cooperative. Their start-up money would only be a loan, to which they had to contribute. But this terrified them. None of them had anything. They needed donations at the outset, not loans, just to get going.

'And then we asked Oxfam for ducks and geese and they said your agency was doing livelihoods in this village, so they would not help.'

Not only had the involvement of three different sectors from my agency – mental health, livelihoods and construction – entirely failed to help the women of this community, we had actually stopped them getting help from elsewhere. The first mistake had been mine: setting up a programme in which I lacked experience, one with multiple components and with no single person in charge, so it fell between the cracks. I was mortified. We had let these women down completely. I was amazed they were even speaking to me.

'Now you are back we hope things will be better,' they all said, smiling.

'I can only apologise and promise you they will,' I replied.

Something has happened to the humanitarian aid business since I began working in the Balkans. In those days agencies specialised. In Goražde, medical agencies like MSF did medical care, development agencies like Oxfam did livelihoods, Save the Children attended to schools and education, and so on. It was a bit like the local high street when I was a child. You went to Boots with your prescription and to get toiletries, W. H. Smith to buy newspapers, the Co-op for food and Marks and Spencer to get underwear. But then I grew up and Marks and Spencer was selling food, you could take your prescription to the Co-op, and some Boots sold everything except newspapers. It became harder and harder to know who did what, as all of them chased 'market share'.

The same thing has happened to aid agencies. During the decade before the tsunami, as agencies ran after donors and money, just like competing high-street stores they extended the range of what they could offer. Here in Aceh, awash with funds, we were all doing everything, but nothing particularly well.

Some agencies had been castigated by the *Washington Post* that May for rebuilding fishing boats using illegally logged wood. They had not realised, because the wood was purchased locally. But we should have known about the trees. Sumatra's pristine forests, full of orang-utans, were a global treasure, and the main protection against future floods and erosion.

'And the *Washington Post* also does not like us giving out fishing nets, apparently,' a colleague from another medical agency told me. They asked, "Why livelihoods and not medicine?"'

The answer was that replacing nets and fishing boats, and so helping men back to sea, was one of the best means to address their psychological distress. It was a truly psychosocial activity. I would much rather prescribe sewing machines and volleyball

courts than amitriptyline. But if agencies worked collabora-
tively rather than competitively we could each stick to doing
what we do best. In my case that would be supporting grieving
people and creating mental health clinics rather than football
fields.

One of the best ways we did help grieving communities was
not our idea at all. It came from the Acehnese themselves. At
one spot on the main road from the airport to Banda Aceh
there was often a lone person standing in prayer or contemplation. It was the site of a mass grave where twenty thousand
people were buried, without names, markers or acknowledgement. Dian and Eddy asked local people what could be
done. They asked for help to build a 'Quiet House', a place
that would provide shelter, privacy and beauty for the relatives of the dead. They wanted to pray and meditate without
the intrusion of traffic from the main road. With agency support they built a traditional wooden structure in less than ten
days. It was landscaped with flowers and trees and decorated
with an inscription: 'From Him [Allah] we come and to Him
we return.' One local worker, who thought his family were
buried there, was in tears: 'Now I can come and talk to them.
We need a place where we can come and feel a sense of loss
and family again, a beautiful house for people to sit and come
together.'

And many came. Other communities with mass graves requested similar 'Quiet Houses'. On one occasion a man came
in to pray for a dead friend. While he was doing so that same
friend came in, very much alive. Some stories have happy
endings.

Somali border, Ethiopia, December 2008

'Psychiatry is not rocket science. Actually you are all psychiatrists.'

The community health workers gathered in the training workshop in Jijiga all giggle. Dr Hassen and I are doing a mental health training workshop for the primary health care staff and volunteers from the two camps, and I always start in this way.

Then I ask them to introduce themselves to their nearest neighbour by having a quick chat. After five minutes I stop them and ask them to write down on a piece of paper all the reasons they think their neighbour is 'normal', or 'not normal'. Everyone laughs but they comply, and as on all previous occasions when I've done this exercise we end up with a neat list that almost matches the basic mental-state examination I was taught to do as a medical student: How does the person appear and behave? Do they make eye contact? Are they listening or distracted? Is their speech fast or slow? Do they make sense or not? Do they understand what you are saying? Are their answers relevant? Do they know where they are and to whom they are talking? . . .

Unlike trying to diagnose appendicitis, which requires young doctors to actively learn how to examine an abdomen and discover the signs of inflammation or rupture in the gut, we grow up making unconscious mental-state assessments whenever we're in the company of others.

'Is he listening to me? Why does he look so angry and distracted?'

'Is she tired, or bored?'

'Why is that man talking to himself and picking up little bits of rubbish in the street?'

The inability to do this is one of the features of autism. So it's not surprising to me that health workers without training, across Africa and Asia, can recognise severe mental illness within their own cultures. This is why Annie got stoned in the marketplace, Amina was left struggling in her *aqal*, and why I and Dr Hassen now use a very simple method of case-finding here in the camps. We give the community volunteers simple case descriptions and ask them to look out for people who might fit:

'Is there anyone in your part of the camp that you see out talking to themselves or behaving oddly. Perhaps they pick up rubbish from the ground, perhaps they don't take care of themselves any more, perhaps they have very strange ideas that you know are not true?'

'Is there anyone who is locked away in their *aqal* and never goes out, because they are too sad or because they cannot think clearly – maybe they prefer not to talk?'

'Is there a child who has not grown in the same way as others? Perhaps she cannot talk or walk, or perhaps she is slow to understand and finds it hard to learn.'

It is important because these are the sort of problems that people don't bring to the clinic. Using this method, Dr Hassen has now already identified and begun treating more than twenty-seven patients with psychosis in one camp. Almost all of them were tied down or chained, many of them had gone years without treatment. We both know we have to start counting.

When I was a medical student I hated statistics. These days I'm an obsessional data collector, bullying Dr Asmamaw and Dr Hassen to log cases. I've finally realised that having numbers at your fingertips matters. They make the invisible visible.

It's not always easy to do. In most of the emergencies where I've worked, the health surveillance systems are geared for acute conditions and communicable diseases; there has either been no category for mental disorder, or the category was inappropriate. In Aceh, on one government form two options were offered: 'psychosis' or 'PTSD'. Bad luck if you were severely depressed. And if you came in with the aches and pains associated with such misery they were logged as arthritis, gastric complaints or headache or whatever, and treated with inappropriate medicines. If a problem is invisible you cannot advocate for the proper treatment.

But since late 2005 I've been part of an international task-force trying to come up with consensus-based guidelines for providing mental health and psychosocial support in humanitarian settings. In particular, I agreed to write the first drafts of two action sheets on providing 'access to care for people with severe mental disorders' and on 'collaborating with local, indigenous and traditional healing systems'. I had no time to research. I spent a couple of exhausting nights in Aceh simply writing out what I had been doing in previous years, as a series of organised steps and principles.

Specifically, I included the practice I had begun with Gabriel in Sierra Leone: recommending that health staff should document mental health problems on primary health care data forms, using simple categories that they would recognise with little instruction. To make things easy I recommended boiling the entire mental-health classification system down to four categories: medically unexplained somatic complaints – those physical ills that had no organic cause and yet took up such a large proportion of the health worker's day; severe emotional distress – to encompass all mood problems including severe grief and severe stress; severe abnormal behaviour – to cover psychosis, epilepsy and other neuropsychiatric problems all of which should be documented in the locally understood terms for 'madness'- like *kpowa*, for example; and alcohol and substance abuse.

I was astounded to discover that none of the approximately sixty experts around the globe to whom the action sheets were sent for comment had any substantial quarrels with them. The *Inter-Agency Standing Committee Guidelines on Mental Health and Psychosocial Support in Emergency Settings* was published in 2007. Since then a group of us, in discussion with UNHCR, have extended the four categories to seven, splitting abnormal behaviour into psychosis and epilepsy, and including intellectual disability and 'other psychological complaints'. This last is a catch-all for all the misery and distress that does not meet the criteria for mental disorder and probably applies to half the people in this camp.

The categories have been included in the 'UNHCR Health Information System for Camp Settings' and we are using them for the first time here on the Somali border. Asmamaw has pinned a large copy of the list and their definitions to the clinic wall, to remind staff. I am astonished at my own excitement at seeing the figures emerge from the official UNHCR printed data sheets.

When not seeing patients and obsessing over data collection, I am still trying to get to grips with people's social needs. Most continue to struggle. One local NGO is helping some families build their own mud-brick houses, another teaching them how to grow vegetables out of a sack, and another has distributed hens and chickens. These are all great ideas but they are tiny projects for fifty to a hundred people at a time, a thimbleful in a sea of need. The old camp is now ten thousand five hundred people strong, and the small projects create conflict. People don't understand the criteria for selection, rumours grow, and the refugee committees are accused of bias, selecting only their own clan and family members for activities. So new committees get formed and the same thing happens again.

The main sources of income are the ubiquitous small stalls selling *khat*. This is not being taken as an after-lunch stimulant – it's an all-day intoxicant. Women tell me they could not get through the day without it. You come across small groups of young men chewing, laughing and lounging. It's followed by beer or diazepam at night to bring you down. In the vulnerable it can cause psychosis. But there are no other ways to make money.

Yet the truth is, services and conditions are better inside our camps than for many impoverished local Ethiopian Somalis in the surrounding villages, so some of them try to register as refugees. Asmamaw and his colleagues solve this by allowing locals to register at the clinics and the school, and receive food rations if they are malnourished, so the presence of refugees has actually improved basic services a little in this area.

Thanks to Dr Hassen, we are doing the same with mental

health. He has moved his working life to Jijiga and plans to
move his family when he is settled. He has negotiated with the
local hospital to have a small number of mental health beds
and an outpatient clinic here. He wants to combine regular
clinics in town with the training and support programme at
the camps. It means that both local people and refugees will
have permanent access to a psychiatrist and inpatient beds.
Humanitarians always talk about turning crises into opportunities to create something better for the whole community. Dr
Hassen is actually doing it.

It is needed. Amina became sick again. Her brother met a
woman in town and left Amina and the children in the family
aqal. Dr Hassen and I recently visited Amina there and found
her lying on a mat complaining of pain, still perfectly coherent,
but clearly not coping. Her two children looked grubby and
neglected, and uncooked maize grains were scattered over a
filthy floor. Her neighbours crowded in after her.

'She is not managing.'

'She does not feed herself or the children.'

'She shouts at us for no reason!'

None of them wanted to help her, Amina was too difficult.

'We have too many problems of our own.'

While we were talking, Osman brought his mother water in
a cup and held it to her lips. At least that relationship remained
intact, even if the three-year-old son was now the carer. I knew
that if we could not get her fed, clean and back on medication she would become manic again. Dr Hassen said he could
admit her and the children together to the hospital. He had no
other inpatients at that moment and there was a small garden
around the ward. With some intensive care she would be stable
in a few days.

So that's what happened. Amina scrabbled around in a tiny
holdall for clothes for her son that were not torn or unwashed.
In the end she found holey, slightly dirty trousers, in which
she carefully dressed him. Then Dr Hassen took them to Jijiga
and now she is the best I have seen her, back at the camp, attending the mother and baby group with Osman and living an

organised life, with a volunteer calling in to help and to make sure she takes her medication.

And some of my other patients have recovered. A tall man stopped me in the feeding centre yesterday. He had a grip on my arm which suggested a request for resettlement was about to follow, and I'd already started my 'I am so sorry but ...' speech when the nutritionist said: 'Don't you recognise him? You saw him last year, he's much better, he just wants to thank you.'

10: BUILDING BACK BETTER

Diary: Port-au-Prince, Haiti, 24th January 2010
I am back inside the asylum, standing in the men's courtyard at the Mars and Kline Psychiatric Hospital in the
centre of town. Hot sun beats down on concrete. There is
a crevasse in the middle caused by the earthquake. A dirty
naked man lies beside it, eating rice from a bowl. Another
naked man sits rocking in the shade. The sleeping area is a
filthy room with bare iron bedsteads, a few pieces of torn
clothing, and nothing else. There are also two tiny barred
cells. Both are occupied by bearded, ragged-haired, naked,
sad-faced men, who stare at me through the bars. There's
scarcely space to lie down inside them and nothing to lie
upon. Dirt and graffiti cover the walls and they stink of
faeces. There is no working toilet or shower in the hospital, just a bucket in the yard.

You wouldn't cage an animal like this. It is completely unbearable. Luckily, most of the sixty inpatients were
evacuated to their families when the quake struck, but
eleven have come back.

The administrator showing me round can see my distress and I can see his embarrassment. He talks vaguely
of government plans for renovation that came to nothing.
What did I expect? Haiti is the poorest country in the
Western hemisphere. The hospital is Haiti's only mental
health facility, the administrator tells me, there is nothing else, no regional units, no community care, and they
have an outpatient population of 10,000 in normal times.

Right now two doctors, who are sleeping on pavements because their own houses have collapsed, are seeing one hundred and fifty patients a day in tents in the yard. I am ashamed of myself.

The administrator, homeless and without salary like his colleagues, is immaculately dressed in a clean white shirt, beautiful tie and perfectly pressed trousers. He locks the door to the inpatient unit and picks his way delicately across the paved courtyard, leading me back to the out-patient tents. The walls of the hospital collapsed with the quake and for some one hundred families this courtyard is a genuine asylum. They have pitched pieces of plastic or blanket canopies attached to wooden poles around the few scrubby trees, and piled their remaining possessions around them in ice boxes and plastic containers.

I am astonished at the cheerfulness. There are women plaiting their hair, and a man drinking beer and having a pedicure, surrounded by plastic chairs and buckets. Three girls are playing with a skipping rope, while other children chase each other between the canopies. There's also a little girl of about six or seven tied to a wooden arm-chair by bandages around her arms and legs. She wears a bright-blue dress, her hair is neatly parcelled into multiple plaits, each sticking perkily out of her head and finished with a bright bead. An elderly woman boils milk in a saucepan and bottle-feeds her. The girl grabs and clutches the bottle in both hands and drinks greedily. She clearly has some form of developmental delay. At this particular moment, with one million people homeless and most of the city centre destroyed, this is probably the safest place for her to be.

'What do you need?' I ask the administrator. The answer is the familiar one:

'Mattresses, sheets, clothes for patients and staff, buckets, cleaning materials, generator, functioning toilets, tents for the staff to sleep in, a vehicle to get us to work, medications . . .'

I have drugs with me. After a year of lobbying and negotiation, a group of us finally persuaded WHO that including one antipsychotic and one anti-epileptic drug in the Interagency Emergency Health Kit that gets sent to disaster zones is a really good idea, if you want to stop people with serious mental illnesses relapsing because they or their families suddenly cannot get the drugs required. The kit also now includes one antidepressant, a minor tranquilliser and a side-effect drug. For the first time in a decade I hoped I might find the drugs I needed, where I needed them, when I needed them.

Unfortunately, WHO is not using this updated kit in this disaster – don't ask me why. Luckily, untrusting soul that I am, I spent my two days pre-deployment buying the same drugs from Boots at cost price. Amazing what wall-to-wall media coverage of hapless victims will do to the most hardened pharmacist heart. Asmamaw and I spent the night before I flew unpackaging all the drugs, reducing the volume by two-thirds, so that I could get them all into one bag which I now carry around on site visits. I give the administrator half of what I have. I promise to return with more drugs and everything else on the list except Portakabin loos. That will be a challenge. They are like gold dust in this city.

The day I arrived, Dina, our director of emergencies, said: 'Give me a list of whatever you need and you can have it. We have the money.' This is because the Haiti earthquake has followed all my how-to-make-your-disaster-noticeable-and-profitable rules: this is not the Karakoram Mountains.

The epicentre of this earthquake (measuring 7-plus on the Richter scale) was just ten miles south of Port-au-Prince, a capital city where some three million people live, a hop, skip and a jump from one of the richest countries in the world. The numbers are mind-boggling: in 35 seconds it killed more than 200,000; injured 300,000; made one and a half million people homeless and destroyed government ministries and the presidential palace. The UN calls it the most destructive urban disaster in recent history. And the timing is perfect, just after Christmas; the population is definitively non-Muslim (50 per cent still using voodoo just adds to the exoticism); and there is still access to nice beaches in every direction. CNN have taken every room at the only structurally sound hotel with a swimming pool. The *New York Times* are following me about and promising to do a story on people with severe mental disorders.

The paradox is that in the midst of all this devastation, sleeping in a tent in a concrete yard, kept awake by the snoring of colleagues in the next tent, sharing a bathroom with minimal water pressure with sixteen other people who never de-clog the plughole, and eating our logistician's idea of a good diet – which seems to consist totally of cheesy Wotsits and bottled water – I am happy. I feel useful. There is something I can do and the money to do it.

And that's the dirty secret. Everyone loves a good emergency. Not the tiresome kind that goes on for years and years, in obscure, dusty places that no one has ever heard of, where it's so difficult to really know who are the good guys and who are the bad. Accident and Emergency is now reality TV. Can someone name a prime-time television programme made about any chronic illness? Never mind one about schizophrenia.

To tell the truth, in some senses I've been tapping my fingers since the tsunami and the Pakistan earthquake. I have been here ten days and I know there's at least a million dollars in unallocated funding from private donors, to address any needs I wish without even writing a proposal. Apparently, a film star will visit us shortly and be photographed looking compassionate. This will bring in yet more money. Of course, that's great for the Haitians, but as always I am nagged by the knowledge that all the money and celebrities being thrown at this disaster are at someone else's expense. One big government funder has

said it is cutting donations to other countries that it usually supports by 22 per cent so as to address urgent needs
in Haiti. Last year, in spite of a televised appeal with Dr
Hassen and a celebrity, the donors were not even slightly interested in the mental health of Somali refugees in
eastern Ethiopia. We could not get the quarter of a million dollars needed to continue our programme. Then Dr
Hassen died of cancer. I miss him terribly and I know his
patients in Jijiga and the camps miss him even more.

Why is it that human beings can be mobilised by
sudden and catastrophic loss, but remain unmoved by the
drip-drip-drip of chronic suffering? This peculiar psychological fact has turned us all into ambulance chasers. I
have learnt that if I move fast, I can use the spotlight of
media and donor attention to open doors into dark and
ugly places that never saw the light before, and maybe
they can be cleaned up a bit, and things can be improved
for a few people who have been living lives of unbearable
degradation. My only hope is to get it done in a way that
will survive the swivel of the spotlight as it turns away to
the next disaster, the next tragic scene.

Port-au-Prince, Haiti, 2010

Every disaster has its own imprint. People ask me whether after
all these years 'in the field' one emergency doesn't simply fade
into another and the misery become a continuous blur. But
quite the reverse seems to happen. The images and sensations
endure in my mind long after I have gone home. If anything,
they sharpen. When I think of Aceh after the tsunami, it's of a
landscape stripped and scoured, accompanied by silence and
an overwhelming sense of loss. When I think of Haiti after the
earthquake, it is of clutter, chaos and the raucous clattering of
a mass of people all struggling to get on their feet at once.

That first early morning in late January when we drove
into Port-au-Prince I was astonished to see people everywhere,

smoke rising over breakfast fires and the streets packed. In the Central Square, traffic passed incongruously around and through an enormous tented camp that had sprung up under the statue of Henri Christophe, the first black president of the country, on his horse, in his Napoleonic hat. People had hung their washing on the railings of what was once the presidential palace, now an iconic collapsed dome and crumpled white masonry. 'Tented' is the wrong word. There were no tents – just close-packed, homemade constructions of sheets and sticks.

Over the following weeks I became accustomed to this cheek-by-jowl juxtaposition of normality and devastation. The Mars and Kline was still standing, but around the corner the nursing school had collapsed, killing almost a hundred students. On the upper floor their intact lockers hung open.

It was the same all over the city. One moment you'd wind down a street of untouched villas, then turn a corner past the ruins of a brand-new shopping centre that had crushed all its customers. In another street one house would be standing intact and the next tilted to one side, so that you longed for a large hand to give it a little shove back into alignment. Or a front wall was missing, exposing the inside living area, with furniture still arranged and pictures hanging, like an oversized doll's house opened for display. In the downtown area, nineteenth-century wooden and brick houses with their corrugated-iron roofs, turrets, pointed towers and balustrade balconies were mostly still unscathed, while their more cheaply constructed twentieth-century neighbours had pancaked. Each house was a grave where the unknown and uncounted lay entombed. And every single empty space – parking lot, roundabout, traffic island, wasteland – had become a refuge for the living, makeshift camps and markets marooned in a sea of almost stationary traffic.

Most of that traffic was created by us, the incoming international humanitarian community, either delivering relief goods in trucks or sitting ensconced in our four-wheel drives, tapping on Blackberries and trying to get to meetings. The UN, having lost its headquarters and more than one hundred staff, was camped out under canvas at the airport and running the coordination system from there. It took at least an hour to get to a meeting from almost any point in the devastated city. I tried not to think about whether the carbon footprint created by all our vehicles, not to mention the vast numbers of plastic water bottles that kept us all hydrated, was causing more long-term damage to the environment than the earthquake itself. But we had to go.

This is another paradox of complex emergencies: there is always a tension between working and coordinating. Work provides the immediate satisfaction of helping people; but possibly the wrong people, and not for very long; or the same people get helped repeatedly because they are the ones who are easy to reach, and others in need get left out. So you have to meet other agencies in order to coordinate. But then there's the question: which meetings? In 2005 the UN introduced a new coordination mechanism for emergencies: the 'cluster system', which was supposed to be much more accountable and more interconnected than the old sectoral approach. And the word 'cluster' was attractive, suggesting some kind of chocolate-nut confection or friendly groups of people clustering together. In reality it meant far more meetings.

And we now had those *Inter-Agency MHPSS Guidelines* that I'd helped to write. Among other things they state that mental health is a cross-cutting issue. For example, good mental health for women living in the makeshift camps depends partly on ensuring good lighting and secure access to showers and toilets, so they don't get raped. So arguably I needed to attend the health, protection, water and sanitation and camp management clusters, just to raise that one issue.

Clinical work was a relief. Our agency was responsible for emergency triage in the devastated university hospital in the centre of town. Although half destroyed in the first days after the earthquake, it had been a magnet for the injured and dying. Volunteer medical staff saw at least three hundred patients a day. The inpatients stayed in large, logo-bedecked tented wards, as the hospital buildings were considered unsafe. Even larger numbers of needy people clustered outside the main gates, but young soldiers with crew cuts and sunglasses from the US 82nd Airborne acted as crowd control in the yard, and as traffic cops and security in the streets. Before the earthquake, Haiti had been one of the gangster capitals of the world; the soldiers were keeping us safe.

I attended to whatever was thrown at me: a man who had taken to wandering around the hospital naked after the surgeons had done an external fixation on his fractured tibia and fibula; tearful and confused old ladies; a woman who hadn't spoken since she was pulled out of the rubble; another man refusing amputation even though his foot was badly injured and in danger of developing gangrene, because he believed the cause was witchcraft, not the earthquake.

Some people were beyond my abilities. A plump young woman with pale skin and dyed red hair lay in one of the medical tents, completely paralysed. She had been repeatedly examined and no organic injury could be found, but she seemed in remarkably good spirits despite her inability to move a single limb. Her appetite was unaffected and a supportive family were in constant attendance, feeding and fanning her. Haitians recognise *sezisman*, or 'seizing up', as an understandable response to shock. When treated with herbal teas and support and attention from loved ones, it usually resolves in a few days, but not in this case. Each time we passed, the family asked when we could arrange a medical evacuation to the United States, given that no one in the hospital could cure her. They knew others with severe traumatic injuries had been evacuated, particularly in the first days, so why not them? My suggestion that the woman had converted her shock and distress at the earthquake into paralysis, and that perhaps with a visit from a traditional healer and physio (the hospital was awash with volunteer physiotherapists) she would recover in time, was met with complete astonishment and disbelief.

This was not what was wanted. I saw no chance of recovery while the medical evacuation flights continued. Nor did I know what to do when the Red Cross referred a dirty, 'demented' or 'possibly psychotic' man in torn clothes. Twenty minutes' conversation established that he was perfectly sane. The grounds had become a refuge for the homeless and the indigent. There was no way I was going to put him out on the street.

On other days I worked with the volunteers and the Haitian doctors and nurses who provided primary health care to all comers in churches, community centres and tented clinics in the devastated towns and villages along the Mirogoan coast. Some turned up simply because they were overwhelmed with the practical difficulties of daily life in the midst of chaos. Others came because they felt the ground shaking all the time. They felt dizzy, had palpitations, could not sleep, were terrified they might be having a heart attack, were terrified of going indoors This was not surprising, given the repeated warnings that another major quake might come soon. I heard the same pattern of symptoms repeated so often I started calling it 'earthquake shock'.

A few months after leaving Aceh, I had gone sea-kayaking. I was surprised how unnerving I found the sight of the very large waves we encountered off the west coast of Canada. At night, camped out on a small island, I would listen to the swell caused by passing cruise ships on their way to Alaska and find myself plotting where to run if we were overwhelmed. I had not been directly exposed to the tsunami, but working with its after-effects and constantly discussing safety strategies had reset my own alarm threshold. I had to sort out sounds and images in my mind and actively explain to myself that they were not dangerous. I had had a similar experience with the sound of back-firing cars after leaving Sarajevo during the war there. I had to keep telling myself this was not gunfire. Many of my tsunami patients found looking at big waves unnerving and were dogged by intrusive images. Earthquake victims in Haiti imagined tremors and felt their hearts beat faster in response.

Each disaster creates its own imprint on the body and on the mind, not just on the landscape. So I was back on familiar territory: teaching health workers not to diagnose these problems as mental illness unless they persisted and prevented the person from functioning, but to educate their patients on how the body responds to stress, and how breathing and relaxation can help to reset the oversensitive fire alarm.

And amidst all the chaos and fearfulness there were stories of extraordinary courage. Five-year-old Michael had been at home with his two older brothers, celebrating their father's birthday, when the earthquake struck. Their uncle had run round to find the house completely collapsed but had somehow managed to dig out the two older boys, one of whom had been lying beside their dead father. He could not find Michael or his mother and had given up. Nine days later he had returned to look for the bodies so he could bury them. He had seen a small arm sticking out. It moved, and he dug Michael out, alive and uninjured. His mother was dead but Michael insisted that she had brought him milk and juice every day.

Neil, our medical director, happened to be driving by at the moment Michael was found, and had taken him to the hospital. While there he became very attached to an American volunteer nurse, and the media became very attached to Michael and the nurse, and so for a while he was quite a celebrity. Then the media lost interest and the volunteer nurse returned home, handing the family over to me. I visited regularly. All the boys were doing well. The family had been given a proper tent in a reasonably organised camp within a school yard. The children went to play every day in a 'child-friendly space'. They didn't cry or have nightmares or palpitations; they slept well, ate normally when food was available, and played and chatted happily with me and my puppets whenever I came to visit. In those first weeks Michael made no mention of his mother, or of being buried alive, so neither did I. It was his call.

There is a transitional moment in all emergencies. The twenty-four-hour news channels are packing up to go. The cluster meetings are switching from daily to twice-weekly. The mapping exercises – trying to pin down who is doing what, where, with whom and for how long – are beginning to make a little sense and our 'local counterparts' (NGO-speak for the people who were actually running things before disaster struck) have picked themselves up, dusted themselves down and started reasserting their authority.

I knew we were reaching that moment in Haiti when I heard the Haitian health ministry representative at the health cluster say wearily, politely, and for at least the third time, that while the government greatly appreciated all the people who had come in to help, they would now be grateful if those with only a fortnight to offer would stop coming, and if those who did come would work with the Haitian government to make longer-term plans. Emergency relief was giving way to 'early recovery' and everyone was talking about 'building back better'.

Meanwhile, at the airport the UN were replacing tents with air-conditioned containers, and I was doing my best to work within a 'relief-to-development framework'. That meant not just seeing patients but trying to create some kind of mental health response that might be useful to Haiti in the longer term. Things were not going so badly. Sabah had joined us from Pakistan and was establishing 'baby tents' in various camps, where trained Haitian facilitators encouraged mothers to come with their babies and young children and play, while learning about nutrition, hygiene and early child development.

We had one mini-cluster in which the handful of agencies interested in helping people with severe mental disorders met with Haitian colleagues and the government representative. This person changed each week, so we often had to repeat ourselves. Peter, a colleague and friend, had joined me from the UK. With the help of Kettie, an elegant and unflappable Haitian psychologist, we had set up a daily psychiatric liaison service in the General Hospital. In the mobile teams we ran emergency mental health clinics and provided regular training to all the Haitian primary health care staff employed by our agency, and any others who wanted to attend.

All well and good, except that 'building back better' raises a number of awkward questions, starting with: Who is doing the building? The answer to which in part depends on the answer to: Who is running the country? This is not the place to detail the tortured history of rebellions, foreign occupations, coups d'état and dictatorships that have plagued Haiti since its slave population astonished the world by successfully throwing off their French masters in 1804. Suffice to say that the Haiti parliament abolished its own armed forces in 1995 (perhaps tired of endless coups), but this did not prevent yet another armed rebellion, fomented by outsiders, leading to the forced resignation and exile of President Jean-Bertrand Aristide in 2004. Since then, the United Nations Stabilisation Mission in Haiti has been present. Although a new president was elected in 2006, UNSTAMIH repeatedly extended its mandate, to address pervasive gang violence and the humanitarian consequences of various catastrophic hurricanes.

The parliamentary and presidential elections due in February 2010 had understandably been postponed. Tragically, the main social democratic opposition leader had died of his injuries a day and a half after the earthquake, as had the archbishop and large numbers of civic leaders.

Who owned and controlled the current aid effort was clearly demonstrated down at the UN logs base at the airport. I worked with Haitians every day but it was Peter or I who went to the main cluster meetings. And apart from nominal Haitian ministers, very few Haitians were to be seen except those holding positions with international NGOs. Local self-help groups and neighbourhood associations lacked the knowledge, transport and credentials to make it to the site, and through the UN security system. Practitioners of the traditional healing systems – the priests, pastors and herbalists to whom the vast majority of Haitians turned for help – were not invited.

The next question is: Are you building what Haitians want? The administrator at the Mars and Kline wanted a new mental asylum and was becoming increasingly fed up with international NGOs. Things had started out well. The Mars and Kline staff were very pleased with the donations of clothing, mattresses, bedding and cleaning materials. We dropped off more drugs and arranged for a vehicle to transport their staff to work. At their request, we started weekly seminars on disaster psychiatry and brought in pizza for lunch. But our relationship grew more fraught as the weeks passed.

Some of the agencies at the health cluster complained that patients they sent to the Mars and Kline outpatient clinic were being charged for drugs, even though the government had announced that medical care should be free for at least three months after the earthquake. The administrator assured us that he was not selling the donated drugs, but that he had to sell the ones he had purchased before the earthquake to cover debt. Mars and Kline depended on the sale of drugs to survive. So severely distressed outpatients simply had to guess that free medication was available, and be calm and assertive enough to ask for it.

And there were other concerns: Peter's lectures on how to give less toxic combinations of psychotropic medication and use less punitive means of containment and control had no impact on the underpaid and exhausted nurses, or on the truncheon-wielding guards. On one occasion Kettie and I arrived to find a psychotic patient we had sent over from the hospital left naked in the yard, un-medicated and begging for food and water.

Rebuilding the asylum was way beyond the means of an emergency humanitarian organisation, even one that believed in 'relief to development'. And we had a better idea. A third British psychiatrist, Nick, had joined us as a trainer, and we now supervised eight Haitian physicians running weekly mental health clinics across the earthquake-affected region, including two in the outpatient departments of district hospitals. In addition, a Haitian psychologist or nurse trained and supported a network of volunteers working in the same communities. Some of these clinics were in remote rural areas that had never had access to medical care before. We dreamt of establishing a new model for delivering accessible mental health care to the wider community.

'Dream' is the appropriate word. We didn't think it through. In Kosovo and Aceh we had integrated mental health services into an established, state-funded primary health care system by training the existing staff. But in Haiti there was no Western-style primary health care system. The four out of five Haitians who lived below the poverty line depended on a limited number of state-run hospitals in urban areas, and on a tiny number of charitable services in rural ones. At least 40 per cent of rural Haitians had no access to modern health care at all, depending completely on religious leaders, herbalists and family. Asmamaw, who had joined me in Haiti that March, was running a mobile medical clinic near Jacmel. One day their team met a group of farmers high up in the mountains, all shoeless and clad in torn clothes. When Asmamaw introduced himself the farmers were amazed. 'We have never seen a doctor in our lives before.' They refused his offered hand. 'You are a doctor! We don't want to make you dirty,' they said.

There was endless discussion in cluster meetings about the need to create a public primary health care service, but there was no way of predicting if and when that might happen. This meant that we were creating a 'model' and 'building capacity' for community mental health services that might not be possible, while ignoring the request to improve the existing psychiatric facility.

And how should we respond to the request to rebuild orphanages? There were at least six hundred in the country with some fifty thousand children living in them, although most of these 'orphans' had at least one living parent whom they visited regularly. UNICEF had assessed more than two hundred and fifty of the institutions and found that they lacked drinkable water or functioning latrines, that the children were malnourished and infectious diseases were rife.

Madame Simone showed me round one that she had set up with her husband, in a large villa in Port-aux Prince. She had become upset about the abandoned children in the neighbourhood and taken them in. Then more and more parents had begged her to take their children. Fifteen lived there now and another twenty attended her school. She chatted away as we climbed the steep unbanistered stairs and looked into one of the unpainted and dilapidated bedrooms.

'All the children share beds,' Madame explained apologetically. 'Or they sleep on the floor.'

Two very small boys, one about two years old and the other four, sat on one of the beds. They were dressed in greying, torn underwear and looked unwell.

'Their mother gave them over to me five days ago. Her house was destroyed in the earthquake and she does not want them any more. We went to the police and signed the paper. It is all legal.'

We continued walking round. All the paintwork was cracked and dirty, the one toilet waterless and full of faeces, but the older children didn't seem unhappy, playing and joshing with one another. Out in the yard, next to an empty kitchen shed, three more children crouched, unsupervised, around an open fire.

We gave Madame the two portable covered stoves we had brought with us. She thanked us, but what she wanted, she said, was money to build a bigger and better orphanage. So did the woman looking after twenty children living under canvas beside an avalanche of rubble, where nine bodies were still buried. And the couple with some fifteen children sleeping on mats in a car park and cooking in a stairwell. All the children told us calmly they were beaten when they misbehaved. They thought it normal.

What was to be done? The desperately understaffed Department of Social Welfare completely lacked the resources to check on conditions. There were concerns about child exploitation, abuse and trafficking. Some Americans had already been arrested for trying to smuggle children over the border.

UNICEF and all the agencies involved in child protection were totally opposed to the building of new orphanages. They wanted to reunite the children with their families, or arrange adoption or fostering within Haiti. They argued that if we improved conditions in the old institutions, as their owners requested, such orphanages would continue to offer an attractive solution to homeless and impoverished parents, weighed down by the burdens of childcare. Yet lifting families to a living standard where they were not tempted to give away their children in order to improve their life chances would require massive social change. I didn't think we could leave children in punitive and inhumane living conditions while we worked for de-institutionalisation. I asked for money to deliver food supplements, do some essential temporary repairs and provide staff training in physical and emotional care. I got the funds.

We were allowed to build back, but not to make it too much better.

The communities where we provided health clinics were not completely satisfied, either. Take the 'boat clinic', so called because it was run in a small fishing village of some two hundred families that could only be reached by water. I had a favourite patient there, an elderly, skinny woman called Joanna with unkempt grey hair, dressed in an oddly youthful T-shirt and full skirt, who had kept striding in and out of the tent where I held my first clinic. She talked to herself or to us, laughed and interrupted all the patients. She told me that she had lived up the mountain alone because she liked to shout. Somehow we had persuaded Joanna to move into a tent in the village where the community kept an eye on her and gave her medication. She had transformed into the smiling, calm, neatly dressed woman who came to greet me at each visit.

But health care was not the only thing this village wanted. From the sea, the half-moon of huts and banana trees by turquoise water beneath a steep cliff looked idyllic. When you stepped out onto the beach, though, you were confronted with the reality: abject poverty and no work. One of my patients explained that her main source of stress was not knowing where her next meal was coming from. All the fish had disappeared. The boats were coming back empty.

The community leader sat me down in the yard outside her thatched hut, pulling chairs out of her own and neighbouring houses to seat the other elders and our team:

'We are very happy you are doing this health clinic, but we have so many other needs. You are the only agency who has been here since the earthquake. We need houses, we need food, we need latrines.'

Fifty per cent of the houses were unsafe or destroyed. They were all terrified of the stones coming down from the mountain. No one had enough to eat. There was water, but it was filthy. I noted down all the problems, explaining that as a health agency we could not address them directly but I would take them to the relevant cluster meetings. I told myself that basic needs were still unaddressed because the village was remote. Except that Michael and his family were having similar problems in Port-au-Prince.

I visited them every week. Uncle George had told the children that their mother was in hospital. Now they were asking when she would come home. I suggested George answered the children's questions about death honestly, and he promised he would. But he had other worries: the family and their neighbours had been told they must move out of the camp when the schools reopened. George had no money and no idea how to house or feed any of the children. Before the earthquake he had worked in a factory, which was now destroyed. They were scraping by on handouts from friends. The last food distribution by the World Food Programme had been fifteen days previously but no one knew how it worked, who got it, or when the next would be.

They were not the only ones. A few days earlier I'd been confronted by an angry and hungry crowd of residents from the camp in the Mars and Kline yard. The administrator wouldn't share the hospital food with them, and no one else was distributing any. I was bewildered by the food distribution set-up myself. Young mothers coming to the baby tents told Sabah they had no idea where to find their next meal. One reported being asked to give sex for food coupons, while others told us they were asked to pay for them.

'Nothing new there. These abuses are bound to occur and thank you for reporting them, but now we're changing the system,' said the friendly woman at the World Food Programme container in the UN compound. I had gone to ask where the mothers, my patients, and the people outside the Mars and Kline building should go for food.

'In the last distribution we fed five hundred thousand families. In future a local committee involving the mayor, selected NGOs and the WFP in each area will identify the most vulnerable families, and these are the ones who will get direct support. Those you identify as vulnerable should go and register with them. There will be no more coupons.'

Coupons or not, the system still seemed complex and wide open to abuse. It is just as easy to sell places on a register as it is to sell coupons. What's more, you have to have the means to go and register. The most vulnerable, like the grandmother with the small girl tied to a chair, were the least likely to be able to do that.

'We are not in the position to feed all of Haiti. It just cannot be done, however much it may be needed,' the kind woman continued with a weary sigh.

Some things were improving. In many areas rubble had been shifted from the heaps that blocked the street to the neatly piled stacks of smaller rocks at the roadside. Some agencies were now giving out 'cash for work', and men in masks and jerkins made their way through the debris hacking and sorting. Spray-painted signs appeared on houses: 'For demolition' or 'For renovation'. Neatly framed plastic and wood shelters sprouted in the gully along the road into town where, previously, shattered houses had piled up, one on top of another. But whole families still lived under bits of cloth that would wash away in the next major storm, and the hurricane season was on its way.

I found it hard to sleep at night. The heavy rains were starting. I would wake to the sound of it on my tent roof and lie fretting over all the people I now knew were still sleeping on cardboard. At the UN Amanda, who led the protection cluster, told me the national staff were up in arms because, unlike their international colleagues, they still had not got tents. She and a number of others had stood up and said they were ashamed to come to work.

'Our priority is to go to other clusters and discuss the urgent need for food and proper shelter,' said Amanda when she chaired the next mental health sub-cluster meeting. She brandished our *Guidelines* with their clear list of 'Dos and Do nots', including 'Do not focus solely on clinical activities in the absence of a multi-sectoral response.' Those attending just stared at her.

'We are much too busy,' said one. 'We are here to do trauma counselling; we have no staff for this.'

'You are busy counselling stressed people because you have failed to make advocacy for their basic needs – that is food, water and shelter – part of your work plan, and it should be!' Amanda snapped back.

I think it was at this point that I realised we were failing, or rather that what we were trying to do was impossible. This was not twenty thousand refugees in a tidy encampment run by UNHCR (the Somali border), or the Pakistani Army (Balakot), or NATO (Kosovo). This was more than one and a half million survivors crowded into one of the poorest, most corrupt and congested capital cities in the world, with its infrastructure in ruins and without a functioning government. Here, the homeless were living in backyards, on roundabouts, on wasteland or in tiny forgotten villages in the countryside. They were indistinguishable from their impoverished neighbours whose tin shacks might still be standing but were utterly degraded. The queues at the emergency room and outside our mobile clinics comprised people like those farmers near Jacmel. Most had never seen a doctor before. Many of the mothers in our baby tents were illiterate teenagers with neither partners nor work.

The catastrophe was not the earthquake, the catastrophe was Haiti itself, and the inequity, corruption and environmental degradation that kept the majority of Haitians destitute and struggling. The causes were not geophysical, they stretched back some two hundred years to the determination of French slave owners to make Haitians pay ninety million gold francs (twenty-one billion dollars at today's prices) for the impudence of throwing them out.

This started Haiti on a cycle of indebted vulnerability that has still not ended. More recent foreign meddling in the form of neo-liberal structural adjustment policies had wiped out public jobs and infrastructure, while free-trade agreements had flooded Haiti with cheap imported rice from the US, driving bankrupted Haitian farmers off the land and into the crowded gullies around Port-au-Prince where they had been most vulnerable to the earthquake. There was nothing natural about this 'natural' disaster. Like the Guatemalan earthquake in 1976 that so discriminatingly killed twenty-three thousand largely indigenous highlanders, it was a 'class quake'.

There was no way to distinguish the sources of destitution. If people were serious about helping Haiti, the fundamental issues had to be addressed. Haitians' views on how that ought be done varied. One of our logisticians thought we should bring back the Duvaliers He was referring to Papa and Baby Doc, who had ruled Haiti as their personal fiefdom from 1957 to 1986, killing and torturing thousands and driving hundreds of thousands more into exile. He was driving a particularly potholed stretch of road when he raised this: 'Twenty years ago everything worked, we had good roads, good hospitals. Nothing works any more; it is not just the earthquake. You know, Haitians really only understand dictatorship.'

'But weren't people terrified?' I asked.

'The thing about the Duvaliers: if you left them alone, they left you alone. Democracy is good, of course, but these people don't understand democracy. Politicians just see it as a way to get rich. Twenty years of Aristide, Préval, Aristide, Préval . . . not a single thing got better . . . nothing. Unless it was done by someone else.'

Others shared his desire for 'someone else' to take over, although not Papa Doc.

'What we want is the Monroe Doctrine,' one of our drivers told me. In an earlier life he had been a policeman, and a lecturer at the now collapsed police academy. When I expressed surprise at his desire for US interference and for the country to be treated as a cheap source of commodities and labour, he explained that no one in his country had the competence to run things. That was why they needed a wealthy benign foreign power to take over. 'Please make us a colony!' he continued. 'It must be better.'

On his last night we took Neil for dinner in Pétionville, the smartest part of Port-au-Prince where lovely villas untouched by the earthquake were interspersed with art galleries, beauty salons and nightclubs. The little tree-lined streets outside the restaurant were jammed with aid worker vehicles. Inside, tables were scattered through terraced gardens. Very few black faces were to be seen in the beautiful white-painted dining room. We ate very good, very French food off very big china plates with heavy cutlery, laid out on linen tablecloths. We drank wine from perfect glasses. Then we came home to a security meeting because two international doctors from another NGO had been kidnapped earlier in the evening from their clinic in the Pétionville camp.

I had been wondering how long it would be before Haitians saw right through our inconsistencies and simply turned on us, saying: 'Forget all this stuff about sustainable futures and capacity building, just hand over the vehicles! Even better, stay at the wheel while we get your bosses to pay for your release!'

Perhaps that was the point at which most of us should have gone home, handing over our money unconditionally, not to the gangsters but directly to the thousands of small communities and family groups with whom we worked. But those are not the rules of the game. The international NGOs are not accountable to the disaster victims we had come to help. Joanna and George had no means of checking on whether I was spending the money fairly and appropriately on their behalf. We are accountable to the donors. Of course, the donors expect me to go and ask people what they need and want, and then to go back and check that they are satisfied with what they got. But if you turn up in your white vehicle with your interpreter and ask someone who has just lost everything, or who never had much in the first place, if they are happy with what you're doing, they are not going to say 'No, no!' You are the only life-line to whatever they do need, so they are unlikely to send you off with a flea in your ear.

We stayed. Asmamaw still slept in a tent outside a villa/office in Jacmel, but my own living situation improved. I no longer slept in the yard. I now had a room of my own with a bed, a chest of drawers and an en suite bathroom, in a shared house with four others. The house was in a garden full of flower-ing bushes and trees set around a tiny bright-blue swimming pool. Inside the house there were sofas with silk cushions and coffee tables with knick-knacks, and dining tables laid for six-teen with full dinner service, candles, silver and crystal. All of this was overlooked by tasteful pictures of poor Haitian peas-ants toiling in the fields and of rebellious Haitians engaged in bloody uprising. We boxed it all up, as I was terrified of break-ing something.

Our landlady was delighted to rent her house to an NGO paying a competitive rent, and had moved into her second home in the countryside. Meanwhile, she had asked us to retain her maid, who cooked and cleaned for us, and her gardener who hosed the plants lavishly every day and tended the generator that supplied us with power. The garden was in a guarded and gated community in the middle of Port-au-Prince. No rubble in sight, because everyone living here was sufficiently wealthy enough to build structurally sound houses and pay for the security at the gate. So I felt safe enough to sleep indoors at night and go running along flowery avenues beside upper-class Haitians in the early morning. My agency had taken two other houses for staff in the same estate.

Moving made sense. It meant I no longer had to try to write up notes at the end of the day perched on a step because every desk space was covered in crumpled paper, dirty cups, maps and open laptops, while every chair had a further pile of paper, or laundry, or an actual person on it. How else could we organ-ise large-scale programmes and work long hours if we couldn't sleep, or live securely? We now had seventy Haitian primary health care staff to train, as well as ten Haitians running the orphanage programme and ten others running the baby tents. We still camped in the field sites. We needed a base to come home to wash and do our laundry. We needed reliable power and computers to write our reports.

And it was growing more insecure. The 82nd Airborne had gone home. Kidnappings were on the rise again. In addition to the always unnamed and uncounted Haitians, eight expatriate aid workers had been kidnapped within a month. There were reports of break-ins into aid worker compounds and attempts to steal vehicles. As predicted, some Haitians had worked out that aid agencies were a great target.

I mapped the changing seasons through what sold on the street: tangerines gave way to heaps of mangoes. There were cherries in the garden in Jacmel and the heat was growing by the day. We interviewed Haitian psychiatrists with a view to their joining the expanding programme. The idea was that they would eventually take it over. As we did not wish to undermine public services, we recruited from the private sector only. One question we asked at interview was what changes they would like to see at the Mars and Kline, where all had worked at some point:

'More doctors and nurses.'

'A laboratory.'

'Better drug supply,' they answered.

Not unreasonable things in themselves, but I was surprised that no one said:

'Getting the patients out of the iron-barred cells.'

'Stopping patients being beaten.'

'Running water, clean toilets.'

'Dignified clothes.'

'Perhaps after a while you just fail to see it,' Nick said.

Perhaps that's why I really was more comfortable sleeping in a tent in the yard. It reminded me of where I was. If you distance yourself, you lose empathy and anger. I no longer lay awake at night when heavy rain fell, worrying how colleagues and patients were faring on the street, but I did make notes that our bedrooms needed bedside lights and rubbish bins.

'The question is,' Nick said one day, 'would you be comfortable if a picture of where we live now was back-projected behind you while you saw patients in the clinic?'

My answer was no. I had never felt more separate from the people I was trying to help and had never been more aware of the close similarity between the humanitarian enterprise in which we were all engaged and its imperial roots. Michael Barnett, a historian of humanitarian affairs, criticises my generation of humanitarian actors for failing to see two important and related aspects of our work. Firstly, that we have turned compassion into a status symbol that feeds suffering, and indeed requires it to continually exist, so that humanitarian actors can feel good about themselves. Secondly, we have failed to recognise the degree to which an increasingly professionalised, centralised and bureaucratised humanitarian order is disempowering those it claims to assist and replicating the paternalistic habits of our imperial forebears: all those missionaries bent on ending slavery and 'enlightening the natives', while relying on the colonial state to provide security.

I see all my humanitarian friends throwing up their hands in horror. So many of us come from rebellious, anti-political backgrounds and regard humanitarianism as one step on the way to achieving those supposedly universal and apolitical values of justice, equality, a life free from want and oppression. There is nothing imperial about that project. Except . . .

Down at the airport the UN jungle of tents was now an organised city of containers with ventilation and power. It was an industrial landscape, the industry being the exercise of compassion and the imposition of a more just world order. It was the central hub for an army of well-meaning and well-paid foreign workers, sustaining the mission that had brought it to Haiti a few years earlier. Never mind the earthquake, Haiti's permanent state of political corruption, and its serial hurricanes (whose increased frequency was largely due to the imperialists' carbon-based economy), justified permanent intervention by unelected bureaucrats and an army of 'experts'. Meanwhile, the locals cooked our meals, cleaned our homes, drove our transport and provided security.

Arguably, Haiti was already the 'colony' that my driver longed for it to be. Over the previous six years, the Bush administration's lack of confidence in the Haitian government had resulted in a deliberate policy of funding NGOs and church agencies that had undermined the central government and created a parallel system. The earthquake had simply intensified the process to the point where the collapsed ministries and presidential palace were more than just symbolic. But foreign NGOs and churches cannot run a country and are not accountable. At the airport that July, some sixty NGOs elected a steering committee to ensure better coordination. No Haitian agencies were there, so none was included.

Pétionville camp provided a nice example of what was happening. Before the earthquake, it was a golf course with a 1930s clubhouse, tennis courts and pool, all secure behind wrought-iron gates. For years there had been a running battle between the American owners of the club and impoverished squatters who had glared with envy at the rolling green hills in the middle of their congested city. After the earthquake, some sixty thousand people just moved in and set up their shelters on the steep hillsides. As the 82nd Airborne had established a logistics base in and around the clubhouse, the squatters didn't actually burn down or occupy the buildings. Then film star Sean Penn's NGO took over the camp management, the troops moved out, and the American owners renovated the clubhouse, making it a very pleasant place for aid workers like me to have meetings and conduct training before wading out to address the needs of the huddled masses beyond the fence at the bottom of the hill. Revolution stopped in its tracks by charity.

But for all the contradictions of the aid business, it still enabled me to see people with mental illnesses who had never had effective care before. By now the 'earthquake shock' patients had given way to those with psychosis, epilepsy and developmental delay. Sometimes I had to sort out the complex mixtures of medication that patients had been prescribed by a series of private doctors, or bought over the counter to no effect. Sometimes, as with Joanna in the boat clinic, we were treating for the first time.

There was the young schoolteacher who had become mute after the earthquake but who had been behaving very oddly for the previous year, isolating herself, talking to people no one else could see, not turning up for class. Her mother said medication had brought back her daughter. There was a boy of ten who had been fitting since a bad bout of malaria at the age of two and needed anti-epileptics; and a girl who was 'unteachable', bullied and harassed at school and beaten for bad behaviour at home. Sometimes it was just advice that was needed. A woman brought in her sister because she talked and prayed too much and too loudly. But what was too much prayer in Haiti, and what was too loud? The sister was forbidding the woman to go to church. We suggested gently that if allowed to go to church, she might pray less at home. None of these patients had ever had the chance to get help before. Now there was somewhere to go.

And then there were the problems we could not solve. Four months after the earthquake the ER staff no longer rang us about post-operative confusion or distressed amputees. What came through the door was a direct result of the violence of people's daily lives. What should they do with a child with multiple abrasions, severely sexually abused, probably by the father who wanted to take her home? Or the child with a broken arm, when they were certain the mother was the abuser? UNICEF was working with the social services and the police to help them create a protection system, but in the meantime such children ended up going home.

Evangelina was referred to Kettie and me because she had taken an overdose. She did not live at home – she was a *restavek*. She had parents in a small impoverished village in the south and had been sent to the city to live with an 'aunt'.

This was a common system, where the child worked for free and in return was supposedly cared for and sent to school. The aunt had brought her in because she had taken a deliberate overdose of antibiotics.

Sitting in our tiny office, Evangelina told us the story in nervous, whispered fragments. She was thirteen. One day a boy in their shared courtyard had pulled her into his room and forced her to have sex. Although she had shouted no one came. She got pregnant. A girlfriend gave her a drink that caused an abortion. Then she got an infection and her aunt brought her to the hospital, where doctors had given her tablets. When she got home – now a canvas tent in the middle of the rubble-strewn courtyard – she decided to take all of them at once.

'And why did you take all the tablets?' we asked.

'I wanted to get better faster.'

'Were you thinking of hurting yourself in any way?'

'No, not at all!'

'Did you have any thoughts about dying or wishing to end things?' She shook her head vehemently.

'And where would you like to go now?'

She shrugged.

'If you go back to this family, what will happen?'

'They will beat me.'

'What about your own family?'

'I would like to go back to them.'

This seemed clear enough. And for once I thought I could help. There was an NGO that worked specifically on returning *restaveks* to their families. I said that I could arrange for someone to come and interview her to fix this. When I explained to the aunt that Evangelina wanted to go home to her parents, she looked very put out.

'She tells us nothing. She won't explain anything. I do everything I can to take care of her!'

'And you have done a great job, so now we really want to follow her wishes and it seems that she would like to go home.'

'Do you want to go home?' the aunt asked accusingly. Evangelina shook her head.

'I would like to stay with your family.'

'You see! She wants to stay with us!'

What I could see was that Evangelina looked terrified. I suggested she have a sleep while we waited for Rick from the NGO to come and clarify her wishes. We took Evangelina into the small, cluttered back office that had a bed in it.

Once she was alone, Kettie asked her again: 'Do you really want to go back to your aunt and uncle?'

She shook her head vehemently. 'But if I say no she will beat me. And if I go home I am afraid my mother will beat me for returning, and my father for going in the first place.'

We left her to sleep while I went to see the red-haired paralysed lady who was still in the hospital. I could see her moving one arm to arrange her clothes while I approached the bed, but when I examined her it was as floppy as before. When I got back, Rick had talked with Evangelina and made a plan for her to stay in their children's village while she decided what she wanted and they talked to her family. By now both uncle and aunt were at the hospital. They were very unhappy.

'We have responsibility for her,' said her uncle.

'Are you happy about what has happened to her in the last few months?' Kettie asked. 'While in your care she has been raped, got pregnant, had an abortion and been beaten, and she is only thirteen.'

'Not beaten by us – by my mother!' Aunt protested.

'But you were unable to protect her,' Kettie said.

'She never does what we say, she is always running off with bad people, we cannot control her.'

'That would suggest that her living there with you is not safe. Would you not like her to be in a safe place with other children until she can go back to her mother and father?' Evangelina looked happier than she had all afternoon and I had a small moment of hope, that for once we might be getting it right.

But a week later Rick told me that after crying for three nights Evangelina had asked to go back to her uncle and aunt. Of course, they let her. He was checking on her and she seemed all right.

Evangelina taught me that we still knew nothing. When humanitarians dream of changing the world they do so in their own language, without recognising their own limitations. Michael Barnett again. I thought I had listened to Evangelina and understood her needs, but the truth was I had simply increased her distress by exposing her to the impossibility of her situation. Rick had already explained that while UNICEF was keen to reunite families, there was no system to support those families so that they could take proper care of their returned children. Evangelina clearly missed her parents, but she knew they would probably beat her and send her back. So why not save herself grief and return to the 'uncle and aunt'? So much for interfering white women trying to rescue child slaves.

I made my last visit to Michael. There had been growing fights over land as the schools opened and empty spaces were reclaimed by the businesses that owned them. There were new camps, but not of the size required. George decided to move the whole family back to his father's house. I say 'house': it was actually a shell of a building with the red scribble indicating 'due for demolition'. But George had put a big white tent in the yard and furnished it with camp beds and kitchen stuff. Outside, only one wall remained standing in their street. Someone had sprayed 'Adieu Agathe, Michel, Pierre, Marie' onto it in bright-red paint. Next door a squashed car was visible beneath a collapsed floor. Michael's old home was now just a neatly stacked pile of rocks. His parents were buried in a small graveyard nearby. As in Aceh, the children liked being close to where they had lived before.

George had told me a couple of weeks earlier that one of the boys had been crying at night and asking for his mother. He had taken my suggestion of explaining simply what had happened, and he told the children she was in heaven. Then he had taken them to see their old home and they had climbed all over it. They were planning a large Catholic ceremony for everyone, when relatives came from the States. All three boys were back in school and doing well – a testament to what loving continuous care can do. George pulled out some photos and albums he had dug out from the ruins: portrait photos of the children, Michael with dreadlocks, a plastic folder of pictures of mother and father. Then we played with the puppets and told stories as usual. I had to go. George thanked me very formally and said how good it was that we had kept coming, when the government hadn't helped them at all.

It was time to leave. Peter was staying to help the new psychiatrist coming to replace me. We had mental health funding until the end of the year. But one donor was saying they could not continue funding the primary health care clinics beyond July. They regarded their job as restoring things to the status quo ante – that being the situation in which more than half the population had no access to any kind of health care. In this they were for once in harmony with the Haitian government. A Haitian ministry of health representative at the Jacmel cluster had recently asked when the free primary health care clinics, run by NGOs like ours, were going to pack up and go home, as they were depriving local private doctors of their incomes.

My country director wheeled me into a donor meeting to explain how, after a disaster, 'emergency' mental health (a) requires functioning primary health care and (b) takes a minimum of two years to achieve anything sustainable.

'Expect a tidal wave of depression next January,' I predicted gloomily, 'as people see they are still without shelter, jobs or security. You will need mental health services more than ever.'

I was pathologising the whole of Haiti in order to raise money for community mental health services; but calling for revolution and discussing ordinary Haitians' extraordinary courage and capacity to cope would not get funding. How stupid is that?

Pemba, Cabo Delgado, Mozambique, February 2013

First it was floods. In January our local tailor lost his nine-year-old son, drowned in a flash flood up the coast – unbearable. Further south it was worse, seven killed in Nampula, electrocuted when water swept them away. Roads were cut off, schools destroyed. Now it is fever: more deaths, rumours and violence follow as surely as bacilli grow in the dirty water that fills the ditches in the countryside; almost three hundred cholera cases in the local districts and two deaths in the last two weeks. A community leader was beaten to death in one district at the end of January, suspected of spreading the disease because he gave out information about it.

The problem is that in the eyes of local people in the countryside, health workers, public officials and NGO staff who try to educate about the disease are all seen as responsible for spreading cholera. Foreknowledge is a magical power. In one community, a leader was accused of spreading it by throwing powder in the air. He must have done, because shortly after his talk someone died of the illness. So he too was beaten up.

My agency is not immune, even in communities where it is well known, building home gardens, running nutrition programmes, providing education. Jane was out doing the food survey with a team of local investigators last week. All the proper procedures were followed: meetings with the community leaders in advance, explanations given, permissions granted, and the afternoon interviews went well. At night the group camped in the yard of the village chief, at his suggestion, and went to bed around 8 p.m. They were woken at 1.45 a.m. by a machete-wielding, torch-bearing crowd, threatening to attack them because they were suspected of bringing cholera into the village.

The group decided that staying in the compound was safer than trying to escape in their vehicle. The chief himself was nowhere to be seen – he was later discovered to be spending the night with his second wife – so they called the programme coordinators in Pemba to get the police to come and rescue them. They then sat tight for an uncomfortable two hours while the mob walked up and down the main road screaming and waving their clubs and machetes, insulting the group and threatening to set things on fire. Jane told me the worst thing was the sound of them actually sharpening the machetes on stones. The cavalry finally arrived, dispersed the crowd with shots in the air, got the team out and arrested all the perpetrators.

This week it was Macomia, the Makonde-speaking area up in the north of the province. Our district coordinator had already pointed out that it was really stupid for the agency to come into a village to do health-information training on diarrhoea and cholera, while at the same time providing food for those attending the training. The villagers immediately became suspicious and assumed the agency was trying to spread the disease through the food.

Some thirty people with suspected cholera are at the local hospital and at least five from one family are known to have died. The figures for the area are probably higher, as people don't want to take sick relatives to the health posts because they don't trust them. They don't trust any of the authorities. The agency is suspect because it built two water pumps in that particular neighbourhood two years ago. These are now broken and don't work. So local people use the faeces-infested river, which is thought to be one source of contamination. The fact that it is a local government responsibility to maintain the pumps is irrelevant. For the villagers we are all the same: outsiders or locals with power, privilege and information.

Things came to a head on Sunday morning when an angry group marched from the funeral of one of the dead family members to ask various local leaders where the cholera came from. One leader had fled, so the group broke down his doors, stole all his belongings and burnt down the house. A second leader was at home with his wife, who was head of the local women's committee. Both were confronted:

'Where does all the diarrhoea come from?'

'We don't know.'

Not a satisfactory answer. By now the crowd was in a rage, so they beat the couple up and burnt down their house as well. The police were called and arrested twelve, but not before they had burnt down four more houses, threatened our agency security guard, broken the hospital windows and started to march on the home of the district administrator. The beaten-up village leader is in a coma in hospital. Everything is suspect, even the bicycles we give to local health volunteers are accused of spreading cholera from one village to another. So our staff are all pulled back to Pemba and no one is allowed to work in these communities at the moment.

I think this reaction to cholera here in Mozambique is partly related to the recent news on the radio, that the UN will not pay compensation for its Nepalese peacekeepers having introduced cholera into Haiti six months after the earthquake. To date, almost eight thousand people have died in that country and almost one in every sixteen Haitians has been affected.

The facts in Haiti are not really in dispute. Cholera has not been present on the island for more than a century and full genome-sequencing has identified a strain of cholera that is present in Nepal. The UN has agreed that inadequate sanitation at its barracks in Mirebalais, sixty kilometres north-east of Port-au-Prince, might have been a source of the bacterium, but it claims immunity and blames a 'confluence of circumstances'. This argument adds up to: because you are poor and vulnerable and have almost no public health infrastructure, we are not to blame if we infect your water system with a lethal bug, and we are too powerful to sue.

And now the problem has come full circle. It is information, not the bacillus, that is infectious. Aid is now a globalised business with globalised risks. Local people in Mozambique listen to the radio and draw their own conclusions. Beware of strangers bearing gifts.

Asmamaw and I left Haiti four months before the cholera epidemic began. He had a place on a Masters course at Tufts

University in Massachusetts to study Humanitarian Assistance, and I had a writing fellowship at Harvard. For a year we filled our shelves with books whose titles – *Do No Harm*, *The Road to Hell*, *Condemned to Repeat* – told their own story. All challenged the modern humanitarian aid business: competing for 'market share' from government-associated donors with their own political agendas; 'scattering aid like confetti', to quote Linda Polman in her aptly named polemic *The Crisis Caravan: What's Wrong with Humanitarian Aid?*

David Rieff asked if humanitarianism was a waste of hope? I thought probably not, but I liked the confetti analogy. Perhaps the time had come to stop being a nomad and try to address what both Asmamaw and I felt was the fundamental emergency: poverty. So when a development agency offered me a position as early-child-development adviser in Mozambique, I took it.

The lovely thing about working on early child development is that it touches on everything. To raise a child well requires good health, nutrition, protection and love. I am expected to develop this holistic approach within the organisation. Asmamaw has also found a job here, with a small foundation on one of the islands off the coast, directing a nutrition programme. No cholera there – it is one of the places where I can work freely.

So we are back on a beach, renting a two-room cabin that overlooks thick banks of seaweed, rubbish and a murky sea full of plastic bottles, chewed-up rubber flip-flops and other filth. For weeks there has been rain and thunder every afternoon and a hot wind blowing through the house at night. But recently squads of bare-footed women have appeared with hoes and rakes, and buried all the seaweed and rubbish in trenches. Now the sky is blue, the wind has gone and the sea is clear and millpond-calm.

This beach is both highway and public park. Schoolchildren in uniform walk back and forth to town; small boys do back flips into the water, while older ones play football. The Chinese workers sit and drink at the Mar e Sol, and now and then swim earnest laps in the water. On Sundays in the early morning, groups from the evangelical churches stand in circles waist-deep in the water, clapping, praying, singing and baptising. Then half the town comes down to party. Music blares out from open stages and sleep is impossible. The trouble is, it should still be raining. Now the talk in the countryside is of crop failure, poor harvests and real hunger coming.

11: THEM AND US

Ibo, Cabo Delgado, Mozambique, 2013

If I were a scriptwriter I would set a movie here, starting with my hero wandering down the sand-filled Rua da República between the crumbling houses, all abandoned by the Portuguese when Mozambique became independent in 1975.

He stops to talk to a family who have set up home in the ruined rooms and are sprawling in the deep shade of a pillared veranda. Dogs and cats doze in the dust of the main street, small boys play marbles on the smooth concrete base of the Monument to Workers.

He reaches the main square: there are benches between beds of succulents, beneath shady trees. The large and elegant governor's residence on one side is now a health centre. There is also a school, and the white-painted eighteenth-century church. But the square is entirely empty. There is nowhere to go and nothing to do, so he continues on to the jetty, where I can put him on a dhow. And with help from his friends he unfurls the graceful sail. It is late afternoon with an offshore wind, so the sail billows between the perfect triangle made by the lines of boom and boat, and catches the rose-coloured light. The sea is where life is: children playing in the shallows, men with outrigger canoes, other men with dhows, women searching for crabs. *Mwani* means 'people of the beach', and that is what these people are. Arabs, Indians and Portuguese have come and gone, traded in slaves and spices, built forts, churches, graveyards. All are now abandoned, while the people here still live as they have been doing for five hundred years.

Well, now I'm stuck because I feel I need a storyline as

opposed to just a scene, and while the views are beautiful, the stories are the old, sad ones.

I know by now that the young man in the dhow is charming and handsome, and went to the school on the edge of the square. He speaks the local language, Kimwani, as well as Portuguese and English. He works in one of the guest houses, running the bar. And he has a girlfriend and she has a baby and is pregnant with another. She is sixteen now, but she got pregnant at thirteen and dropped out of school. She speaks only Kimwani and is unable to read or write. She studied four years in school, but the teachers only cared whether she could copy correctly and never bothered to find out if she understood.

She and her baby still live with her mother in a small house made of coral and mud on the edge of the town, as her boyfriend has not yet built her the house he promised. Nor has he married her and given her the TV, promised along with the house, when she first agreed to have sex with him. He has told her he wants to look for work in Pemba and she can come there when he finds it. If they do marry, the girl believes, the boy has the right to beat her if she does not do what he wishes. Her mother has taught her the rules of marriage: to wash clothes, sweep, collect water and firewood, cook, wash up and be available to her husband whenever he wants. Her biggest fear is that he will abandon her for a younger girl when she is in her twenties, with five or six children, just as her father abandoned her mother.

Her mother is thirty-five and has ten children by three different men; the youngest is three years old. The mother and daughter survive by growing maize and cassava on a very small plot of land on the island, and by fishing from the shore, using the bed nets handed out by the health centre. These are meant to protect children from malaria. The women stretch the net between them as they walk fully dressed through the waist-high water at low tide. A younger daughter follows with a basket on her head. Every so often they stretch the net flat to see what is caught. It's just a few tiny fish, which they throw in the basket. If they are lucky they may eat twice a day, but sometimes they go two days without eating. The sadness of this situation is that, try as I might, while I really want it to be the young woman wandering down the street and getting on the dhow, with the sail unfurling in the sunset, I cannot imagine her doing so.

So I will make that younger sister twelve. She too goes to the school on the edge of the square, and she wears a white blouse with short sleeves and a navy skirt, very like my own school uniform when I was a child. The shirt is already tight over young breasts. She has not noticed. She wants to be an electrician. She saw a woman electrician for the first time when they brought electricity to Ibo a few months ago. The woman wore a hard hat and overalls and climbed a pole, and she was beautiful. The men treated her like a man. The girl would love to be like that, so she studies hard. She does not want babies like her sister.

The trouble is, her teacher keeps coming up to her after class and talking to her and asking her if she would 'like to love him'. He has twice followed her home asking her to have sex. She says no and runs away, but the other girls say she is stupid. He will fail her in her exams.

I am too angry to continue this story as it does not have a happy ending.

'What's to be done?' I asked Ronaldo, my translator, how we could help the lovely group of uniformed schoolgirls who had been telling me about their lives and complaining of the constant sexual harassment they suffered from their schoolteachers.

'Nothing,' he replied, 'the teacher goes to the family and says, "Don't report me! I will marry your daughter and pay." The family is poor so they prefer that solution.'

'And then the daughter has a baby and the teacher abandons her and moves on?'

'That's about it.'

'So the girls go to school to lift themselves out of poverty, but because they are harassed, they drop out and remain illiterate, which keeps them poor, which means they and their daughters will continue to be harassed and illiterate, and round and round it goes.'

We were drinking at the bar at Miti Mwini, an eco guest house constructed entirely out of local materials from the ruins of an old mansion. There were no schoolgirls here, only the new invaders: intrepid tourists pleased with themselves for having got this far off the map; NGO staff like ourselves – the lady from the World Wildlife Fund who was full of praise for her local partner NGO for burning those mosquito nets when local people used them for fishing: 'Mosquito nets are too fine,' she said. 'They scoop up everything! It's brutal to burn them but it is the only way to get local people to understand.'

The WWF helped run the national park. We were surrounded by mangrove swamps beyond which whales and dolphins danced in azure seas, but it was under threat. Natural gas had been discovered off the coast, fifteen miles from the Quirimbas Islands. Mozambique had access to more potential oil wealth than Saudi Arabia. 'Development' was coming. I already paid more to rent a cabin on the beach in Pemba than I got for renting out my flat in Cambridge. It could only be a matter of time before the bar was full of oilmen, and all the mansions on Rua da República were restored and replastered.

'There will soon be art galleries selling local crafts and chichi little restaurants doing perfect fish in coconut sauce; small boutiques will sell designer beach bags,' I told Ronaldo. 'Don't worry, it will all be very tasteful, all contributing to the local economy by employing local people as guards, cooks, cleaners and maids. So maybe my schoolgirls will get nice jobs like that. It's a step up from subsistence fishing with mosquito nets.'

Ronaldo shook his head and smiled. He was getting used to me.

We crossed to the island of Querambo at 5 a.m. to catch the tide. Roberto, the local education facilitator, came with us, bringing a heavy sack of beans to celebrate the opening of the pre-school. Two men from the village came to greet the boat and take the sack, then the very pregnant pre-school volunteer teacher joined us, carrying an infant on her back. The men handed her the sack, which she placed on her head, uncomplaining, and we all walked up to the village on the sandy paths between the dunes and mangroves. The tide was retreating, leaving bare mud and scuttling fiddler crabs.

'What are you photographing?' Ronaldo asked. I showed him my picture of three strapping men walking ahead, followed by the pregnant teacher with the infant on her back and the bean sack on her head.

'Does anything about this picture bother you?' I asked. Ronaldo grinned and looked at me knowingly. And note, I didn't take the sack myself. It was hot, I didn't know how to carry large sacks of beans on my head, I didn't want to cause a scene when I was a guest. These were my excuses.

The village houses were constructed of coral, mud and thatch around a wide-open rectangular space. Each had a bamboo-fenced compound. In some, men sprawled, sleeping in the deep shade of the roof, while women pounded cassava and children played everywhere. If you were less than ten this life could be idyllic. There were fish, coconuts and rice, innumerable playmates, very few dangers, and you were surrounded by a community of families and neighbours to watch over you.

But then I visited an eighteen-year-old single mother of two who thought she might be going blind and whose baby had intermittent diarrhoea. She had visited the health centre but they had not solved the problem, nor referred her to Pemba for investigations. She planned to visit the local healer. She went to him before when her other child was feverish. He cured it with drink, massage and an amulet. Now she sat on a torn mat in her compound in the shade of a straw roof, breast-feeding one child while the other played with a coconut shell, banging it down on the sand. She looked far too thin. There was a neat cane fence but no dried corn, no pots or pans. She explained that she got married before she menstruated. She had no idea how one gets pregnant. The two babies came but her husband drank, and beat her badly so she divorced him; so now she was alone with no one to help her, and miserable because of that.

At least she had left her abusive husband.

Another woman on the island told me that if a husband beat a woman it was her responsibility: 'Don't abandon him because he tries to correct you. You made a mistake. It is a normal thing to beat a wife. I accept it because he is trying to correct me. My husband never beats me because I have not made a mistake.'

We were at the end of two months' travelling around Cabo Delgado, the northernmost and poorest province of Mozambique, asking women how they raised their children and what were their main concerns. Oddly, although the agency had embarked on training mothers in child-rearing, they had not actually asked the mothers themselves how they did it. I had been given permission to address this deficiency. But asking mothers 'What problems do you face while trying to raise your babies?' had worried Francisco, one of my colleagues.

'If you ask this question you will create expectations.'

'But I can't not ask them. We can't just arrive with a programme to assist early child development without asking first how they do it and what their own priorities are.'

'I understand, but asking them will mean we are going to address those problems.'

'So we have to fully explain ourselves, what we can and cannot do. Doesn't driving into the village in a large white vehicle create expectations from the start?'

We had a similar argument about 'refreshments'.

'You cannot give them a drink!' Francisco expostulated, when I asked the price of a bottle of Fanta.

'But we will be interviewing or having group discussions for at least two hours and they'll be thirsty, I'll be thirsty – how can we not offer them a drink?'

'You will mess up every other meeting we have in the same community. Every time we meet with someone they will expect a drink!'

'So when you do a training you don't provide refreshments?'

'If the training lasts more than six hours.'

'So yet again we waltz in and ask people to give us their time,

explain their lives and give nothing in return. They are the pro-
viders here, we are the beneficiaries. We need this knowledge.
It is not the same as if you go in and hold a meeting about how
to organise a home garden, or look after cows. Then you are
doing something for *them*.'

'This difference won't be clear to the villagers. They will see
us meeting and giving drinks and assume next time we come
we will give drinks to them, for whatever reason we meet.'

'So we can explain why we give drinks at one meeting, but
not at another?'

'They won't understand and it will damage our relations
with the villagers, it will make it harder to work because we
will create these expectations.'

'That's a bit patronising, don't you think? The villagers are
too stupid to understand the difference between different kinds
of meetings, and they are so demanding that if we give some a
bottle of juice because they were kind enough to talk to us for
two hours, everyone will want one.'

'They will, I promise you! Don't you think you should learn
how we do things first before you criticise and try to change
us?'

Fair point. I backed down. It was Francisco's country. I admired him. He was from the south, had to live away from his
own family to do this job, worked long hours and had been
with the agency for a number of years. And when he came to
the first group meeting, he relented. Perhaps it was listening to
a group of older women castigate their lazy menfolk for stealing their *kaplanas* (the soft cotton wraps they wore as skirts)
to fund their drinking habits, and telling us: 'You have to live
with a man to survive, but they are not useful for anything.' Or
maybe it was hearing them explain that 'development' was to
blame for the increasing number of child marriages. 'Development' meant older men had more money, and they spent it on
tempting younger girls to have sex: 'The girls might not want
to, but a man shows money to the young girl and she is attract-
ed.' While 'democracy' meant there was no way to stop young
girls going to the local 'cinema' (meaning a hut with a DVD

player) and getting into trouble. 'Girls say "We are free." There is a lot of freedom now. Even if you beat them you cannot stop them.'

Not all the mothers thought child marriage was bad, though: one told us she would be happy if her daughter got pregnant at twelve. And the girls themselves explained to me that it was a matter of survival. A good boyfriend paid for soap and underwear, and hospital if you were sick. After a day of listening to these discussions, Francisco allowed me to buy refreshments.

The young mother on Querambo took the offered *refrêsco* and immediately gave it to her three-year-old. We returned to the head man's compound. He sat us both down in the shade, thanked us courteously for coming to learn from his community, and handed Ronaldo and me fresh coconuts, opened, for us to drink the juice.

I had hoped that by shifting from emergencies to development I could get rid of the feeling of 'us' and 'them' that I had felt so strongly in Haiti, but if anything it was more entrenched. *Us* being the 'professionals', both Mozambicans and internationals, who had jobs. *Them* being the beneficiaries, the subsistence farmers on whose behalf we were working but whom we were so wary to consult. We sat in our offices in Pemba, designed programmes and budgets, wrote grant proposals and reports, and then sallied forth in our four-wheel drives to the villages scattered through the forest that stretched in every direction, to do trainings and supervise. Sometimes the sessions were delivered in Portuguese so that half the women in the room, who spoke only the local language, fell asleep. Sometimes we might be the only car that had passed that way in twenty-four hours. Health centres were often twenty-five kilometres distant. But we didn't give lifts unless it was a medical emergency. After all, we were a development agency, not a bus service.

Between us and them, there were others. These were the local coordinators and facilitators, all graduates in health, education or agriculture, who lived in the villages, spoke the local languages and ran the programmes on the ground. And their work depended completely on another group without whom the whole enterprise would collapse: the 'community activists' and 'volunteers' who were supposed to actually implement those plans we wrote in our offices.

Take the pre-school programme. It had funding for pre-schools and playgrounds to be built. We visited some in my first days in the country. In each small village we found a newly built pre-school with cane walls and a thatched roof, swings and climbing frames outside. In some, delightful infants in smocks sang songs, played games and learnt their alphabets. But many were empty. The facilitators accompanying us lamented: the volunteer teachers were all subsistence farmers, they explained, who worked every day with hand-held hoes in the hot sun to feed their families. How could the facilitators insist they put this work aside and run the pre-school for free? The programme could not work without incentives, but none were provided, so many of the pre-schools went unused.

I tried discussing this issue a few weeks later. We were brainstorming how to respond to a 'call' from the World Bank. They would be dishing out large sums of money for nutrition programmes. The government would get the money and would be looking for partners to do the work. My agency was in with a chance. We were told to ready ourselves. I was invited to a discussion, to consider a psychosocial component for the project.

Twenty of us crowded into a small meeting room. We had a technical expert visiting from Geneva and our senior health adviser had flown up especially from Maputo, to present the ministry view. The plan appeared to involve at least four levels of paid government bureaucrat. But the actual job of helping mothers in the community towards a better grasp of nutrition and child development, and better-fed babies, ultimately depended on an NGO partner, hopefully us, training volunteer community activists to train the mothers.

'These would be the same community activists we train to run pre-schools or to do health education, and who already work approximately eight hours a week for nothing, trekking all over their communities, giving up time from their subsistence farms, without a bicycle to ride or a T-shirt to say who they are?'

The health adviser nodded.

'Where will they find the time for this additional work?'

Silence.

'Why can't they be paid for it?'

'How would the pay be sustained? We would create an expectation . . .'

'So here we are again. Well-paid, well-suited government bureaucrats and NGO staff living happy lives on beaches (me) will drive into some of the poorest communities in the world and ask subsistence farmers to volunteer to improve the lives of their neighbours for nothing. And if they say, "Please could I be paid?", we reply, "Well, even if we could find a short-term salary from some donor, there's no guarantee that we could sustain it. So you would get something at the start but it might not continue, and that would – apparently – be worse than not getting anything at all. And what we are really trying to create here is a Republic of Virtue, where we are paid good salaries and given big cars to come and train you to work for nothing at all."'

I knew I was being over-emotional. This outburst was met with another silence.

'Well, we could ask the community to think how they could compensate the volunteers,' someone said. 'People used to volunteer all the time, under socialism.'

'Great! the cooperative Communist dream, except the government here gave up on socialism a while back, and you may have noticed that right now they are all into private enterprise and individual profit and making money from natural gas off the Quirimbas. If they want village cooperatives again, perhaps they should come and join them and model free cooperative labour themselves.'

'Look,' said our senior adviser, 'the Ministry of Health says "Don't pay volunteers"!'

'Yes, and many NGOs simply lie and say they don't, but then they do and then people won't work with us,' Angelo interjected. He was the local health coordinator, a doctor who shared some of my concerns.

'Well, I'm on the side of the liars. Except I think all the NGOs should get together and confront the government on the exploitation of the poorest members of their community. Volunteering happens when you have enough and you want to share and give back, not when you have nothing and are struggling to survive. And can someone tell me why a professional job like pre-school teaching should be done as a voluntary favour? So the school is closed when the infants arrive, because the teacher is unpaid and has to pick mangoes today. I don't think we should be applying for funding that locks us into exploiting people in this way. At home in Britain, my sister-in-law is a professional pre-school teacher, and gets a salary.'

'But if you do give them money they will just drink it! If we give them anything it should be something they need and is worthwhile,' someone else chips in.

'Absolutely. The feckless and ignorant poor, what can we do with them? Certainly we cannot risk giving them cash!'

I knew it was time I shut up. I did, and the discussion progressed as if I hadn't spoken. If there's one golden rule for most NGOs, it's run after the money or die.

Jenny, the visitor from Geneva, came to find me after the meeting. She understood how I felt but did not see how the situation could be changed. She told me a story. She was running a mobile clinic somewhere in East Africa. It was the usual thing, dispensing drugs and advice from the back of a Toyota. They spent the afternoon in a remote community and then packed up to go. The car was running, ready to leave, and as Jenny walked towards it she noticed a woman standing at the back and holding a tiny baby directly into the filthy stream of exhaust, so the baby had no choice but to breathe in the fumes. Jenny rushed over, yelling at the mother, and pulled her and the baby away from the car.

'Don't you realise you can kill her?' The baby was spluttering, crying and coughing, Jenny was praying that not too much damage had been done. The mother turned on her in fury.

'Why are you trying to stop me! You drive here in your big car and we have nothing, and now you won't even let me take the good stuff that comes out of the back of the car for my baby.'

Fortunately, I was mostly out of the office. The cholera epidemic had confined our community work to the northern districts including Ibo, where I had no need of a car. I was dependent on the tides, and either walked to work through the mangrove swamps or caught a boat.

And in spite of all the hassles, I loved the work. It felt like getting back to basics. We know by now that the relationship between a parent and their baby is one of the fundamental building-blocks upon which good mental and physical health depends throughout a person's life. Babies who have loving and stimulating relationships with their parents will be better nourished, healthier, learn better in school and cope much better with stresses and losses in later life than babies who don't. This isn't just rhetoric. I have sat in therapeutic feeding centres in East Africa with listless babies who don't feed and won't cry because they have given up trying to get attention from their exhausted, unhappy mothers; and I have watched the transformative effect of very simple programmes that just get mothers to talk to and play with and show love to their infants for a short time every day.

Many of the younger mothers I talked to here in my first months saw love as something to be expressed through buying things, and play as a luxury for which they had no time. So I helped the facilitators in setting up and running their own mother and baby groups to try and change those views. This month I was helping Roberto and sat with him as the mothers came into the yard with their children on their backs. One was carrying the water container and soap. 'Wash your hands and save your life' was our motto of the moment, and every group began with hand-washing. The previous week we had discussed how to promote a baby's physical development. It was a topic on which most of them were expert, particularly when it came to baby massage. One mother demonstrated: holding her four-month-old baby by her legs, throwing her in the air, rolling her against her own outstretched legs, pulling back both arms. The baby was ecstatic and it ended with a hug and a kiss.

This week we were discussing 'what to do if your child is sick'. Some mothers thought the traditional healer was best. One explained that her seven-month-old got red eyes because of the *Namachula*, a mysterious bird that flew around at night but that no one could see. But another said, 'When your baby is sick like this you must always take her to the health centre.' Roberto was skilled at letting the mothers discuss among themselves and then reinforcing the messages he wanted to get across: 'Take the child to the health centre if they are unwell in any way.'

For brief periods in the mother and baby groups, my sense of us and them almost dissolved. The mothers treated me as a welcome guest and were eager to show and share with me what they knew, and curious for new information. It was easy here to challenge false beliefs because there were usually at least one or two mothers who knew better. So when one young mother said babies are blind and deaf in the first month of life, another sang to her very new baby and the baby turned her head to watch and listen. And when another one said you need to put a key in a baby's mouth and turn it if the child is slow to speak, it was an older mother who explained why that might be dangerous.

But I had to go back to Pemba. There were reports to write and finances to organise. The agency vehicle dropped me off at our home. Three men and a plump, well-dressed woman and baby were sitting on the beach next to my veranda. 'Boa tarde,' they called, and waved. I smiled and greeted them back: 'Boa Tarde.' I opened my front door, put down my things, then turned to find that the woman had followed me inside and was thrusting the very fat baby in my face, holding it uncomfortably under its arms.

'Feed my baby! Give me money!'

I was startled and alarmed, wondering if the men would follow her in. I had no guard and there was no one else around. 'Please go!' I said, 'you cannot come in here!' I knew I looked and sounded angry, and she turned and stomped out, roaring with laughter and calling out to her friends something about the mean *muzungu* ('white person').

Perhaps they had dared her. Pemba was full of well-fed Mozambicans who worked for the oil companies, wore dark glasses, drove pick-ups, partied and drank on the beach at the weekends. They were never hassled, as far as I could see – the supplicants had learnt they would get a sharp dismissal. But my white skin marked me out as an obvious target. I was not a stranger to be made welcome in the country, or an object of curiosity to be questioned as to where I had come from, either of which would have been fine. I was a *muzungu*, therefore I must have surplus wealth to give away, and so the only reason for connecting with me was to get a share.

I have never worked out how to cope with begging. In Cambridge, I simply carried sufficient change in my pocket to give without question to every homeless person I met on the street. I didn't care what they spent it on. It was not for me to decide. But the requests were sufficiently infrequent to make that strategy possible. Here in the poorest part of Mozambique the needs were limitless, and at what point do you stop giving when everyone asks? Walking on the beach alone I learnt to keep my eyes down and not return greetings, because they were always followed by an outstretched hand. The most curious thing was that the very poorest didn't beg: the raggedly dressed women and their straggling lines of dirty children that scrabbled for shrimps and crabs at low tide never asked me for anything, and always smiled and said 'Salama'. It was the plumper, slightly better-off, better-dressed, with shoes and language, who had the confidence to assert themselves.

So what to do? Not giving to the plump woman held a mirror up as to what it meant when I said I was an 'aid worker'. In my head I was already sharing what I had: my noble ideas about working with her rural sisters to promote better childcare, better brain development, children better able to learn, quicker to be literate, staying longer in school, breaking the whole cycle of deprivation.

I took on board all those 'Give a man a fish and you feed him for a day, teach him to fish and you feed him for life' posters of my childhood. Except the waters were fished out a while ago, and the man – or woman – was saying, 'Give me the money and I, not you, will decide if I spend it on fishing lines, or cigarettes, or second wives, or food for my children.' I saw my life as 'simple'. But there was no sign on the veranda of my nice pink *casita* saying, 'Aid worker – don't touch – she has already taken a salary cut, and pays half what she earns in rent to live here, because the oil boom has driven prices through the roof.' What the people on the beach saw was a 'millionaire' who could afford to pay a cleaner and carried a computer bag, and who got picked up for work in a four-wheel drive.

And how to get round this? My education, my job, my freedom to travel and my relative security rest in part on a history of despoliation, slavery and extraction from this continent, and in part on chance. Where are the rules written in the universe that make me entitled, and that woman and her baby not? Nowhere.

The aid business has turned aid into a profession and a career for thousands. The argument is that if you do not create the living conditions that will attract professionals, along with access to leave, schooling, recreation, etc. etc., you will not get the professionals who will do it correctly. But partnership rests on real equality. In emergencies I can see some justification for bringing in outsiders at some expense, as we have to act quickly, and local people are dead or busy with their own affairs. Here in Mozambique we were still replicating the colonial structures that impoverished these countries in the first place. No amount of critical studies of humanitarianism has changed this.

Perhaps the only truly ethical way to help another person is to first of all put yourself in a position of equality with them, but if you do that, the little voices in my head mumble, how will you command the financial resources to create the programmes – school, health care or whatever – to assist them?

Asmamaw's tiny agency offered a possible answer. I envied him. He had found a job on Ibo with a small NGO, as the director of their nutrition programme. In many ways its ambitions were similar to those of my own agency: improving health and nutrition, helping with education, agricultural production and income generation. But in other respects it was entirely different. His NGO concentrated on doing as much as possible in one community rather than dispersing its energies across an entire province. Whilst I spent days and weeks sorting out poorly organised logistics, and travelling vast distances into communities where I might appear just once, like an alien from outer space never to be seen again, Asmamaw walked everywhere and was familiar with every small village on the island. He too depended on volunteers, but these were high-school students eager to learn how to teach, and they were recompensed with computer classes in the evening.

At his community centre women were taught good maternal and child health and how to prepare nutritious meals. In the nursery garden they were taught to take care of vegetables that they could also grow at home. The nursery sold its produce to the guest houses and restaurants. Asmamaw introduced a scheme whereby the women who did the selling got 10 per cent of the profit, the rest going back into the enterprise. There was also vocational training for electricians and carpenters and in IT. The teachers were local professionals who received a small stipend for the extra hours they worked. There was a shop where islanders sold local crafts and tailoring, and plans for a school of tourism. International volunteers came for substantial periods to help with different aspects of the programme. Asmamaw's compensation was a small salary and shared housing. A low-key egalitarianism permeated the whole enterprise. I wondered if we could replicate it.

In my last week in the country I got a kind of answer. Back on Ibo, Roberto was passing on what he had learnt from me.

The health activists had come from all over the province to be trained by both of us in early child development and how to run mother and baby groups. My hope was that he would be able to sustain this part of the programme after I left. After lectures on the first evening I handed out their per diems: 150 meticash for accommodation, plus 100 for an evening meal: 250 (eight dollars) in total, not including their transport money.

Rosa, a health activist from Querambo, looked at the notes in disgust: 'It's not enough.'

'I agree with you, but I can only give out the money I am given and these *are* the rules, everyone gets the same.'

'You know we do this work for nothing! We don't get paid anything!'

'Yes, I know.' I felt deeply ashamed.

After I had dished out the paltry sums and received further disgusted looks from seven more disgruntled activists, the facilitators (who as 'staff' got 400 a day) warned me that people would probably not be very enthusiastic the next day. Then I went to Miti Mwini, the guest house where the staff from the Pemba educational team and two visitors from the Geneva office were dining. Dinner cost 500 per head, so definitely no activists eating here. I wanted to check I had the amounts correct. Yes, I had, I was told over crab salad and chocolate tart. But Roberto had told me that the cheapest accommodation cost 300 minimum. I was glad the Geneva people were buying him dinner.

I rang Angelo to say we had to increase the per diems. He agreed, but wanted an explanatory email. So I sat up late to write it, arguing that the food money was insufficient and that as the accommodation money was pathetic, the activists were all sleeping on mats on the floor at the local office. My agency was very hierarchical: internationals and Pemba office staff stayed in posh B-and-Bs, facilitators (field-based) in office guest rooms, volunteer activists slept 'in the community' – otherwise translated as on someone's floor, if their own 'community' happened to be somewhere else. I was still sharing Asmamaw's room in his guest house.

When I arrived the next morning, I found a note scrawled in biro on a torn-off sheet of paper from one of the notepads given out in the training packs. It said quite simply: 'The activists want to be given their transport money, as the per diem is too little, and they are going home.'

I was impressed. I rang Angelo again and told him the activists were on strike and I might have to abandon the training. Within an unprecedented mere four hours he called me back, when I was in the middle of a discussion on how to teach children moral values and the rights and wrongs of beating. We had just reached agreement that children should be loved, and that they should also understand the consequences of their actions. I was given permission from the office to book somewhere for the activists to sleep, and claim the money back. I could also make a reasonable increase in their food allowance, so I immediately doubled it, enough for a full meal, even if not at the Miti Mwini.

But the activists were having none of it. They wanted money in their hands. They would book their own accommodation. I called the agency again. To my amazement, I was given permission to give them cash: 300 meticash each for accommodation. This was what it was all about. They would continue to sleep on floors to save as much accommodation money as they could for their families. So a small victory for non-violent collective solidarity.

But Asmamaw listened to my phone calls and sighed. 'When will you humanitarians understand the damage you do by not paying people properly for their work, and offering incentives for training instead?' He was right. We were cheating the poorest people in the world into working for nothing, something none of us did, and then when they turned up for a lecture, we 'rewarded' them with money for bed and a meal, so they didn't care what the topic was, just how much they would get for being there.

After the course was finished I went home to Asmamaw's guest house and sat on the small porch facing a dusty garden, where hummingbirds and hoopoes jumped about among the coffee bushes and the small vegetable patch he had planted. Pedro, who had come as a volunteer from Spain to teach carpentry, sat smoking. Asmamaw was cooking shrimp. There were two cats and a small boy waiting for their share, along with a couple of others who turned up whenever we cooked. Pedro's attitude was if you have food, share it with whoever comes for dinner. Rather than saying no to anyone because you cannot give to everyone, you do what you can with what you have. When you run out, you run out, and that's it.

Tacloban, Philippines, January 2014

'Have you ever held a substantive consultant post, Dr Jones?'

The questioner was a representative of the Royal College of Psychiatrists. He and five other people, none of whom I could see, were sitting in a committee room in the United Kingdom. I was sitting in our beach house in Mozambique, wrapped in a *kaplana*, being interviewed over Skype audio. The needs of an ageing parent meant we had to leave Mozambique and return to Britain. So I had applied for a consultant job in the NHS.

'Umm . . . actually no.'

The familiar tight silence. I felt as if I was back in the Allinton boardroom.

'Erm . . . I have set up and run mental health services in places that have never had a psychiatrist before.'

The service user chipped in with a friendly voice: 'Can you sum up your attitude to mental health services in four words or less?'

'Patients come first,' I replied without thinking. They gave me the job.

Six weeks after I begin, Typhoon Haiyan hits the west coast of the Philippines and my old agency asks if I am available to go and help with the mental health response. To my astonishment my boss gives me two months' unpaid leave. So once again I'm sitting in a packed psychosocial cluster meeting, making notes as the agencies introduce themselves and explain how they plan to help. My list reads: trauma healing; training teachers to work with traumatised children; trauma support for teachers; teaching doctors how to take care of their own traumatisation when they talk to others about trauma; training trainers on how to work with grief; identifying and working with children who have lost parents; 'ventilation groups' for people with disabilities (but not including the intellectually disabled) and stress debriefing . . .

Stress debriefing is very popular. At an earlier cluster meeting an official from the regional department of health announced that she wanted every affected family 'debriefed' in the next three months. It is called 'psychosocial processing' in the

Philippines. Health departments in every stricken municipality have deployed teams of volunteer 'processors', who gather people into groups and encourage them to tell their stories and ventilate and process their emotions. This is actually 'critical incident stress debriefing' by another name, and there are now clear WHO guidelines saying that this should *not* be done for everyone in the aftermath of a disaster, because at best it does nothing and at worst there is some evidence of harm.

Some of the 'processing' volunteers at one of the evacuation centres complained to a colleague that they were failing, because the people affected just did not want to get into groups and talk about what had happened, or ventilate any feelings. Filipinos don't want debriefing. They want tarpaulin for shelter, cash, food, or a flight out.

In my first weeks in the Philippines I asked our own staff to list the three things that had helped them most when something terrible happened in their lives. They all wrote down similar things: being with family; getting practical help, like someone taking care of their children or cooking meals; having friends and colleagues who could provide a comforting shoulder to lean on, who could advise, encourage them to restart their lives and give financial support. These were the most important, followed by being able to pray, to do something altruistic, being diverted, entertained, or distracted. No one listed talking to a counsellor, or getting debriefed.

I once went to a talk by a Glaswegian psychiatrist who had gone down to Lockerbie a year or so after the plane fell out of the sky. He systematically asked people what had helped most in the immediate aftermath. And despite the fact that the town was flooded with counsellors who had rushed in to do debriefing, the most helpful intervention was apparently the Salvation Army van, handing out cups of tea, a chat and a familiar shoulder to weep on.

All of us know how to help others after a disaster: comfort them, make them safe, help them get the basic things they need, listen if they want to chat – but not force them to do so – and connect them with others. There is now a manual saying all this. It's called *Psychological First Aid*. My worry is that, by manualising this common-sense approach, we are undermining people's trust in their own empathic responses. We have again created a technology that people think they cannot deliver unless they are trained, rather than empowering people to do what seems natural and right in helping others in distress.

The cluster meeting continues after the introductions. A woman stands up. She apologises for having no mental health knowledge or experience. She has come to this cluster meeting to ask for help. She manages an evacuation centre where they have a woman who has gone mad: the woman is grandiose, excitable, talking all the time, disoriented, overactive. They have taken her to the acute mental health unit where there are only two beds because the rest were washed away, but she was refused admission because she has no care-giver. The Department of Social Welfare have also said they can't help. The camp management don't want to leave the woman unattended because she says she has been raped and continues to be at risk.

'What should we do?' the woman asks. Silence. None of the trauma healers have anything to offer. My agency is running a programme for patients with severe mental disorders, but we are based two hours to the south. As she sits down three more people come in, all dressed in smart red waistcoats, the kind with lots of useful pockets for pens and torches and emergency bits of string.

'Would you like to introduce yourselves?' the very friendly Filipino cluster leader asks.

'We are from the People's Republic of China,' a tall man replies. 'We have come to do crisis counselling.'

Why, two months after the disaster, is the humanitarian community still unable to treat, or protect, a psychotic woman from being raped? What is it about 'trauma' that continues to exert such a pull and fascination in a humanitarian crisis that every NGO and its baby cousin wants to treat it, while at the same time anything remotely resembling real madness is regarded like bubonic plague?

12: THE WAY WE LIVE NOW

Ethiopia, 2015

I am still asking this question two years later, while running a ten-day course on 'Mental Health in Complex Emergencies in Ethiopia'. One of my colleagues has just received a phone call from a local NGO in Serbia working with the influx of refugees from Syria. They want training materials on trauma counselling.

In fact our teaching on traumatic stress has got better. Research continues to show that the most traumatising experiences are those close to home – prolonged torture, and physical and sexual abuse – and that most people in the aftermath of conflict and disaster are resilient. When I went back to Bosnia in 2012 to follow up some of the war-affected children I had studied twenty years earlier, all of them were doing well, even those who had clearly suffered PTSD immediately after the war.

In 2011 I was invited to join a working group to prepare new definitions of stress disorders for the forthcoming eleventh edition of the *International Classification of Diseases* (*ICD 11*). One outcome was the removal from the pathological disorder categories of 'Acute Stress Reaction', in its numerous emotional, behavioural, cognitive and physical manifestations, and its reclassification as a 'non-pathological response to an exceptional stressor that may require therapeutic intervention'. This means that doctors will be able to look it up in *ICD 11* and see that it's not a disease, but that sufferers may need assistance. A small victory for common sense. It means that fainting girls, or those with earthquake shock or tsunami distress or all those children in the Philippines who cried and hid under the bed when the weather was stormy, no longer need to be given a pathological diagnosis if their symptoms are not prolonged. They can be told these are normal reactions to abnormal events and given advice on the simple measures that will help recovery. I think Dr Henry Wilson would be pleased.

There are recommendations that PTSD should be much more tightly defined in *ICD 11*. Non-specific symptoms have been removed, and a person must have been exposed to an event of an extremely threatening or horrific nature; after which they should be 'experiencing the three core elements' to receive the diagnosis. These continue to be: re-experiencing the traumatic event, that is, not only remembering it but experiencing it as occurring again; avoidance of reminders likely to produce such re-experiencing; and a perception of heightened current threat resulting in increased arousal, all of which should limit the individual's ability to function. Simply becoming distressed after exposure to a traumatic event is no longer enough.

But the stigma that surrounds and obscures severe mental disorders continues to be lethal. Here in Ethiopia people with severe mental illnesses are twice as likely to die as those in the general population. They are also likely to die three decades earlier. Peter, head of mental health for UNHCR, teaches the students about the *mhGAP Intervention Guide*, brought out by WHO five years ago as part of a global programme to address the gap in mental health services. It is one of the tools for training district medical officers and primary health care physicians.

I know it works. After Typhoon Haiyan, I used it to train general practitioners in the Philippines. There I accompanied Dr L., one of the trainees, on a visit to a girl who had spent much of the last five years either wandering the neighbourhood, naked, shouting and giggling, and asking for sex, or at home silent, weeping and immovable. When we called, she was lying on a wooden platform in a cardboard shelter attached to a half-destroyed cane house, one side open to the elements. She had deteriorated since her sister had been killed by falling debris in the typhoon. Father was a fisherman, they had no money to go to hospital or buy medicine. She had never been treated. After our visit Dr L. and I sat in the clinic with the *mhGAP Intervention Guide*, and even though we hadn't yet discussed psychosis or bipolar disorder in the training, he was able to follow the simple assess-diagnose-manage model to make a diagnosis of bipolar disorder, and come up with a treatment plan.

One of the reasons the curriculum is straightforward is that the basis for recognising and diagnosing most of the priority conditions is still phenomenological, just as it was thirty years ago when I first started training in psychiatry. We are still arguing over the pathogenesis of schizophrenia, and what are the boundaries of normality in sadness and fear. There are still no blood tests or X-rays or scans that will pin down the underlying biological changes in severe mental disorders. Although the acute organic causes of confusion, such as cerebral malaria, encephalitis or head injuries, need to be excluded, this can usually be done by careful history-taking and clinical examination. There are new medications, but some have troubling side effects and so we continue to use many of the old ones. We are still in the business of making the unbearable bearable, rather than providing a cure.

We have taught this short course for ten years. All the students are professional humanitarians who want to learn how to do better mental health and psychosocial programming. We use part of the time for them to share their own personal histories and motivations. Tadu and Abdulwasi are Ethiopians working in the refugee camps to the south and west. Mahmouda works with refugees in Bangladesh. Many of them have been victims themselves. Alaa's grandparents were Palestinian refugees in 1948. His family still cannot go home. But he works to help Syrian refugees in Jordan. Wafaa left Syria to live in Britain as a young woman, but has chosen to return to her country to help. Boniface was a refugee from the fighting in South Sudan for most of his childhood and now works to help those escaping the new rounds of fighting. Bishnu and Sujen both grew up in conflict-ridden Nepal and are now helping others find the missing victims of that war.

It is humbling to listen to colleagues who work on the problem in their own countries year after year. I sometimes feel international emergency relief workers are dangerously prone to ADHD, as media and funding efforts flit from one devastating disaster to the next: Yazidis in the mountains of northern Iraq, Ebola victims in West Africa, war in eastern Ukraine, then back to Iraq and West Africa, then an earthquake in Nepal – oh, and don't let's forget Syria. Nothing is ever finished.

Haiti continues to haunt me. There have been more than twenty-five thousand cholera cases this year, 2015, alone. Eighty thousand still live in camps, and according to the latest UN summary 3.5 million live in 'informal settlements and precarious urban neighborhoods, facing similar socio-economic deprivation, protection threats [that would be rape, murder, extortion and gang violence] and disaster risks without supportive assistance'. The report goes on: half the population continue to live in poverty and more than 3 per cent cannot meet their basic food needs, while floods, droughts and hurricanes attack the eroded, deforested island with increasing frequency. My old agency left long ago and there's no trace of the mental health programme we began.

In Sierra Leone the Ebola epidemic has destroyed the health infrastructure so painfully recreated a decade ago. Beautiful Kailahun was at the epicentre, and the traditional healers paid the highest price. In Iraq Dr B.'s predicted Sunni–Shia conflict has engulfed the entire Middle East. We have unleashed those latent, uncontrollable institutional and social forces beside which fantasy will pale, just as Faleh Jabar warned. And the fighting in Somalia is never-ending. The camps where Asmamaw and I used to work have swollen to forty thousand. Ethiopia now hosts the largest numbers of refugees on the continent.

And now all these crises have come home to us. Quite literally. At night after classes are finished and the moon rises over its own lovely image in the crater-lake below the hotel, I watch on TV as the hundreds of thousands who have managed to survive treacherous sea crossings, walk up familiar Balkan highways through Croatia and Slovenia, to face fences and tear gas on the Hungarian border. Viktor Orbán, the Hungarian prime minister responsible for those particular fences, was once a friend who stayed in my home, back in the eighties, when we both wanted to bring down the Iron Curtain and create democracy and freedom throughout Europe.

In the airport on the way back to the UK I catch the news on TV. More than twenty staff and patients in a hospital run by MSF in northern Afghanistan were killed when a US plane bombed their hospital. The coordinates of the hospital were provided to all the fighting forces, yet the bombing continued for more than thirty minutes after they raised the alarm. It is unbearable.

Larry lectured on security on the course. It's vital. Three hundred and twenty-nine aid workers were attacked last year: 121 killed, 120 kidnapped and 88 wounded. In 1997 those figures were thirty-nine, twenty-eight and six, respectively. I flick to the magazine section of the *Financial Times*, to stop thinking about it. This is not a paper I usually read but it's all the plane has to offer. I discover that if I have a spare half-billion dollars I can buy a house in Bel Air, California, the size of thirty-six tennis courts, with floor-to-ceiling tropical fish tanks, a four-hundred-foot-square room just to store handbags, and four indoor swimming pools. Meanwhile, Eurotunnel is closed again because of 'a very large, determined and organised group of migrants who burst through the fence and made their way to the terminal'.

Why are we surprised that people want to move to escape misery and improve their lives? Oxfam reported last year that the eighty-five richest people on the planet owned as much as the poorest half of humanity, and that seven out of ten of us live in countries where the gap between rich and poor is widening. Meanwhile, 'a tax of just 1.5 per cent on the wealth of the world's billionaires . . . invested in the poorest 49 countries . . . could fill the annual gaps in funding needed to get every child into school and deliver health services'. Every day between March 2013 and March 2014 the wealth of those eighty-five people grew by 668 million dollars. Every day. So it shouldn't be a problem to find the 405 million dollars the UN says Haiti needs for enduring solutions to all its problems.

Today, there are sixteen billionaires in sub-Saharan Africa, alongside the 358 million people living in extreme poverty. I could not recognise Addis this week. High-rise condominiums, new hotels and designer shops have sprung up all over town. Ethiopia is apparently producing dollar millionaires faster than any country in Africa. Yet in the north, south and east of the country more than twelve million people face famine because of drought and crop failure. What does it take to show that inequality actually damages us all? One of the first films I remember seeing as a child was *A Tale of Two Cities*. There's an unforgettable scene where a child is killed under the wheels of a French aristocrat's carriage. I remember wondering how people could live right next door to abject suffering and poverty and remain unmoved. How did you drive by it, and over it? The consequences of such indifference were clear: the downtrodden took matters into their own hands. They pulled down the walls and gates and executed both the indifferent and those who were not indifferent but had not done much to change things.

Now the downtrodden are at our own gates. And it's not as if Britain is a bed of roses, either: inequality rules here as well. The five richest families apparently have more wealth than the poorest twelve million, and the top 5 per cent have seen their incomes increase while the rest have seen their incomes decline. I only have to look at the food banks in the Co-op at home to know that this is true. There are 3.7 million children living in poverty in Britain, and it's expected to increase by a million in the next five years.

What is to be done? I doze fitfully in the transit lounge in Dubai, trying to make sense of it all. By the time I get to London I am completely awake. I decide I have to go to Calais.

Calais, France, 2015

I drive down a misty M20 in the early morning, snug in my car as it is carried under the English Channel, then drive out of Calais to a toxic-waste dump among the sand dunes now called 'the Jungle'. I know I am on the right route because all along Rue des Gravelines there's a procession of mostly young men in hooded jackets, heading back to the camp after a night of trying to get onto the cross-Channel trains to Britain. Fences, police, dogs, detention, the threat of deportation, the risk of death – nothing stops them. It is impossible to get accurate figures, but perhaps up to three people die in the Tunnel every week, electrocuted on wires or crushed under carriages. Everyone knows that a sixteen-year-old Afghan refugee died a week ago. His body was spread over four hundred metres of rail track.

I spend my first afternoon in what is called the 'family camp'. It has been here only a few weeks, springing up in the Kurdish area on the southern edge of the Jungle, next to the birch trees, beside the road. I meet Hawar and his eight-year-old daughter Samira. Both tried the Tunnel last night, but got turned back by police with pepper spray and dogs before they even got to the fence. The idea of this little girl trying to jump onto a train fills me with horror. The father tells me, 'There is no life here.' They fled from Mosul when ISIS attacked – no life there either. Around us other families are cooking over open fires. Smoke rises in the sunlight. Children play with donated scooters, an infant charges around unsteadily, watched by his mother; a baby cries. It looks benign enough, but what will happen when temperatures drop?

I get an answer the following day. There's a cold rain, no fires, and I spend much of it tramping about in an amazed rage. How is it possible that on the borders of a north European town, some 6,000–7,000 people are camped out in conditions worse than those I've encountered with Somali refugees on the Ethiopian border, Pakistanis after a devastating earthquake, or

Darfuris in the deserts of northern Chad, one of the poorest countries in the world? I pick my way through rivers of mud and between piles of uncollected garbage; try to help a teenage boy get water out of a blocked faucet – water that is apparently positive for *E. coli* – hold my breath while making use of Portakabin loos that no one has cleaned for days, and step over human excrement lying six inches from tent doorways where children play.

Where are the big agencies? I wonder. Médecins du Monde is running a clinic and MSF are cobbling the roads and cleaning the toilets, but otherwise the only help is from small local French charities and a constant flood of British volunteers. The other big NGOs, and UNHCR itself, are noticeable by their absence.

'It's completely political,' Ben, volunteering in his gap year between Eton and Yale, tells me. He is fluent in French and goes to the French coordination meetings. 'The French authorities don't want anything that attracts more migrants, but they don't want it to be so awful it creates a scandal. Possibly in some way we are playing straight into their hands, just preventing things tipping over the edge.'

'You're saying it might be better if there was a mass outbreak of disease or people froze to death?'

'Of course not, but how do we actually get people out of this situation?'

'Invest massively in the health and education and infrastructure of the countries from which they are coming. Fight corruption and human rights abuses in those places. Argue for HMG to come here and sort out asylum claims jointly with the French. That's what the UN are asking them to do.'

'It will never happen. The French don't want this place to be a magnet for refugees all over Europe.'

'They are already coming.'

But another question follows: Are the big agencies actually needed? Because in between the muddy footpaths and bursting bin bags, something else is going on: people are building a community. There are shops and restaurants made of tarpaulin and wood with brightly painted façades. Mosques are being constructed that shelter newcomers at night and create a quiet, clean space for anyone. There's an Ethiopian church, St Michael of the Jungle, complete with tarpaulin tower and hand-painted icons. In the few days I've been here an information centre has sprung up which will provide clear information on people's rights and the asylum process. There's a women and children's centre, where ex-firewoman Liz and other volunteers provide a warm refuge. Soup kitchens feed thousands each night. And there's an extraordinary flowering of creativity, paintings on the plastic walls of the tents, an art school and a theatre space in a dome where I sit and watch Afghan and Sudanese musicians make music together with instruments donated by Musicians without Borders.

In the Jungle Books Library, built by Mujib, an Afghan refugee and a volunteer, English and French lessons are given every day. Galasso, a famous maître d' from the Basque area, incongruously dressed in immaculate blazer and pressed trousers, shows four fascinated young Sudanese how to make cocktails and match the right wine with cheese. He is running a certified course in 'The Art of the Table'. They all hope it will help them find jobs in the future. Galasso's own family migrated to France from Italy in the thirties, to escape hunger and find work, just like his students.

Of course the Jungle has petty crime, a black market, drugs, alcohol and violence, as in any community. I am having a coffee with Mujib in his restaurant in the Afghan area, when he is called because a young, drunk Sudanese man has appeared at the MDM tent with a knife. Mujib gets some other Sudanese to mediate, and sorts it out without any casualties. The remarkable thing is how quickly fights can be de-escalated.

Mujib has spent five years in Europe. He actually got asylum in Italy (after waiting three years), but there was no work. Then he spent a number of years in Norway, until they told him there were no problems in Afghanistan and he should go back.

'I would love to go back. All I want to do is help my people.

It's impossible at the moment. And this is your fault. You made the problems in my country, not me. Look around you: here are Pashtun, Tajik, Uzbek, we all get on, but in Afghanistan there are more than forty-two countries with their guns, making things worse.'

He came to Calais in July to try and get to the UK to find work. He was in hospital for three weeks because of a beating. Now he has stopped trying to cross the Channel and puts his energy into helping his fellow countrymen. He plans to open a more expensive restaurant with good food, where volunteers will eat. He will encourage them to buy attractive cards, then to visit different areas of the camp to see who really needs help. They should give half the card to the vulnerable person, who can then come to the restaurant for a free meal. So Mujib has worked out a neat system of assessing needs, generating income and providing food for the most vulnerable, while using the time and energy of random volunteers. Brilliant.

I go to a volunteers' meeting. They are getting organised. Eva has turned up with a large chart, drawn with a marker pen onto two large pieces of cardboard. She has mapped all the sectors – sanitation, food, shelter, health care, arts and education – and then noted which groups are trying to address which needs in different parts of the camp. It is the who-what-where-when chart beloved of humanitarian communities in emergencies. These volunteers – many of whom have never done anything like this before in their lives – have worked it out for themselves. They have also worked out that they need a code of conduct: for example, no volunteers consuming alcohol or drugs on the site: 'Volunteers getting shit-faced is completely inappropriate,' someone says.

And they want better coordination with the French NGOs who have been working with the migrant community for fifteen years, some kind of security guidelines, as well as guidance on culturally appropriate behaviour. There's a lively discussion going on about how female volunteers should dress. Tifa, an Iranian who works in the women and children's centre, stands up. She's wearing baggy jeans and a loose, long-sleeved top. Her long dark hair is neatly tied.

'This is the way we should dress here. No miniskirts, no tight jeans, no long loose hair, and we have to be careful about touching and hugging. It is not appropriate. For many people here, these things are provocations and misunderstood, and we are not the ones who suffer the consequences, it is the women who live with these men. I understand what the men are saying and it's not polite.'

A woman from the No Borders network disagrees: 'They are coming to Europe – they will be living among women like us. This is a chance to educate them.'

'This is not the place to start, in a vulnerable community of ninety per cent young men. There will be time for that. Right now our job is to protect any women living here from harassment.'

Raul, a Kurdish refugee, is worried that Tifa is suggesting all the men are dangerous.

'Of course not. We are not suggesting this. You have a pure heart and there are many like you, but unfortunately not all.'

The volunteers have broken down the usual barrier between givers and receivers. At many points in the meeting I have no idea if it is a volunteer or a refugee voicing a view. Tom, the chair, announces: 'A volunteer is someone who helps other people. There is no distinction in this respect between volunteer and refugee.' No one disagrees.

'This is all very good,' a tall, thin young man speaks up, 'humanitarianism is essential for people's day-to-day needs, but what people want is to get to the UK and nothing we have discussed here addresses that problem. Blankets won't solve the problem of police violence. Fascist rallies are planned in Calais.'

I don't completely agree. It's clear to me, and to the French authorities, that the existence of this camp is in itself politically threatening; it challenges the whole organised asylum process and exposes all its weaknesses. That is why the mayor of Calais has discussed bringing in the army. In fact, this camp has much more in common with the Occupy movement or Greenham Common Women's Peace Camp than any humanitarian operation in which I have been involved. My own presence here, like many of the volunteers', is as much an act of political solidarity as an offer of practical assistance.

I realise I'm beginning to have the same issues with the word 'humanitarian' that I had with 'trauma' and 'PTSD'. Labelling the social problem as a biomedical one implies it is an individual problem for which there is a technical fix. Similarly, calling large-scale crises 'humanitarian' neutralises them and puts them beyond the ugly, chaotic, complicated political worlds that created them. The interventions required are, thus, humanitarian, be they airstrikes, food aid or shelter. But I am with David Rieff: there are no humanitarian solutions to humanitarian problems. That doesn't mean we shouldn't provide relief. It is essential and lifesaving. In the worst of all possible worlds at the very least we can be there, a companion in the darkness.

We have to respond to distress, but we cannot allow that response to become the excuse for political inaction, as we have in the past. If relief is not combined with political advocacy to challenge fundamental injustices, then as Michael Barnett predicted, we will have humanitarianism without end.

It's dark and late. We sit around Raul's fire. He and a handful of Kurdish friends share a large tent near the south entrance. Raul is twenty-five and was studying literature in Mosul until ISIS came. He tells me this is the first time he's spoken at a meeting, and he is rightly very proud of himself. Wherever I go people greet me with friendliness and invite me to sit at sputtering fires sharing small cups of tea. The stories pour out.

There is seventeen-year-old Adam, who left Darfur because of the fighting: 'I wanted a safe country where I could get an education.' He spent three months getting to Libya, where he worked on a building site for another three months to get the thousand dollars he needed to take a boat with four hundred and fifty others. In Italy he got on a train, hid from the police and made it to France. He has tried jumping onto the Channel

Tunnel train some nineteen times, but he was arrested a week ago and put in jail. When he came up in front of a judge they told him that as he was seventeen, he was free to go.

Fourteen-year-old Abdul and his twelve-year-old friend Jamal fled their village in Afghanistan when it was shelled while they were in class. Neither has any idea where their parents are, or if they are alive. They have been travelling together for the last two months. They play chess with me in the Jungle Books Library, but all they want to do is get to England where Abdul has an uncle in Manchester. He does not know the address. Telling him that life in Britain is not a bed of roses does not put him off.

Twenty-year-old Egid was a history student in Mosul until the arrival of ISIS. 'Then I went to Turkey, but I was not a refugee so everything cost money, so I worked illegally in a factory, but you earn nothing. So I took a boat. If you agree to be captain it's free, although of course you risk a seven-year jail sentence – but we made it to Greece. Then Macedonia, then Hungary. They put us on a bus for Austria, and the Austrians are lovely people, wonderful! They gave us money and food and put us on a bus for Germany where we were in a camp for three days. But I don't speak any German, and in England there is work . . .'

If you needed a selection process to identify the most resilient and most able refugees, one possible way would be to ask them to find their way across either Eurasia and the Middle East or sub-Saharan Africa, to risk their lives in the Mediterranean, and then place them in a toxic-waste dump on minimal handouts, before offering further life-threatening challenges in the form of avoiding electrocution while jumping onto trains, or freezing or suffocating in the back of a lorry. Indeed, I'm amazed these journeys have not yet been franchised as material for some kind of reality TV show in which the public votes for who they want to come in.

As you see, I don't use the word 'migrant'. In my five days here I have not met anyone who is not fleeing a war we started or failed to stop, a genocide we have failed to end, or human rights abuses to which we turn a blind eye. What shines through is intelligence, courage, concern for one another and a deep admiration for Britain. I would welcome any of the people I have met as my neighbours.

Asylum. What does that word mean? If you offer genuine sanctuary to those who are desperate and in need, what happens? This summer I went back to Kosovo and met up with Saranda. After she and her cousins were medically evacuated to Britain in 1999, they were granted asylum along with their fathers. I had not seen them since that trial in Belgrade of one of the perpetrators of the massacre of their families. The children had completed their education. Both Saranda and her sister went on to art school and to become practising artists.

The cousins' continuing search for justice has resulted in the trial and conviction in Serbia of four more of their families' killers. In 2013 Saranda returned to live in Kosovo, accepting a job as Director of Culture, Youth and Sports for the municipality of Prishtina. I sat one afternoon with this extraordinary, talented, multilingual young woman, watching her run a meeting with the press and the representatives of all the regional sports clubs. I walked round the peace park she had built outside her home town with help from friends in Manchester. Every summer there are peace camps here, where Albanian children and international volunteers work together creating art and drama. I looked at the exhibition brochure for the extraordinary piece of installation art that she and her cousins had created: an 'artistic and visual response to the massacre' and 'a homage to all the families and victims of war'. It had recently been exhibited in Belgrade. This is what can happen if you offer asylum: justice and creativity, and the possibility of returning with hope and imagination to rebuild your country.

And what happens if we continue to lock ourselves inside our fortress? While I'm sitting in Mujib's restaurant I get talking to Tawab, one of the boys helping out. He is nineteen, and he left Afghanistan when he was ten. His parents were killed when the Taliban bombed his village, and he ran away to avoid recruitment by them. After nine years of wandering around

Europe, including fourteen months in a camp in Italy, getting to the UK once, being deported, and spending three months in a French detention centre, he has asked the French government to help him get back to Afghanistan.

'I want to go back and help my country, I don't care about money, I don't care about Europe. I did not see any human rights here. And when I get home I will ask for ten minutes on Afghan TV and I will tell them what I experienced here. And I will say yes, there are some good people, but when Americans and British come to our country, without passports and with guns, we should kill them.'

He sees the shock on my face.

'You don't know human rights but you teach them in Afghanistan! Why do you think I left Afghanistan? Because if I had not they would have forced me to join a group! It was the only way to survive. There are no human rights there, the government fucks people up. It's impossible to be a normal person in Afghanistan, the Taliban is everywhere and now we have ISIL. In Italy I was in a camp for fourteen months. But what can I do with asylum in Italy when there is no work, no housing, no benefits – and yes, I know it's the same in the UK, I know that now, that is why I'm going back . . .

'And tell me this. How can you come and work in my country, when I cannot work in yours? How can you come with a Kalashnikov and no passport, when I'm not allowed in yours? Your soldier: he is born in England, he comes to my country, he walks my roads and mountains and villages with his Kalashnikov, and we give him tea, we give him everything. I don't have a Kalashnikov. I'm not like you. I'm just a donkey – Afghan, Iraqi, Syrian, we are all kicked. You see me as a dog, but I'm a human being and all humans are the same. We understand the law, just like you, we don't break laws.

'So now, when I get home I will go on TV and tell people: when you get to Europe, they fuck you up, they beat you and put you in prison, they hate you, so if they come here, you have to kill them.'

Sitting in the mud in Calais, I finally realise that I am the one in the madhouse. This asylum looks a bit like my lovely home in Haiti, in its flowery, guarded compound; except it is called northern Europe, and outside the gates, half the world is clamouring to come in. The Jungle confronts us with a question. We have one planet. Will we share its resources equitably and take care of it together, or will those of us with more firepower build ever higher fences to try and protect ourselves from those 'marauding swarms' trying to escape the poverty, violence and injustice that we are complicit in creating? The recent bombings in Paris show there are no fences high enough. On the contrary, Tawab's despair suggests that by rejecting those fleeing terror and seeking democracy we foster the very thing we fear.

We can delude ourselves that this global flight has nothing to do with the centuries of exploitation and theft through which we have enriched ourselves; that our high-consumption, high-carbon-exuding lifestyle and our endless demand for 'growth' have no relation to the expanding deserts in sub-Saharan Africa; that our ill-thought-out military interventions have brought peace and stability all round; and that the neo-liberal structural adjustment policies, imposed on all for the last thirty years, are making things better for everyone, rather than enriching a few while impoverishing many.

The fundamental issue is not who we let in or who we keep out, but whether those of us who have more than we need will share with those who have less, wherever they live. What we fail to realise is that it is not just migrant mothers and babies who are drowning as overcrowded inflatable rafts founder beneath the waves. We are all on the same sinking ship. This is the real mental health emergency. I think I have to attend to it now.

AFTERWORD

Syracuse, Sicily, November 2016

Sadiq cannot believe I have pictures of Jijiga on my computer. He stares at the photos of the dusty town on the Somali border, in eastern Ethiopia.

'A *tuk tuk*,' he cries delightedly, 'the water!' It seems we both loved that reservoir outside the town. 'I think I know this man! . . . Look, this is how we build houses!'

He wants his friends, Mohammed from Ghana and Fazil from Egypt, to see everything. Fighting broke out in Sadiq's village in eastern Somalia when he was seven years old. He escaped alone across the border into Ethiopia. Jijiga was his home for the next six years. We have worked out that we must have been there at the same time, when I was working in the neighbouring refugee camp.

Now he is living in a small children's home in Syracuse with eleven other migrant children aged between twelve and eighteen. He has just finished morning school, followed by prayers, and is having lunch. Mohammed volunteers to translate while Sadiq tells me his story in Arabic. It is both heartbreaking and extraordinary. When the fighting started, his father was killed and his two brothers were lost, never to be seen again. He ran away in the confusion, following some people over the border into Ethiopia. While sleeping on the streets in a foreign city he worked out how to survive.

'Some people say they want shoe-cleaning. So I see one man with a car and I say I want to help, and the man says "OK" and gives me some water and I clean his car and he gives me some money, and I go to a shop and buy some stuff to clean shoes. When people have seen what I have seen, it makes you older than your age. Because I was small and I did not have a mother or a father, so I had to be my own mother and father. I went to the market and found people who could help me. So every day I was in the market cleaning shoes and cleaning cars all day.'

He slept on the street for a year, until he had saved enough to rent a room. Then he got another job helping a woman make coffee and run a market stall.

'And I cleaned shoes and I cleaned cars and I kept all the money from cleaning. I saved as much as I could and only used a little for the food and the house. I did this for another year until I was nine years old. After that I could buy clothes and I took a house alone.'

By the time he was eleven he was in a position to help three other boys who came from Somalia.

'I showed them how to work like me and I let them live in my house. I didn't ask them for money because I knew what it's like for them. If I'd had more I would've given it to them. At that time, I had three jobs, so I shared the work with them so they could see how to do it. I was happy to help them.'

But then the effects of the conflict spilt across the border and his life was directly threatened by an inter-clan feud. So twelve-year-old Sadiq and his friends decided the only solution was to leave and go to Europe. They caught a bus and headed across Ethiopia and Sudan. In Libya they were kidnapped. Sadiq was trapped for a year in a house with forty other Somalis. They were beaten daily, starved and threatened with death unless they phoned their relatives to send money.

'This man had one phone. He said, "Call your family to send money." And they start beating you, so your family knows it is going badly. We told him, "We don't have money. We don't have any people to send money." And he said, "If you don't have money I will kill you." So we told him, "We don't have money, so kill us." We did not have a place to go to the toilet, nowhere to shit, nothing, it was like a prison.'

At this point in the telling, Sadiq is crying and Mohammed is crying, saying he never heard this story before. I tell Sadiq there is no need to continue, but he insists that he wants to tell the whole story.

'I thought my life was ending and I would escape this room.' But then finally he managed to locate someone who found his mother. 'So Mother went to the city to beg for money.'

Sadiq, with tears running down his face, mimes his mother holding out her apron, a mother he has not seen for eight years. I am crying now as well.

'She begged and she was weeping, saying, "My son is dying in Libya," and she got a small amount and she sent it to me. Then they threw me out, because they were worried I might die in Libya, because I was very sick. So they took me to the seaside, to some people with a boat. They said, "We don't want this dead boy in Libya. We don't want this boy dying here." The boat man called his boss saying, "One Somali boy is going to die today or tomorrow." So the boss says, "If he is going to die today or tomorrow, throw him on the boat. He can die at sea." I stood on the boat for two days. There was no room to sit. There was no food, so I did not need to shit or pee. God is wonderful.'

Cornwall, 29 January 2017

I wish President Trump could meet Sadiq. All he wants to do is become a mechanic and send money to his mother and sister in Somalia. He is just one of the 65.3 million forcibly displaced people in the world today – the highest number on record, more than after the end of the Second World War and greater than the entire population of the UK. These figures are a better indicator of the state of things than any of the other frightening (and easily verifiable) facts. But some are worth listing.

The world has just experienced its hottest year ever for the third time in a row. 'Natural' disasters are becoming more common and the human cost ever more apparent – and not just from floods in Cumbria and wildfires in California. The drought in Ethiopia last spring was the worst for fifty years and drove eighteen million towards starvation. In October 2016 yet another hurricane in Haiti has left 1.5 million on the brink. Drought threatens Ethiopia again this year. Meanwhile, according to the *Daily Mail*, Ivanka Trump is moving her shoe factory there from China, because five Ethiopians can be employed for the cost of one Chinese worker. The gap between rich and poor widens and the concentration of wealth increases. The combined wealth of just eight men now equals that of half the population of the planet.

Our ship is still sinking and yet the solution offered is to throw those not quite like us overboard. The most powerful democracy on the planet has elected as president a racist, misogynistic bully who fails to understand that the best way to inspire hatred and terror around the world is to bring back torture, build walls, ban refugees and Muslims and cut international aid. Trump should read Auden and meet Tawab, the teenage Afghan refugee who found no human rights in Europe and was going home to tell his countrymen to kill Americans and Brits.

Before Trump's election, three eminent US psychiatrists asked President Obama to order a neuropsychiatric evaluation of the President-elect. They stated:

> Professional standards do not permit us to venture a diagnosis for a public figure whom we have not evaluated personally. Nevertheless, his widely reported symptoms of mental instability – including grandiosity, impulsivity, hypersensitivity to slights or criticism, and an apparent

inability to distinguish between fantasy and reality – lead us to question his fitness for the immense responsibilities of the office.

The evaluation did not happen. So this is the man who now has his finger on the nuclear button. There are no checks and balances and the fact that the missile, once launched, might fly in the wrong direction provides little comfort. Nor is it possible to see how such missiles work to deter the next angry, embittered, dispossessed man who has discovered from social media that HGV trucks are lethal weapons. 'Mismanagement and grief: / We must suffer them all again.' Auden's poem is prescient.

And there is something else just as frightening as Trump. It is watching those who previously called his behaviour indefensible now say, 'Well, of course it is indefensible, but . . .'

In *Rhinoceros*, Ionesco's absurdist drama written in the fifties, the citizens of a small French town are initially outraged by a rampaging rhinoceros that kills a cat. They insist it should not be allowed. A rhinoceros is dangerous and inhumane, yet one by one each finds a reason for transforming himself. I played Botard in a school production, an office worker who argued that people were too intelligent to succumb to 'rhinoceritis', before changing into a beast himself. 'Humanism is dead,' declares another, before he too changes.

The indefensible is indefensible. The only choice is not to capitulate. What gives me hope is that this is exactly what is happening. I am not just talking about the millions of women, men and children who turned out around the world the day after Trump's inauguration to demonstrate their opposition to everything he stands for, inspiring as that was. I am talking about all those I encountered in 2016, working with the displaced across France, Italy and Greece.

In Lesbos in Greece last March there was a Japanese man who had travelled thousands of miles at his own expense to sit with some Norwegians on a cliff trying to help stop refugees drowning. Across the island some local Greeks and international volunteers, horrified by the barbed wire, the grim conditions and the bureaucracy that faced arriving refugees, rented land to create a more humane and welcoming camp. Jim, a retired GP from Scotland volunteering in the health post there, told me it was the first time he had done anything like this.

'I am usually a spectator,' he said. 'But you sit at home. You watch John Wayne shoot Indians on the telly, then you watch Homs being blasted to smithereens on the same screen, then you walk the dogs in the park, up to the pond, round the church, and you think about those two sets of images on the same screen and it's like it's not happening. It's not enough. I needed to come. If I am brutally honest we did not give a monkey's when we invaded their countries, we paid no attention to their borders. We chose the boundaries of the Middle East and Africa to suit ourselves. If you believe what goes around comes around . . . the sins of the Fathers . . . I'm left with what responsibility do we bear because of what we have allowed our governments to do?'

And there was Konstantin, who ran the Park Hotel near the closed Greek–Macedonian border, turning it into a refuge and organising centre for volunteers and refugees alike: 'Solving the problems of one person can give happiness to another. We are all brothers and sisters. If people have love they can see we are all the same, all one.'

The people of Riace in Calabria, southern Italy, have gone even further. When some Kurdish migrants arrived on the beach in 1998 the local mayor, Domenico Lucano, had the simple idea that if he helped them, they would help revive the fortunes of his tiny hilltop village which, like so many in the area, was being abandoned by the locals fleeing in search of work. So the mayor offered the migrants accommodation in local empty flats, and created projects to teach them work skills while they waited for their documentation. The village blossomed and continues to do so.

'At the beginning it was difficult,' Angela told me. She is a local artist who runs a weaving project. 'We had no experience with foreigners. We did not even know where Kurdistan was. Now it's completely normal. We treat everyone as one. You don't look at colour, you see people like brothers and sisters. For me we are all the same. I don't understand why some people say we are white, they are black, we are European, they are African. We are all the same blood, we are all one and I think we can live as one.'

The primary school was closed when Angela was a teenager. Now it has reopened and half the children are migrants from twenty countries. Ghanaians, Somalis, Syrians and Afghans speak Italian with the local accent. Neighbouring villages have also made them welcome: mutual aid for the benefit of all.

But the people who give me the most hope are the refugees themselves: like Soloman, the lay preacher who built and organised St Michael's Church in the Jungle, Calais. He stayed to look after the constantly changing community of Eritreans and Ethiopians instead of trying to cross to the UK. On the last night before the eviction in October 2016, I took him to buy petrol for the church generator and beer for his friends.

'What have I been doing for the last year?' he asked me.

'Holding a community together, keeping it safe and peaceful, helping people stay sane, helping people express their faith. There are so many people who would not have survived here without you, Soloman. You were needed here. You still will be, wherever people go.'

Or there is Housam and his friends, young Syrian refugees in northern Greece who, to quote their Facebook page, 'decided to use our skills, knowledge and capacity to serve our community'. They now work with refugees in Athens helping to renovate community spaces and shelters and providing activities and training.

And there is Sadiq, who used his intelligence to make something out of nothing and then, as soon as he had a little, shared it with friends in need.

These are tiny examples but they are a fragment of something much bigger – a realisation that humanitarianism is not something apolitical done by others, somewhere else.

Humanitarianism is the small, continuing everyday acts of mutual aid, carried out wherever we live and in whatever situation we find ourselves. These actions are our best forms of resistance to the idea that greatness can only happen when one person or country does well at the expense of another. Mutual aid is infectious. Such actions overcome borders, and challenge and undermine fear as well as both political and corporate greed. Mutual aid can also keep us happy and sane.

This is the real meaning of globalisation. It is not about the free movement of capital in its endless quest for the cheapest labour, the lowest taxes and the least regulations, never mind the cost to the planet and to those who produce the goods. True globalisation must mean global solidarity and global justice; that is, the equitable distribution of rights, wealth, environmental protection and security. True globalisation must mean us working together so that a child born in Afghanistan or on the Somali border has the same opportunities for education, health, free movement and a productive life as a child in Western Europe.

We can help Sadiq or we can create more Tawabs. That is the choice. It is that simple.

NOTES

[xii] To admit any hope . . . working for it: D. Graham (ed.), *Letters of Keith Douglas* (Carcanet, 2000).

1. Inside the Asylum

{3} I saw a documentary . . . *The Tribe that Hides from Man*: A. Cowell (director), *The Tribe that Hides from Man* (film, 1970).

[5] In 1973 . . . schizophrenia in remission: D. L. Rosenhan, 'On Being Sane in Insane Places', *Science* 179 (1973): 250–8.

[5] There were particularly . . . their British counterparts: R. E Kendell, J. E. Cooper and A. G. Gourlay, 'Diagnostic criteria of American and British psychiatrists', *Archives of General Psychiatry* 25 (1971): 123–130.

2. Why Are You Here?

[30] I wrote an article . . . stick to my patients: L. Jones, 'The Medicine of Misery', the *Guardian,* 27 November 1987.

[38] I am against war . . . the threat of force: L. M. Jones, 'The Peace Movement's Moral Failure in Bosnia', *Peace and Democracy News* (Summer 1993): 23–8.

Somali Border, Ethiopia, October 2007

[45] The Islamic Courts Union was a group of Sharia courts in Somalia that wanted to promote Islamist rule in Somalia. They united and challenged the Transitional Federal government, gaining control of most major cities in the southern half of the country by the autumn of 2006.

3. On a Front Line

[63] Some of the most powerful . . . become relief workers: D. Rieff, *A Bed for the Night* (Simon and Schuster, 2002):123–54.

[64] Alain Destexhe . . . making them possible: B. Simms, *Unfinest Hour: Britain and the Destruction of Bosnia* (Allen Lane, 2001): 35–6

4. Trauma Tales

[74–5] A 1941 article . . . evacuation, etc.: P. E. Vernon, 'Psychological effects of air-raids', *The Journal of Abnormal and Social Psychology* 36 (4) (1941): 457–76.

[75] They were all told . . . next nine months: H. Wilson, 'Mental Reactions to Air-Raids', *Lancet* (1942): 284–7.

[75–6] In line with . . . reaction: World Health Organisation, *The ICD 9 Classification of Mental and Behavioural Disorders* (WHO, 1978).

[76] Accident neurosis . . . might be improving: H. Miller, 'Accident Neurosis', *British Medical Journal* 1 (1961): 992–98.

[76] They proposed . . . DSM III: American Psychiatric Association, *Diagnostic and Statistical Manual of Mental Disorders,* 3rd edition (1980)

[80] One researcher found . . . the criteria for PTSD: R. Goldstein, 'War Experiences and Distress of Bosnian Children', *Journal of Pediatrics* 100 (1997): 873–8.

[80] Researchers in other . . . disorder requiring treatment: D. J. Somasundaram, 'Post-Traumatic Responses to Aerial Bombing', *Social Science & Medicine* 42 (1996): 1465–71.

[80–81] One side . . . treatments on offer worked: D. A. Summerfield, 'A Critique of Seven Assumptions behind Psychological Trauma Programmes in War-Affected Areas', *Social Science & Medicine* 48 (1999): 1449–62.

[81] To make a drama . . . in my opinion priceless: F. de Vries, 'To Make a Drama out of Trauma Is Fully Justified', *Lancet* 351 (1998): 1579–80

[81] Dr Vries alludes . . . is not pathology: D. A. Summerfield, '"Trauma" and the experience of war: a reply', *Lancet* 351 (1998): 1580–81

[81] A simple medical fix . . . traumatic reactions: J. T. Mitchell, 'When disaster strikes . . . The critical incident stress debriefing', *Journal of Emergency Medical Services* 8 (1983): 36–39. A. Dyregrov, 'The Process in Psychological Debriefings', *Journal of Traumatic Stress* 10 (1997): 589–605.

[84–94] Elderly Mrs Babić . . . south, to Kosovo: Lynne Jones, Republic of Yugoslavia: 'Each Scar is Different', *Aeon* (22 May 2014). https://aeon.ce/essays/the-more-we-label-every-traum a-with-ptsd-the-less-it-means; L. Mastnak. 'Diary', *London Review of Books,* 21 August 1997. www.lrb.co.uk.

[87] In the late nineteenth . . . constricted the blood supply: J. M. Da Costa, 'On Irritable Heart: A Clinical Study of a Form of Functional Cardiac Disorder and Its Consequences', *American Journal of the Medical Sciences* 61 (1871): 18–52.

[87] When doctors recognised . . . effort syndrome: E. Jones and S. Wessely, 'Psychological Trauma: A Historical Perspective', *Psychiatry* 5 (2006): 217–20. B. Shephard, *War of Nerves: Soldiers and*

Psychiatrists in the Twentieth Century (Harvard University Press, 2002).

[88] The men with . . . exercises and relaxation: S. G. Potts, R. Lewin, K. Fox and E. C. Johnstone, 'Group Psychological Treatment for Chest Pain with Normal Coronary Arteries', *Quarterly Journal of Medicine* 92 (1999): 81–6

[92] One of the sickest . . . the daughter recovered: L. Jones, *Then They Started Shooting: Children of the Bosnian War and the Adults They Become* (Bellevue Literary Press, 2012).

[93] The revision . . . witnessed it on television: American Psychiatric Association, *DSM-IV. Diagnostic and Statistical Manual of Mental Disorders,* 4th edition (1994).

5. Fight or Flight

[105–18] After going to see Fejza . . . nothing is going to happen: L. Mastnak, 'Why are you leaving?': a child psychiatrist records the daily round in Kosovo before and since the bombing', *London Review of Books,* 27 May 1999. www.lrb.co.uk

6. Neutral and Impartial

[123–4] Central to its work . . . interest in the conflict: International Committee of the Red Cross and International Federation of Red Cross and Red Crescent Societies, *Handbook of the International Red Cross and Red Crescent Movement* (2008).

[124] This first incarnation . . . the human condition: C. Craig, 'The imperative to reduce suffering', in *Humanitarianism in Question: Politics, Power, Ethics,* ed. M. Barnett and T. G. Weiss (Cornell University Press, 2008): 73–97.

[124] However, this kind . . . humanitarian military interventions: D. Rieff, *A Bed for the Night* (Simon and Schuster, 2002).

[124] Dorothea Dix endlessly . . . almshouses: D. Dix, *Memorial. To the Legislature of Massachusetts [protesting against the confinement of insane persons and idiots in almshouses and prisons. Jan. 1843]* (Munroe and Francis, 1843). http://collections.nlm.nih.gov/catalog/ nlm:nlmuid-101174442-bk.

[124] Dorothea Dix described . . . southern United States: D. Gollaher, *Voice for the Mad: The Life of Dorothea Dix* (Free Press, 1996).

[125] Wilberforce was moved . . . improve their own lives: W. Hague, *William Wilberforce: The Life of the Great Anti-Slave Trade Campaigner* (Harper Press, 2007).

[125] In 1942 the International . . . compromise Swiss neutrality: B. A. Rieffer-Flanagan, 'Is Neutral Humanitarianism Dead? Red Cross Neutrality: Walking the Tightrope of Neutral Humanitarianism', *Human Rights Quarterly* 31 (2009): 888–915.

[125] Ojukwu, the Biafran . . . prolonged the conflict: F. Terry, *Condemned to Repeat? The Paradox of Humanitarian Action* (Cornell University Press, 2002).

[125–6] The ICRC made . . . humanitarian principles: J. Kellenberger, 'Speaking Out or Remaining Silent in Humanitarian Work', *International Review of the Red Cross* 86 (2004): 593–609.

[127–31] Today's shift at the medical . . . put back on: ibid., 27 May 1999.

[131–6] Airstrikes ended in June 1999 . . . much as psychotherapy: L. Mastnak, 'Not Much Tolerance, Not Much Water: the last nine months in Kosovo', *London Review of Books,* 30 March 2000. www.lrb.co.uk

[134] Some evidence that . . . some people worse: S. Rose, J. Bisson, R. Churchill and S. Wessely, 'Psychological Debriefing for Preventing Post Traumatic Stress Disorder (PTSD)', *Cochrane Database of Systematic Reviews* (2002). DOI:10.1002/14651858.CD000560.

[135] Over the next . . . service today: L. Jones, A. Rrustemi, M. Shahini and A. Uka, 'Mental health services for war-affected children: Report of a survey in Kosovo', *British Journal of Psychiatry* 183 (2003): 540–46.

Dire Dawa, Ethiopia, January 2008

[139] This was the first conflict . . . many tens of thousands: R. Baudendistel, *Between Bombs and Good Intentions: The Red Cross and the Italo-Ethiopian War, 1935–1936* (Berghahn, 2006).

[140] Emperor Haile Selassie . . . morality which is at stake: 'Stock Footage – 1936 NEWS: EMPEROR HAILE SELASSIE OF ETHIOPIA ADDRESSES LEAGUE OF NATIONS' (MyFootage. com, uploaded 9 April 2012), https://www.youtube.com/watch?v=oyX2kXeFUlo.

7. Interventions

[143] Our attempts at curing . . . almost every complaint: R. Porter, *The Cambridge Illustrated History of Medicine* (Cambridge University Press, 2001).

[143] We have whirled . . . the rest of the brain: R. Porter, *Madness: A Brief History* (Oxford University Press, 2003).

[143] Would it not . . . every grade of natural life: A. K. Strahan, 'The Propagation of Insanity and Allied Neuroses', *Journal of Mental Science* (1890): 325–38.

[144] After all, it was . . . hygienists of the day: 'Buck v. Bell: 274 U.S. 200' (1927) https://www.law.cornell.edu/supremecourt/text/274/200.

[144] The compulsory sterilisation . . . into the 1960s: M. H. Haller, *Eugenics: Hereditarian attitudes in American thought* (Rutgers University Press, 1984).

[143] German psychiatrists enraged. . . Hippocratic oath: R. J. Lifton, *The Nazi Doctors: Medical Killing and the Psychology of Genocide* (Basic Books, 1986).

[143] The United States Department . . . outcry in the seventies: S. B. Thomas, 'Light on the Shadow of the Syphilis Study at Tuskegee', *Health Promotion Practice* 1 (2000): 234–7.

[143] doctors have among other things . . . with dementia: S. Krugman, 'The Willowbrook Hepatitis Studies Revisited: Ethical Aspects', *Clinical Infectious Diseases* 8 (1986): 157–62. B. Roberts and L. W. Roberts, 'Psychiatric Research Ethics: An Overview of Evolving Guidelines and Current Ethical Dilemmas in the Study of Mental Illness', *Biological Psychiatry* 46 (1999): 1025–38. A. Gercas, 'The Universal Declaration on Bioethics and Human Rights: Promoting International Discussion on the Morality of Non-Therapeutic Research on Children', *Michigan Journal of International Law* 27 (2006): 629–56.

[143–4] Dietrich Bonhoeffer . . . concrete responsibility: D. Bonhoeffer, *Letters and Papers from Prison* (Simon and Schuster, 2011).

[144] If we tear up . . . genocide with impunity: L. M. Jones, 'Upholding the Rule of Law', *Peace and Democracy News* (summer 1994): 36–40.

[144] On the brink . . . ethnically partitioned Bosnia: B. Simms, *Unfinest Hour: Britain and the Destruction of Bosnia* (Allen Lane, 2001).

[144] After NATO airstrikes . . . one hundred thousand fled: Independent International Commission on Kosovo, *The Kosovo Report: Conflict, International Response, Lessons Learned* (Oxford University Press, 2000).

[144–5] Today in Kosovo . . . 35–49 per 1000 births: J. Harding, 'Saved and Depoliticised at One Stroke: The Dangers of Intervention', *London Review of Books* 30 (2008): 5–8.

[145] Rwandan Genocide. . . community to procrastinate: D. Rieff, *A Bed for the Night* (Simon and Schuster, 2002).

[146] Bombing them to . . . supported the idea: A. Travis, '2 in 3 back air strikes', *Guardian,* 18 September 2001, https://www.theguardian.com/world/2001/sep/18/september11.usa7?INTCMP=SRCH

[148] David Rieff . . . imposed by force: D. Rieff, *A Bed for the Night* (Simon and Schuster, 2002).

[148] Michael Walzer . . . the hand of Saddam: M. Walzer, *Arguing about War* (Yale University Press, 2005).

[148–9] He argued that . . . risk untold consequences: F. A. Jabar, 'Opposing War Is Good, But Not Good Enough', *The Progressive,* January 2003 20–22. https://www.globalpolicy.org/component/content/article/167/35171.html.

[152–3] directed against . . . prosperous and free' George W. Bush, 'Full text: Bush's speech: A transcript of George Bush's war ultimatum speech from the Cross Hall in the White House', *Guardian*, 18 March 2003, http://www.theguardian.com/world/2003/mar/18/usa.iraq.

[154] An estimated 3,000 . . . 7,000 to 8,000 Iraqi combatants: C. Conetta, *The Wages of War: Iraqi Combatant and Noncombatant Fatalities in the 2003 Conflict. Research Monograph #8* (Project on Defence Alternatives, 2003). http://www.comw.org/pda/0310rm8.html

[154] The Iraqis are sick . . . I'll just kill him: M. Franchetti, 'US Marines turn fire on civilians at bridge of death', *The Sunday Times*, 30 March 2003.

[155] Colin Powell . . . find new partners: N. de Torrente, 'Humanitarian Action under Attack: Reflections on the Iraq War', *Harvard Law School Human Rights Journal* 17 (2004).

[171] No one mentioned that . . . 793 in August: Iraq Body Count, https://www.iraqbodycount.org/.

[176] Aristotle described. . . that started in 1980: A. V. Horwitz and J. C. Wakefield, *The Loss of Sadness: How Psychiatry Transformed Normal Sorrow into Depressive Disorder* (Oxford University Press, 2007).

[177] A study of 160 . . . significant anxiety symptoms: Z. Rasekh, H. Bauer, M. Manos and V. Iacopino, 'Women's Health and Human Rights in Afghanistan', *Journal of the American Medical Association* 280 (1998): 449–55.

8. Healers

[203] There is now . . . physical ills are neglected: G. Thornicroft, 'Physical Health Disparities and Mental Illness: The Scandal of Premature Mortality', *British Journal of Psychiatry* 199 (2011): 441–2.

[205] I always kept . . . *Where There Is No Psychiatrist*: Vikram Patel, *Where There Is No Psychiatrist: A Mental Healthcare Manual* (Gaskell, 2003).

Jijiga, Ethiopia, November 2008

[209] Winter had begun in earnest . . . was no compensation: L. Jones, 'Diary of a Disaster', *O, the Oprah Magazine*, June 2006.

9. After the Wave

[213–23] The story my landlord . . . clearing in the forest: L. Jones, 'Love Among the Ruins: Rebuilding After the Tsunami', *O, the Oprah Magazine*, July 2005.

[231] Some agencies had been . . . was purchased locally: M. Casey, 'Tsunami Boosts Illegal Indonesia Logging', The Associated Press,

5 August 2006, http://www.washingtonpost.com/wp-dyn/content/
article/2006/08/05/AR2006080500421_pf.html

Somali Border, Ethiopia, April 2008

[235] consensus-based guidelines . . . in humanitarian settings:
Inter-Agency Standing Committee (IASC), *IASC Guidelines on
Mental Health and Psychosocial Support in Emergency Settings*
(2007), http://www.who.int/mental_health/emergencies/guidelines_
iasc_mental_health_psychosocial_june_2007.pdf. DOI:10.1037/
e518422011-002.

[235] discussion with UNHCR . . . applies to half the people in this
camp: United Nations High Commission for Refugees (UNHCR),
Health Information System (HIS) Toolkit, http://www.unhcr.org/uk/
protection/health/4a3374408/health-

10. Building Back Better

[244] The *New York Times* . . . promising to do a story: D. Sontag,
'In Haiti, Mental Health System Is in Collapse', *New York Times*
19 March 2010, http://www.nytimes.com/2010/03/20/world/
americas/20haiti.html

[258] More recent foreign . . . it was a 'class quake': J. Díaz,
'Apocalypse: What Disasters Reveal', *Boston Review,* 1 May 2011,
http://bostonreview.net/junot-diaz-apocalypse-haiti-earthquake. P.
O'Keefe, K. Westgate and B. Wisner, 'Taking the Naturalness out of
Natural Disasters', *Nature* 260 (1976): 566–7.

[262] Michael Barnett . . . to provide security: M. N. Barnett, *Empire of
Humanity: A History of Humanitarianism* (Cornell University Press,
2011).

[262] Never mind the earthquake . . . an army of 'experts': O.
Cunningham, 'The Humanitarian Aid Regime in the Republic of
NGOs', *The Josef Korbel Journal of Advanced International Studies* 4
(2012): 103–26.

Pemba, Cabo Delgago, Mozambique, February 2013

[271] Cholera has not . . . 'confluence of circumstances': R. R. Lall and
E. Pilkington, 'UN Will Not Compensate Haiti Cholera Victims,
Ban Ki-moon Tells President', *Guardian,* 21 February 2013, https://
www.theguardian.com/world/2013/feb/21/un-haiti-cholera-victim
s-rejects-compensation.

[272] shelves with books . . . *What's Wrong with Humanitarian Aid?*: D.
Moyo, *Dead Aid: Why Aid Is Not Working and How There Is Another
Way for Africa* (Penguin, 2009). M. Maren, *The Road to Hell: The
Ravaging Effects of Foreign Aid and International Charity* (Free Press,
1997). F. Terry, *Condemned to Repeat? The Paradox of Humanitarian
Action* (Cornell University Press, 2002). L. Polman, *The Crisis
Caravan: What's Wrong with Humanitarian Aid* (Picador, 2011).

[272] David Rieff asked . . . a waste of hope: D. Rieff, *A Bed for the Night* (Simon and Schuster, 2002).

11. Them and Us: Tacloban, Philippines, January 2014

[294] WHO guidelines . . . some evidence of harm: World Health Organisation, *Psychological Debriefing in People Exposed to a Recent Traumatic Event* (2012), http://www.who.int/mental_health/mhgap/evidence/other_disorders/q5/en/.

[294] There is now a manual . . . *Psychological First Aid*: World Health Organisation, War Trauma Foundation and World Vision International, *Psychological First Aid: guide for fieldworkers* (WHO, 2011)

12. The Way We Live Now

[296] Research continues . . . conflict and disaster are resilient: G. A. Bonnano, C. R. Brewin, K. Kaniasty and A. M. La Greca, 'Weighing the Costs of Disaster: Consequences, Risks, and Resilience in Individuals, Families, and Communities', *Psychological Science in the Public Interest* 11 (2010): 1–49. W. Tol et al., 'Mental Health and Psychosocial Support in Humanitarian Settings: Linking Practice and Research', *Lancet* 378 (2011): 1581–91.

[296] When I went back . . . immediately after the war: L. Jones, *Then They Started Shooting: Children of the Bosnian War and the Adults They Become* (Bellevue Literary Press, 2012).

[297] There are recommendations . . . is no longer enough: A. Maercker et al., 'Proposals for Mental Disorders Specifically Associated with Stress in the International Classification of Diseases-11', *Lancet* 381 (2013): 1683–5. J. Bisson, S. Cosgrove, C. Lewis, 'Post Traumatic Stress Disorder', *British Medical Journal* 351 (2015), *doi: http://dx.doi.org/10.1136/bmj.h6161*

[297] Here in Ethiopia . . . die three decades earlier: A. Fekadu et al., 'Excess Mortality in Severe Mental Illness: 10-Year Population-Based Cohort Study in Rural Ethiopia', *British Journal of Psychiatry* 206 (2015): 289–96.

[297] *mhGAP Intervention Guide* . . . primary health care physicians: World Health Organisation, *mhGAP Intervention Guide for Mental, Neurological and Substance Use Disorders in Non-Specialized Health Settings* (2010). http://www.who.int/mental_health/publications/mhGAP_intervention_guide/en/. World Health Organisation and United Nations High Commission for Refugees, *mhGAP Humanitarian Intervention Guide* (2015), http://www.who.int/mental_health/publications/mhgap_hig/en/.

[299] There have been . . . with increasing frequency: United Nations Office of the Humanitarian Coordinator, *Haiti Transitional Appeal*

2015/2016 (2015). http://reliefweb.int/sites/reliefweb.int/files/
resources/haiti-TAP_exec_summary_0.pdf.

[300] Three hundred and twenty nine . . . and six, respectively: The Aid
Worker Security Database, https://aidworkersecurity.org/.

[300] The *Financial Times* . . . indoor swimming pools: H. Cox, 'Yours
for $500m – Los Angeles Builds Big', *Financial Times*, 1 October
2015, http://www.ft.com/cms/s/0/56f75f06-6398-11e5-9846-
de406ccb37f2.html.

[300] Oxfam reported last year . . . in extreme poverty: E. Seery and
A. Caistor Arendar, *Even It Up: Time to End Extreme Inequality*
(Oxfam International, 2014), http://policy-practice.oxfam.org.uk/
publications/even-it-up-time-to-end-extreme-inequality-333012.

[301] Ethiopia is apparently . . . than any country in Africa: D.
Smith, 'Ethiopia Hailed as "African Lion" with Fastest Creation
of Millionaires', *Guardian*, 4 December 2013, http://www.
theguardian.com/world/2013/dec/04/ethiopia-faster-rate-million
aires-michael-buerk.

[301] The five richest families . . . seen their incomes decline: S.
Dransfield, 'A Tale of Two Britains' (Oxfam GB, 2014), http://
policy-practice.oxfam.org.uk/publications/a-tale-of-two-britains-
inequality-in-the-uk-314152.

[301] There are 3.7 million . . . the next five years: Child Poverty Action
Group, *Child Poverty: Facts and Figures* (2015), http://www.cpag.
org.uk/child-poverty-facts-and-figures.

[307] David Rieff . . . to humanitarian problems: D. Rieff, *A Bed for the
Night* (Simon and Schuster, 2002).

Afterword

[312] I and the public . . . evil in return: W. H. Auden, *Collected Poems*
(Random House, 1976).

[315] He is just one . . . population of the UK: UNHCR media centre:
Global forced displacement hits record high, press release (20 June
2016) http://www.unhcr.org/uk/news/latest/2016/6/5763b65a4/
global-forced-displacement-hits-record-high.html. UNHCR *Global
Trends 2015* (2016).

[315] The world has . . . third time in a row: Met Office news release,
'2016 Record breaking year for global temperature (18 January
2017) http://www.metoffice.gov.uk/news/releases/2017/2016-recor
d-breaking-year-for-global-temperature

[315] 'Natural' disasters are . . . ever more apparent: Sam Jones,
'World heading for catastrophe over natural disasters, risk expert
warns', *Guardian*, 24 April 2016, https://www.theguardian.com/
global-development/2016/apr/24/world-heading-for-catastroph
e-over-natural-disasters-risk-expert-warns

[315] The drought in Ethiopia . . . population of the planet: Aisling Laing, 'Ethiopia struggles with worst drought for 50 years leaving 18 million people in need of aid', *Telegraph*, 23 April 2016, http://www.telegraph.co.uk/news/2016/04/23/ethiopia-struggles-with-wors t-drought-for-50-years-leaving-18-mi/. UN News Centre, 'Three months after Hurricane Matthew, 1.5 million Haitians face hunger – UN agencies report', 18 January 2017, http://www.un.org/apps/news/story.asp?NewsID=55998#.WIzBKn9FrDo Chris Summers, 'Inside a Trump Chinese shoe factory: 100,000 pairs of footwear branded with Ivanka's name have been made at huge facility (but now it's moving to Africa!)', Mailonline and AFP (6 October 2016) http://www.dailymail.co.uk/news/article-3824617/Trump-factory-jobs-sen t-China-never-come-back.html#ixzz4X4e6Jtv8

[315] The combined wealth . . . of the planet: Deborah Hardoon, 'An economy for the 99%' (Oxfam GB, 2017), https://www.oxfam.org/en/research/economy-99

[315] Before Trump's Election . . . did not happen: Richard Greene, 'Is Donald Trump Mentally Ill? 3 Professors of Psychiatry Ask President Obama To Conduct "A Full Medical And Neuropsychiatric Evaluation"', *Huffington Post*, 20 December 2016, http://www.huffingtonpost.com/richard-greene/is-donal d-trump-mentally_b_13693174.html

[316] In *Rhinoceros* . . . he too changes: Eugène Ionesco, *Rhinoceros*, translated by Martin Crimp (Faber and Faber, 2007).

BIBLIOGRAPHY

Aid Worker Security Database, https://aidworkersecurity.org/.

American Psychiatric Association, *DSM-III. Diagnostic and Statistical Manual of Mental Disorders,* 3rd edition (1980).

American Psychiatric Association, *DSM-IV. Diagnostic and Statistical Manual of Mental Disorders,* 4th edition (1994).

Auden, W. H. *Collected Poems* (Random House, 1976).

Barnett, M. N. *Empire of Humanity: A History of Humanitarianism* (Cornell University Press, 2011).

Baudendistel, R. *Between Bombs and Good Intentions: The Red Cross and the Italo-Ethiopian War, 1935–1936* (Berghahn, 2006).

Bisson, J., Cosgrove, S. and Lewis, C., 'Post Traumatic Stress Disorder', *British Medical Journal* 351 (2015), *doi: http://dx.doi.org/10.1136/bmj.h6161*

Bonhoeffer, D. *Letters and Papers from Prison* (Simon and Schuster, 2011).

Bonnano, G. A., Brewin, C. R., Kaniasty, K., and La Greca, A. M., 'Weighing the Costs of Disaster: Consequences, Risks, and Resilience in Individuals, Families, and Communities'. *Psychological Science in the Public Interest* 11 (2010): 1–49.

'Buck v. Bell: 274 U.S. 200' (1927) https://www.law.cornell.edu/supremecourt/text/274/200.

Bush, George W., 'Full text: Bush's speech: A transcript of George Bush's war ultimatum speech from the Cross Hall in the White House', *Guardian,* 18 March 2003, http://www.theguardian.com/world/2003/mar/18/usa.iraq.

Casey, M., 'Tsunami Boosts Illegal Indonesia Logging', The Associated Press, 5 August 2006, http://www.washingtonpost.com/wp-dyn/content/article/2006/08/05/AR2006080500421_pf.html

Child Poverty Action Group. *Child Poverty: Facts and Figures* (2015), http://www.cpag.org.uk/child-poverty-facts-and-figures.

Conetta, C., *The Wages of War: Iraqi Combatant and Noncombatant Fatalities in the 2003 Conflict. Research Monograph #8* (Project on Defence Alternatives, 2003), http://www.comw.org/pda/0310rm8.html

Cowell, A. (director), *The Tribe That Hides from Man* (film, 1970).

Cox, H., 'Yours for $500m – Los Angeles Builds Big', *Financial Times*, 1 October 2015, http://www.ft.com/cms/s/0/56f75f06-6398-11e5-9846-de406ccb37f2.html.

Craig, C., 'The imperative to reduce suffering', in *Humanitarianism in Question: Politics, Power, Ethics*, ed. M. Barnett and T. G. Weiss (Cornell University Press, 2008): 73–97.

Cunningham, O., 'The Humanitarian Aid Regime in the Republic of NGOs', *Josef Korbel Journal of Advanced International Studies* 4 (2012): 103–26.

Da Costa, J. M., 'On Irritable Heart: A Clinical Study of a Form of Functional Cardiac Disorder and Its Consequences', *American Journal of the Medical Sciences* 61 (1871): 18–52.

de Torrente, N., 'Humanitarian Action under Attack: Reflections on the Iraq War', *Harvard Law School Human Rights Journal* 17 (2004).

de Vries, F., 'To Make a Drama out of Trauma Is Fully Justified', *Lancet* 351 (1998): 1579–80.

Díaz, J., 'Apocalypse: What Disasters Reveal', *Boston Review* (1 May 2011), http://bostonreview.net/junot-diaz-apocalypse-haiti-earthquake.

Dix, D., *Memorial. To the Legislature of Massachusetts [protesting against the confinement of insane persons and idiots in almshouses and prisons]. Jan. 1843* (Munroe and Francis, 1843), http://collections.nlm.nih.gov/catalog/nlm:nlmuid-101174442-bk

Dransfield, S., 'A Tale of Two Britains' (Oxfam GB, 2014), http://policy-practice.oxfam.org.uk/publications/a-tale-of-two-britains-inequality-in-the-uk-314152.

Dyregrov, A., 'The Process in Psychological Debriefings', *Journal of Traumatic Stress* 10 (1997): 589–605.

Fekadu, A., et al., 'Excess Mortality in Severe Mental Illness: 10-Year Population-Based Cohort Study in Rural Ethiopia', *British Journal of Psychiatry* 206 (2015): 289–96.

Franchetti, M., 'US Marines turn fire on civilians at bridge of death', *The Sunday Times*, 30 March 2003.

Gercas, A., 'The Universal Declaration on Bioethics and Human Rights: Promoting International Discussion on the Morality of Non-Therapeutic Research on Children', *Michigan Journal of International Law* 27 (2006): 629–56.

Goldstein, R., 'War Experiences and Distress of Bosnian Children', *Journal of Pediatrics* 100 (1997): 873–8.

Gollaher, D., *Voice for the Mad: The Life of Dorothea Dix* (Free Press, 1996).

Graham, D. (ed.), *Letters of Keith Douglas* (Carcanet, 2000).

Greene, R., 'Is Donald Trump Mentally Ill? 3 Professors of
    Psychiatry Ask President Obama To Conduct 'A Full Medical And
    Neuropsychiatric Evaluation'', *The Huffington Post*, "20 December
    2016, http://www.huffingtonpost.com/richard-greene/is-donal
    d-trump-mentally_b_13693174.html
Hague, W., *William Wilberforce: The Life of the Great Anti-Slave Trade
    Campaigner* (Harper Press, 2007).
Haller, M. H., *Eugenics: Hereditarian attitudes in American thought.*
    (Rutgers University Press, 1984).
Harding, J., 'Saved and Depoliticised at One Stroke: The Dangers of
    Intervention', *London Review of Books* 30 (2008): 5–8.
Hardoon, D., 'An economy for the 99%' (Oxfam GB, 2017), https://
    www.oxfam.org/en/research/economy-99
Horwitz, A. V. and Wakefield, J. C., *The Loss of Sadness: How
    Psychiatry Transformed Normal Sorrow into Depressive Disorder*
    (Oxford University Press, 2007).
Independent International Commission on Kosovo, *The Kosovo
    Report: Conflict, International Response, Lessons Learned* (Oxford
    University Press, 2000).
Inter-Agency Standing Committee, *IASC Guidelines on Mental Health
    and Psychosocial Support in Emergency Settings* (2007), http://www.
    who.int/mental_health/emergencies/guidelines_iasc_mental_health_
    psychosocial_june_2007.pdf. DOI:10.1037/e518422011-002.
International Committee of the Red Cross and International Federation
    of Red Cross and Red Crescent Societies, *Handbook of the
    International Red Cross and Red Crescent Movement* (2008).
Ionesco, E., *Rhinoceros,* translated by Martin Crimp (Faber and Faber,
    2007).
Iraq Body Count, https://www.iraqbodycount.org/.
Jabar, F. A., 'Opposing War Is Good, But Not Good Enough', *The
    Progressive,* January 2003, https://www.globalpolicy.org/component/
    content/article/167/35171.html.
Jones, E., and Wessely, S., 'Psychological Trauma: A Historical
    Perspective', *Psychiatry* 5 (2006): 217–20.
Jones, L., 'The Medicine of Misery', *Guardian,* 27 November 1987.
— 'The Peace Movement's Moral Failure in Bosnia', *Peace and
    Democracy News* (summer 1993): 23–8.
— 'Upholding the Rule of Law', *Peace and Democracy News* (summer
    1994): 36–40.
— 'Love Among the Ruins: Rebuilding After the Tsunami', *O, the
    Oprah Magazine,* July 2005.
— 'Diary of a Disaster', *O, the Oprah Magazine,* June 2006.
— *Then They Started Shooting: Children of the Bosnian War and the
    Adults They Become* (Bellevue Literary Press, 2012).

—'Each Scar is Different', *Aeon* (22 May 2014). https:/aeon.ce/essays/
the-more-we-label-trauma-with-ptsd-the-less-it-means.

Jones, S., 'World heading for catastrophe over natural disasters, risk
expert warns', *Guardian,* 24 April 2016, https://www.theguardian.
com/global-development/2016/apr/24/world-heading-for-catastroph
e-over-natural-disasters-risk-expert-warns

Kellenberger, J., 'Speaking Out or Remaining Silent in Humanitarian
Work', *International Review of the Red Cross* 86 (2004): 593–609.

Kendell, R. E., Cooper J. E., and Gourlay A. G., 'Diagnostic criteria of
American and British psychiatrists', *Archives of General Psychiatry*
25 (1971): 123–30.

Krugman, S., 'The Willowbrook Hepatitis Studies Revisited: Ethical
Aspects', *Clinical Infectious Diseases* 8 (1986): 157–62.

Laing, A., 'Ethiopia struggles with worst drought for 50 years leaving
18 million people in need of aid', *Telegraph,* 23 April 2016, http://
www.telegraph.co.uk/news/2016/04/23/ethiopia-struggles-with-wors
t-drought-for-50-years-leaving-18-mi/

Lall, R. R. and Pilkington E., 'UN Will Not Compensate Haiti Cholera
Victims, Ban Ki-moon Tells President', *Guardian,* 21 February
2013, https://www.theguardian.com/world/2013/feb/21/un-hait
i-cholera-victims-rejects-compensation.

Lifton, R. J., *The Nazi Doctors: Medical Killing and the Psychology of
Genocide* (Basic Books, 1986).

Maercker, A., et al., 'Proposals for Mental Disorders Specifically
Associated with Stress in the International Classification of
Diseases-11', *Lancet* 381 (2013): 1683–5.

Maren, M., *The Road to Hell: The Ravaging Effects of Foreign Aid and
International Charity* (Free Press, 1997).

Mastnak, L., 'Diary', *London Review of Books,* 21 August 1997.

— 'Why are you leaving?': a child psychiatrist records the daily round in
Kosovo before and since the bombing', *London Review of Books,* 27
May 1999.

— 'Not Much Tolerance, Not Much Water: the last nine months in
Kosovo', *London Review of Books,* 30 March 2000.

Met Office news release, '2016 Record breaking year for global
temperature' (18 January 2017) http://www.metoffice.gov.uk/news/re
leases/2017/2016-record-breaking-year-for-global-temperature

Miller, H., 'Accident Neurosis', *British Medical Journal* 1 (1961): 992–8.

Mitchell, J. T., 'When disaster strikes . . . the critical incident stress
debriefing. *Journal of Emergency Medical Services* 8 (1983): 36–9.

Moyo, D., *Dead Aid: Why Aid Is Not Working and How There Is
Another Way for Africa* (Penguin, 2009).

O'Keefe, P., Westgate K., and Wisner, B., 'Taking the Naturalness out of
Natural Disasters'. *Nature* 260 (1976): 566–7.

Patel, Vikram, *Where There Is No Psychiatrist: A Mental Healthcare Manual* (Gaskell, 2003).

Polman, L., *The Crisis Caravan: What's Wrong with Humanitarian Aid* (Picador, 2011).

Porter, R., *The Cambridge Illustrated History of Medicine* (Cambridge University Press, 2001).

— *Madness: A Brief History* (Oxford University Press, 2003).

Potts, S. G., Lewin R., Fox K., and Johnstone E. C., 'Group Psychological Treatment for Chest Pain with Normal Coronary Arteries', *Quarterly Journal of Medicine* 92 (1999): 81–6.

Rasekh, Z., Bauer H., Manos M., and Iacopino V., 'Women's Health and Human Rights in Afghanistan', *Journal of the American Medical Association* 280 (1998): 449–55.

Rieff, D., *A Bed for the Night* (Simon and Schuster, 2002).

Rieffer-Flanagan, B. A., 'Is Neutral Humanitarianism Dead? Red Cross Neutrality: Walking the Tightrope of Neutral Humanitarianism'. *Human Rights Quarterly* 31 (2009): 888–915.

Roberts, B., and Roberts L. W., 'Psychiatric Research Ethics: An Overview of Evolving Guidelines and Current Ethical Dilemmas in the Study of Mental Illness'. *Biological Psychiatry* 46 (1999): 1025–38.

Rose, S., Bisson J., Churchill R., and Wessely S., 'Psychological Debriefing for Preventing Post Traumatic Stress Disorder (PTSD)'. *Cochrane Database of Systematic Reviews* (2002). DOI:10.1002/14651858.CD000560.

Rosenhan, D. L., 'On Being Sane in Insane Places', *Science* 179 (1973): 250–58.

Seery, E., and Caistor Arendar, A., *Even It Up: Time to End Extreme Inequality* (Oxfam International, 2014), http://policy-practice.oxfam.org.uk/publications/even-it-up-time-to-en d-extreme-inequality-333012.

Shephard, B., *War of Nerves: Soldiers and Psychiatrists in the Twentieth Century* (Harvard University Press, 2002).

Simms, B., *Unfinest Hour: Britain and the Destruction of Bosnia* (Allen Lane, 2001).

Smith, D., 'Ethiopia Hailed as "African Lion" with Fastest Creation of Millionaires', *Guardian,* 4 December 2013, http://www.theguardian.com/world/2013/dec/04/ethiopia-faster-rate-million aires-michael-buerk.

Somasundaram, D. J., 'Post-Traumatic Responses to Aerial Bombing'. *Social Science & Medicine* 42 (1996): 1465–71.

Sontag, D., 'In Haiti, Mental Health System Is in Collapse', *New York Times,* 19 March 2010, http://www.nytimes.com/2010/03/20/world/americas/20haiti.html

'Stock Footage – 1936 NEWS: EMPEROR HAILE SELASSIE OF ETHIOPIA ADDRESSES LEAGUE OF NATIONS' (MyFootage. com, uploaded 9 April 2012), https://www.youtube.com/watch?v=oyX2kXeFUlo.

Strahan, A. K., 'The Propagation of Insanity and Allied Neuroses', *Journal of Mental Science* (1890): 325–38.

Summerfield, D., 'A Critique of Seven Assumptions behind Psychological Trauma Programmes in War-Affected Areas', *Social Science & Medicine* 48 (1999): 1449–62.

Summers, C., 'Inside a Trump Chinese shoe factory: 100,000 pairs of footwear branded with Ivanka's name have been made at huge facility (but now it's moving to Africa!)', Mailonline and AFP, 6 October 2016, http://www.dailymail.co.uk/news/article-3824617/Trump-factory-jobs-sent-China-never-come-back.html#ixzz4X4e6Jtv8

Travis, A., '2 in 3 back air strikes', *Guardian,* 18 September 2001, https://www.theguardian.com/world/2001/sep/18/september11.usa7?INTCMP=SRCH

Terry, F., *Condemned to Repeat? The Paradox of Humanitarian Action* (Cornell University Press, 2002).

Thomas, S. B., 'Light on the Shadow of the Syphilis Study at Tuskegee', *Health Promotion Practice* 1 (2000): 234–7.

Thornicroft, G., 'Physical Health Disparities and Mental Illness: The Scandal of Premature Mortality', *British Journal of Psychiatry* 199 (2011): 441–2.

Tol, W., et al., 'Mental Health and Psychosocial Support in Humanitarian Settings: Linking Practice and Research', *Lancet* 378 (2011): 1581–91.

United Nations High Commission for Refugees, *Health Information System (HIS) Toolkit,* http://www.unhcr.org/4a3374408.html

— *Global Trends: Forced Displacement in 2015* (2016), http://www.unhcr.org/uk/news/latest/2016/6/5763b65a4/global-forced-displacement-hits-record-high.html

United Nations News Centre, 'Three months after Hurricane Matthew, 1.5 million Haitians face hunger – UN agencies report', 18 January 2017, http://www.un.org/apps/news/story.asp?NewsID=55998#.WIzBKn9FrDo

United Nations Office of the Humanitarian Coordinator, *Haiti Transitional Appeal 2015/2016* (2015). http://reliefweb.int/sites/reliefweb.int/files/resources/haiti-TAP_exec_summary_0.pdf.

Vernon, P. E., 'Psychological effects of air-raids', *The Journal of Abnormal and Social Psychology* 36 (1941): 457–76.

Walzer, M., *Arguing about War* (Yale University Press, 2005).

Wilson, H., 'Mental Reactions to Air-Raids', *Lancet* (1942): 284–7.

World Health Organisation, *The ICD 9 Classification of Mental and Behavioural Disorders* (1978).

— *mhGAP Intervention Guide for Mental, Neurological and Substance Use Disorders in Non-Specialized Health Settings* (2010), http://www.who.int/mental_health/publications/mhGAP_intervention_guide/en/.

— *Psychological Debriefing in People Exposed to a Recent Traumatic Event* (2012). http://www.who.int/mental_health/mhgap/evidence/other_disorders/q5/en/.

— and War Trauma Foundation and World Vision International, *Psychological First Aid: guide for fieldworkers* (2011).

— and United Nations High Commission for Refugees, *mhGAP Humanitarian Intervention Guide* (2015), http://www.who.int/mental_health/publications/mhgap_hig/en/.

ACKNOWLEDGEMENTS

My thanks to the Radcliffe Institute for Advanced Study at Harvard University for the Fellowship that enabled me to start this book, to the *Lancet* for permission to quote from the article by F. de Vries: 'To Make a Drama out of Trauma is Fully Justified' (1998), and to Faled Jabar and the *Progressive* to quote from his essay: 'Opposing War Is Good, But Not Good Enough' (2003). I would also like to thank the *London Review of Books* for permission to reuse material that first appeared in Diaries published under the name Lynne Mastnak in 1997, 1999 and 2000; *O, the Oprah Magazine* for permission to reuse material that appeared in articles in 2005 and 2006; and *Aeon Magazine* for publishing an early version of Chapter 4. (Full details of all pieces are given in the bibliography.)

Over seven years of writing there are many people who have helped. My fellow Fellows at the Radcliffe all inspired and encouraged. Christopher Frugé and Rachael Goldberg were amazing research assistants. Rachel Holmes, Mark McCrum and Hannah Pool were all inspiring teachers of memoir writing. Kristin Brown, Patrick Burke, Mark Cousins, Shkumbin Dauti, Neil Joyce and Ben Shephard all read early drafts and gave invaluable feedback. Karl French at TLC was a thoughtful and encouraging first editor. Nick Tregenza provided a 'writing room' with no distractions.

Thanks to my agent Chris Wellbelove for his enthusiasm and support for this book, and to Alan Samson, Lucinda McNeile, Sue Phillpott and all at Weidenfeld & Nicolson for such scrupulous care over publication.

I would like to thank Larry Hollingworth, Peter Ventevogel, Mark van Ommeren and Willem van der Put for more than a decade of friendship and discussions on mental health and humanitarianism. Kevin and Brendan Cahill and everyone at the Institute of International Humanitarian Affairs at Fordham University gave me further opportunities for reflection by supporting the Mental Health in Complex Emergencies Course for the last twelve years. Most importantly I would like to thank all my patients, friends, colleagues and students in so many different parts of the world. It is your lives, courage and companionship which have inspired me and taught me so much. I hope our shared histories are accurately reflected here.

INDEX